FOUNDATIONS OF THEORY FOR ANCIENT CHINESE MEDICINE

by the same author

Discussion of Cold Damage (Shāng Hán Lùn)
Commentaries and Clinical Applications
Guohui Liu
Foreword by Dr. Henry McCann
ISBN 978 1 84819 254 6
eISBN 978 0 85701 200 5

of related interest

Acupuncture and Chinese Medicine
Roots of Modern Practice
Charles Buck
Foreword by Barbara Kirschbaum
ISBN 978 1 84819 159 4
eISBN 978 0 85701 133 6

Heavenly Stems and Earthly Branches—TianGan DiZhi
The Heart of Chinese Wisdom Traditions
Master Zhongxian Wu and Dr Karin Taylor Wu
Foreword by Fei BingXun
ISBN 978 1 84819 151 8
eISBN 978 0 85701 158 9

Gold Mirrors and Tongue Reflections
The Cornerstone Classics of Chinese Medicine Tongue Diagnosis—The Ao Shi Shāng Hán Jin
Jing Lu, and the Shāng Hán She Jian
Ioannis Solos
Forewords by Professor Liang Rong and Professor Chen Jia-xu
ISBN 978 1 84819 095 5
eISBN 978 0 85701 076 6

Essential Texts in Chinese Medicine
The Single Idea in the Mind of the Yellow Emperor
Richard Bertschinger
ISBN 978 1 84819 162 4
eISBN 978 0 85701 135 0

Foundations of Theory for ANCIENT CHINESE MEDICINE

Shāng Hán Lùn and Contemporary Medical Texts

GUOHUI LIU

Foreword by CHARLES BUCK

SINGING DRAGON

LONDON AND PHILADELPHIA

First published in 2015
by Singing Dragon
an imprint of Jessica Kingsley Publishers
73 Collier Street
London N1 9BE, UK
and
400 Market Street, Suite 400
Philadelphia, PA 19106, USA

www.singingdragon.com

Library of Congress Cataloging in Publication Data
Liu, Guohui, 1956-
Foundations of theory for ancient Chinese medicine : shang han lun and contemporary medical texts /
Guohui Liu.
pages cm
Includes bibliographical references and index.
ISBN 978-1-84819-262-1 (alk. paper)
1. Medicine, Chinese. 2. Medicine, Chinese--History. 3. Herbs--Therapeutic use. I. Title.
R601.L67964 2015
615.3'21--dc23
2014047511

British Library Cataloguing in Publication Data
A CIP catalogue record for this book is available from the British Library

ISBN 978 1 84819 262 1
eISBN 978 0 85701 211 1

Printed and bound in Great Britain

CONTENTS

Foreword by Charles Buck 7

Acknowledgments 11

Preface. 13

Chapter 1 The Concept of Shāng Hán 17

Chapter 2 Brief Introduction to Zhang Ji and His Works 24

Chapter 3 Exploration of the Cultural Landscape for Writing Discussion of Cold Damage 27

Chapter 4 School of Cold Damage and School of Studying Discussion of Cold Damage 44

Chapter 5 Six Conformations, Six Conformations Diseases and Six Conformations Disease Differentiation . . . 79

Chapter 6 The Theory of Qi Transformation in Six Conformations in Discussion of Cold Damage . . . 106

Chapter 7 Half Exterior and Half Interior, Harmony and Shao Yang 155

Chapter 8 Nutritive Qi, Defensive Qi, Tai Yang Qi and Their Treatments 185

Chapter 9 Exploration of the Resolving Time for Diseases in Six Conformations. 209

Appendix 1: Chinese Dynasties and Historical Periods 237

Appendix 2: Authors of Chinese Medicine Books 238

Bibliography 243
Subject Index 263
Author Index. 272
Classic Texts Index 274
Herb and Formula Index 277
Pinyin Index 279

FOREWORD

When, in 1983, I first attempted to read Hong-yen Hsu's English language translation of the Shāng Hán Lùn I was already aware of the line in the Yijing that reads "go hunting without the forester and you will soon be lost in the forest." Not for a moment did it occur to me that, with the resources available to me at the time, it would be near impossible to simply read and understand this cornerstone of classical Chinese medicine. Indeed, I had no inkling that I was actually lost in the forest—in the beginner's blissful ignorance I imagined it possible to find my own way.

At that same time, on the other side of the world, I guess that Guohui Liu was also wrestling the Shāng Hán Lùn for its secrets. His linguistic and cultural proximity to the primary sources meant that he was in a very much better position to do so. In addition, Liu's own father was a respected Chinese medicine scholar. If further qualification were needed we could note also that, as a long-standing faculty member of the Oregon College of Oriental Medicine, Professor Liu is accustomed to communicating the ideas of Chinese medicine to English speakers. Evidence of this we have already seen in an earlier English language masterwork, his *Warm Diseases: A Clinical Guide*.[1]

As all serious students of this medicine know, the Shāng Hán Zá Bìng Lùn is the very foundation stone of scholarly Chinese herbal medicine practice and is the source of roughly a quarter of the core formulary taught to undergraduates. All undergraduates learn the rudiments of these formulas in the early years of our studies, but if we aspire to high-level practice we need to fully understand their use in the context of the

1 Guohui Liu. *Warm Diseases: A Clinical Guide*. Seattle, WA: Eastland, 2001

explanatory models used by the Shāng Hán Lùn author Zhang Ji (aka Zhang Zhong-Jing c. +150 to 219).

Despite its pre-eminent position in Chinese medicine, the Shāng Hán Lùn has not been without its critics. I first stumbled across these controversies when, on a clinical trip to Shanghai in 1990, a senior physician assured me that the Shāng Hán formulas, despite their elegance, mostly do not work today as our patients differ from those in the Han Dynasty. This seemed a challenging thing to say. Later I became aware that he was stating his position in a very longstanding debate wherein some Ming Dynasty practitioners asserted that the ancient classical formulas style did not suit illnesses suffered by patients in their era. We might say that this debate continues today and has, alongside the increased sophistication of practitioners and scholars in the here, spread to the West.

To hold an informed position in this requires that we have a proper overview of the complexities of scholarly literature over the past thousand years—the insider's understanding of Shāng Hán theory that Professor Guohui Liu provides here. So, by explicating the story for us, and presenting his personal scholarly interpretation, he allows us to more properly understand the issues. Liu is our forester offering guidance through the dense Shāng Hán literature forest.

When we have learned to read the language and structure of the classic Chinese herb formulas, we gain the sense that those from the Shāng Hán Lùn possess a characteristic elegance and luminosity. Here we find numerous exemplars on the use of contrasting properties such as matching the cold, sinking effect of *shí gāo* with the *xuan*-dispersing effect of *xing rén*, or the warm pungent dispersal of *guì zhī* with the cool contracting nourishment of *bái sháo*. We can sense the focus his formulas have on specific energetic niches in the body and the way he applied the *three methods* (exterior release, emesis, precipitation). In addition, we can appreciate in the Shāng Hán formulas his specific adjustment of the body's *qi mechanism* and his sophisticated insight into the *ba gang* principles long before the idea had been formally distilled from the classic texts. If we are reasonably adept in Chinese medicine we can appreciate these aspects but, as we learn from this book, it is possible to peer deeper into Zhang Ji's mastery.

As an aside, it is sometimes forgotten that a significant facet of the historical practice of Chinese medicine is the fight against epidemic and pestilential disease and there is confusion about the dual use of Shāng Hán Lùn theory inside and outside of this context. In modern times we can get a diluted sense of the dread associated with these diseases by reflecting on the realities of words such as plague, Ebola and cholera but few of us have actually witnessed first hand the darkness of such fatal pandemics. The three-millennia-old Shang and Zhou Dynasty *jià gǔ wén* writings on tortoiseshell and bone mention "disease years" and everything under the sun must have been tried to save life by combating these diseases. In his foreword to the Shāng Hán Zá Bìng Lùn, written in about +219, Zhang Ji wrote that he had witnessed the death of the majority of his relatives in an epidemic and this motivated his life quest for a medical system that was more effective in combating such strife. He adopted a schema taken from the *Sù Wèn* that outlined the day-by-day progress of febrile disease and refined this on the basis of his medical scholarship and experience. Some of the herb formulas he used were probably self-penned, whereas others, such as *guì zhī tāng,* are believed to have been in existence in the medical traditions that existed in centuries prior to his own, traditions that are now lost.

Zhang Ji's Shāng Hán Zá Bìng Lùn text might also have been lost had it not been for the pulse diagnosis master Wang Shu-he, who recovered the writings from bamboo slats and re-ordered to these into two texts, the Shāng Hán Lùn and the Jīn Gùi Yào Lüè. In the few centuries after this rescue work it became a text that was rarely transmitted, it was tersely written, difficult to understand and so it was difficult to convey its meaning to students. Then, in the Song Dynasty it was found in the Imperial library archives and attracted interest because of its potential as a resource to help tackle the epidemics of the time. With imperial sponsorship a great deal of high-level scholarship was applied to the text and, decade by decade progress was made in unravelling its meaning. This work continued through the subsequent Jin-Yuan, Ming and Qing dynasties and has carried on right up to modern times.

As a result of this thousand-year scrutiny, the Shāng Hán Lùn has inspired a vast body of literature intended to discuss, analyze and interpret its meaning—work that is formidable both in volume and complexity. Literally thousands of books and articles are in existence and debate continues in specialist journals today. As we see from Liu's account of the debate, the style of the historical discourse differs from modern scholarship. It presupposes a high level of understanding of the dense forest that is traditional scholarship which itself is one reason that so very few native Westerners are in a position to access this source literature in a meaningful way. Without the right guidance such as this we are lost.

One key difficulty is making sense of the *six conformations* (*liù jīng*) schema. Does it refer to the *jīng luò* system? The *zang fu*? Is it a theoretical energetic construct built upon concepts of the *qiji* (qi mechanism) or is it rooted in the traditional Cosmology theories? Liu carefully unravels the *six conformations* for us. What classical Chinese models can we best apply to its interpretation—*ba gang*? Traditional chronobiology? To what extent is Shāng Hán Lùn theory applicable in general medical practice outside the context of *cold attack*? In examining the issues Liu guides us through the complex journey the Shāng Hán Lùn has taken spanning the writings of the various commentators from the Song Dynasty through to modern times and explains the ideas that they developed.

In addition to explaining the Shāng Hán scholarly narrative Professor Liu details his own approach to its use in practice including a detailed discussion on the understanding of *tai yang* and *shao yang* layers. This is very valuable—Professor Liu is a guide in this forest, allowing us to deepen our understanding into the way we can apply Shāng Hán Lùn theory clinically in the modern world. With access to this understanding we will also be better placed to consider the relationship between Shāng Hán and Wēn Bìng (Warm Disease) theory.

Charles Buck
Chester, UK
May 2015

ACKNOWLEDGMENTS

I would like thank my father Lu-yan Liu, my mother Yi-xin Liu and my brother Liang-hui Liu, who taught me Chinese medicine and Chinese culture when I was a child. Also, I would especially like to thank Junlan Cai and Ruolan Liu for their boundless love, support and forgiveness in keeping me in line throughout this very long project.

I also would like to thank Ran Pin-Zhen, my mentor in my graduate study 33 years ago, for his wonderful teaching and guidance. It was he who inspired me to continually study these Chinese medical classics.

Because English is my second language, it has been a big challenge for me to translate ancient classics and write this book. It has also been quite difficult for me to find the references for this book, especially when I am outside China. Without help from the following people, this book could not have been written. I am very grateful to Mr. Wang Sen for his translation of the name and dates of Japanese scholars related to Discussion of Cold Damage and his efforts to collect several ancient Chinese medical books that relate to this classic. I am indebted to David Frierman for providing some feedback for Chapter 7 of this book.

I deeply appreciate the support from Oregon College of Oriental Medicine and the patience, enthusiasm, and encouragement from my students in this school. Also, I appreciate the excellent foreword for this book written by Charles Buck.

Finally, I would like to thank Jessica Kingsley, who is so passionate about publishing Chinese medical classics. I would also like to thank all the editors at Singing Dragon for editing my manuscript. Without their support and help, this book would not have gone to print.

PREFACE

Everyone who begins to study Chinese medicine has probably heard of, and maybe even partially read, Discussion of Cold Damage (傷寒論 *shāng hán lùn*), as this classic book lays out the basic framework for Chinese medicine in the regard of disease differentiation and treatment. The formulas the book records are still widely applied to treat various kinds of diseases or disorders, which is a testament to its modern-day relevance. This is why Discussion of Cold Damage is considered as one of the most important texts on Chinese medicine from which everyone in this field must learn. It can be compared to the steps of a palace that holds many treasures: to get to these treasures, one must first climb many steps.

Studying Discussion of Cold Damage is no easy task, however, because there are many concepts that are either hard to understand or confusing. Without understanding these concepts, it is difficult to grasp their clinical applications. Among these concepts are: (a) the concept of tai yang qi, (b) the concept of qi transformation, (c) the relationship between the defensive qi and the nutritive qi, (d) how to harmonize the defensive qi and the nutritive qi, (e) the meanings of the half exterior and the half interior, (f) how to harmonize shao yang and (g) why each disease in three yin diseases and three yang diseases resolve at particular times. For more than 900 years, scholars and practitioners have offered many good answers and formulated various theories related to these concepts in Discussion of Cold Damage.

I have spent more than 30 years studying these concepts and theories, and the outcomes of my research are presented in Chapters 1 and 5 to 9 of this book. Chapters 2 to 4 were written in order to help readers deeply understand Discussion of Cold Damage and the history of studies done on this classic.

The first question raised by readers might be: What is the concept of *shāng hán*? Chapter 1, "The Concept of *Shāng Hán,*" answers this question. In that chapter I present *my* interpretation, which is slightly different to common ideas from ancient and contemporary scholars, based on the information in the preface written by Zhang Ji and the application of the term "*shāng hán*" in Discussion of Cold Damage. I strongly believe that my interpretation is very close to the original meaning of this concept since it is based on the original materials of this classic instead of on ancient and contemporary clinical application of the theories and formulas therein.

Historically, both ancient and contemporary scholars have shared the same ideas about how Discussion of Cold Damage has been passed down over the centuries. I have collected this information in Chapter 2, "Brief Introduction to Zhang Ji and His Works."

To understand the original meaning of Discussion of Cold Damage, one has to consider what the background—especially the philosophical and cultural landscape—was when Zhang Ji wrote his work, because Chinese medicine is deeply rooted in traditional Chinese culture in the regard of basic theory, academic contexts, ways of thinking and so on. Surprisingly, past scholars have failed to systematically explore the cultural landscape associated with the writing of Discussion of Cold Damage. However, in this book, Chapter 3, "Exploration of the Cultural Landscape for Writing Discussion of Cold Damage," discusses Zhang Ji's era and the great influence that Confucianism and Daoism had on his work. I have also adapted some doctrines from the Book of Changes (易經 *yì jīng*) and River Map (河圖 *hé tú*) to explain some of the content from *shāng hán lùn*, though analysis of the content of these classics does not necessarily lead to the conclusion that Zhang Ji applied them.

Chapter 4, "School of Cold Damage and School of Studying Discussion of Cold Damage," was written to demonstrate the specific contributions past and present scholars have made to the development of the theories contained in Discussion of Cold Damage and the kinds of approaches they have used for studying the book, because these theories and approaches are still important for our understanding and study of this classic.

There is general agreement that the theory of six conformations (六經 *liù jīng*) is key to understanding Discussion of Cold Damage; therefore, I have dedicated a lot of space to Chapter 5, "Six Conformations, Six Conformations Diseases and Six Conformations Disease Differentiation."

In the history of studying Discussion of Cold Damage, scholars have adapted many approaches. These approaches include employing the theory of channels and collaterals, the zang-fu organ theory, the theory of qi and blood, and the theory of qi transformation. Among these approaches, the qi transformation theory has been largely ignored by scholars and practitioners in the West. According to my studying experience, the theory of qi transformation is the only one that can integrate all of the theories mentioned above, and it serves as an indispensable tool in applying disease differentiation and treatment approaches from Discussion of Cold Damage in our practice. In other words, without studying the theory of qi transformation, it would be very hard to understand the theories and treatment approaches in this classic and apply them widely in a clinical setting. Therefore, Chapter 6, "The Theory of Qi Transformation in Six Conformations in Discussion of Cold Damage," helps the reader to comprehend this theory. (For some explanations, based on this theory, for many lines in Discussion of Cold Damage, see my book Discussion of Cold Damage (Shāng Hán Lùn): Commentaries and Clinical Applications.[1])

Because shao yang is located in the half exterior and the half interior, and plays an important role in communicating qi between the exterior and interior, and in expelling pathological factors, Chapter 7, "Half Exterior and Half Interior, Harmony and Shao Yang" discusses the concepts and theories related to shao yang.

Tai yang is the first layer to defend the body. Its two types of qi, i.e. the defensive qi and the nutritive qi, play an important role in fulfilling this goal. Zhang Ji dedicated almost half of the volume of his writings to discussing disorders in tai yang disease; therefore, it is extremely important to understand qi in tai yang and its treatment. The discussions related to these concepts can be found in Chapter 8, "Nutritive Qi, Defensive Qi, Tai Yang Qi and Their Treatments."

The time it takes for each disease to resolve has been a long-standing mystery. I have tried to make the theories related to certain assumptions more clear. The discussions related to these theories can be found in Chapter 9, "Exploration of the Resolving Time for Diseases in Six Conformations."

There are a total of 14 formulas from Rhymed Formula for Keys to Employ Herbs According to Zang-fu Organs (輔行訣臟腑用藥法要 *fǔ xíng jué zàng fǔ yòng yào fǎ yào*) when discussing the cultural landscape associated with writing Discussion of Cold Damage. In order to keep distractions to a minimum, reference information is not provided for any of these formulas, because the works cited herein are dedicated mainly to theoretical study and historical review. Furthermore, I do not provide any reference information regarding the ingredients for those formulas for the

1 Guohui Liu. *Discussion of Cold Damage (Shāng Hán Lùn): Commentaries and Clinical Applications.* London: Singing Dragon, 2015

same reason; however, the reader can get some sense of those ingredients from Table 3.1 in Chapter 3.

In order to give a clear idea of how these developments in Chinese medicine took place in the regard of writer and time, often I have put the honorific name and/or alias, as well as the dates, in parentheses after the name of the scholar. This way, the reader can quickly get a sense of when a cited book was first published and know the context of the development of such explorations instead of having to check back and forth between a given chapter and Appendix 2, "Authors of Chinese Medicine Books."

Although I have put much thought and hard work into bringing this book to fruition and making it accessible and useful to students as well as practitioners, due to my limited knowledge and experience, I feel that I simply could not do complete justice to this classic book, Discussion of Cold Damage. There are still many questions and some theories that are not so clear in six conformations, though I have done some research on them. I strongly believe that at least some of these questions eventually will be answered by other scholars engaged in profound research.

1

THE CONCEPT OF SHĀNG HÁN

When one studies Discussion of Cold Damage (傷寒論 *shāng hăn lùn*), the first question one has is what the term "傷寒 *shāng hán*" means, because the book is named after this term. The term "傷寒 *shāng hán*" was first recorded in Chapter 31 of Basic Questions of The Yellow Emperor's Inner Classic (*huáng dì nèi jīng sù wèn*),[1] which is one of the important classics Zhang Ji referred to when he wrote his work. The first book that implies there are two types of "傷寒 *shāng hán*," i.e. *shāng hán* in a broad sense and *shāng hán* in a narrow sense, is Difficult Questions (難經 *nàn jīng*).[2] In Chapter 58 of Difficult Questions, it is recorded that "there are five types of *shāng hán* [all externally contracted diseases], which include *zhòng fēng* [wind stroke], *shāng hán* [cold attack], damp-warm disease, febrile disease and warm pathogen disease. And they have different clinical presentations." According to research from Guan Qing-Zeng and colleagues, the topic of *shāng hán* is put forward by contemporary scholars, though studies in ancient books related to Discussion of Cold Damage have addressed this subject.[3] According to my resources, the first person who clearly stated that there are two types of concepts for the term "傷寒 *shāng hán*" was the famous scholar Huang Qian (also known as Huang Zhu-Zhai, 1886–1960), who states:

> The term "傷寒 *shāng hán*" recorded in the ancient book can be classified into two types, i.e. one in a broad sense and one in a narrow sense. In a broad sense, it refers to all externally contracted diseases due to wind,

1 Wang Bing. *Basic Questions of The Yellow Emperor's Inner Classic* (*huáng dì nèi jīng sù wèn*). Beijing: People's Health Publishing House, 1963: 183

2 Nanjing College of Traditional Chinese Medicine. *Annotation and Explanation for Difficult Questions* (*nàn jīng jiào shì*). Beijing: People's Health Publishing House, 1979: 128

3 Guan Qing-Zeng et al. *Ancient and Contemporary Study for Discussion of Cold Damage* (*shāng hán lùn gŭ jīn yán jiū*). Shenyang: Liaoning Scientific and Technological Publishing House, 1994: 77

> cold, summer heat, damp, dryness and heat… In a narrow sense, it is an exclusive term for the disease due to invasion of cold.[4]

Historically, there are three interpretations of this term, i.e. all diseases, all externally contracted diseases and an externally contracted disease due to invasion of wind-cold, based on how the character "寒 *hán*" is understood in this term. These three interpretations can be classified into two categories, i.e. *shāng hán* in a broad sense and *shāng hán* in a narrow sense.

Shāng hán in a broad sense

All diseases

According to my resources, the first person who clearly pointed out that the term "傷寒 *shāng hán*" refers to all diseases was Koretada Nakanishi (1724–1803), a Japanese scholar. In his book, Study on Discussion of Cold Damage (傷寒之研究 *shāng hán zhī yán jiū*), he states:

> The term "傷寒 *shāng hán*" refers to injury due to pathological factors. The reason to interpret the character "寒 *hán*" as being related to pathological factors is based on its meaning in ancient literatures… although pathological factors can come from outside or be generated inside; all diseases they induce are called "傷寒 *shāng hán*."[5]

Nakanishi's interpretation is echoed by Lü Zhen-Ming (also known as Lü Jian-Xun and Lü Cha-Cun, 1796–1852) and Ren Ying-Qiu (1914–1984). In his book, Search the Source for Discussion of Cold Damage (傷寒尋源 *shāng hán xún yuán*), Lü writes that "ten thousand diseases fall into the category of *shāng hán*."[6] Ren Ying-Qiu found further evidence to support Nakanishi's interpretation based on the study of ancient Chinese literature. Ren points out that the character "寒 *hán*" should be interpreted as being related to pathological factors instead of being limited to cold. He cited a sentence from Mencius's work, which was written between 372 and 289 BC, to demonstrate that the character "寒 *hán*" must be interpreted as

4 Huang Qian. "What I have learned from studying Discussion of Cold Damage and Miscellaneous Diseases by Zhang Zhong-Jing." *Shanghai Journal of Traditional Chinese Medicine*, 1955 (7): 24

5 Koretada Nakanishi. *Study on Discussion of Cold Damage* (*shāng hán zhī yán jiū*). Beijing: People's Health Publishing House, 1957: 5, 16

6 Lü Zhen-Ming. *Search for the Source of Discussion of Cold Damage* (*shāng hán xún yuán*). Changchun: Continent Publishing House, 1942: 1

the character "邪 *xié*," which means "evils" in the following sentence in Mencius's work: "吾见（齐王）亦罕矣，吾退而寒之者至矣（*wú jiàn yì hǎn yǐ, wú tuì ér hán zhī zhě zhì yǐ*)." There is general agreement that the character "寒 *hán*" should be understood as the character "邪 *xié*" and that the whole sentence should be translated as "I have few chances to meet King Qi. After I have left King Qi, the evil villain will appear in front of King Qi." Based on this research, Ren states that "the term '傷寒 *shāng hán*' means injury by pathological factors and suffering from diseases. Understanding the term in this way can give this term a broader meaning…in sum, this book discusses all diseases."[7]

It is absolutely right that the character "寒 *hán*" in the sentence from Mencius's work should be translated as "evil villain," but it is hard to convince one that Zhang Ji indeed read this book and used this meaning for the term "傷寒 *shāng hán*" in his book. According to my study, Zhang Ji used the character "寒 *hán*" 27 times to describe pathology in Discussion of Cold Damage, and all such occurrences refer to cold, harmful cold fluid or cold phlegm instead of all pathological factors that lead to various kinds of disease. Interesting, he also recorded the character "邪 *xié*" 12 times to talk about etiology, and none of those occurrences exclusively refers to cold. Rather, "邪 *xié*" refers to all pathological factors including wind, fire, phlegm and so on. Obviously, from Zhang Ji's point of view, the characters "寒 *hán*" and "邪 *xié*" bore quite different meanings when he wrote his book, though they do refer to pathological factors.

All externally contracted diseases

Scholars who have put forward this concept of *shāng hán* have cited a sentence from Chapter 31 of Basic Questions of The Yellow Emperor's Inner Classic to support this interpretation. The sentence is that "all febrile diseases fall into the category of *shāng hán*."[8] As stated in the preface of his work, Zhang Ji did take this classic to be one of the important reference sources when he wrote Discussion of Cold Damage. And it is absolutely right that when one wants to explore the concept of *shāng hán*, one must consult Basic Questions of The Yellow Emperor's Inner Classic. However, if one does further research on Chapter 31, one may find that

7 Ren Ying-Qiu. *Classified Explanation for Differentiation and Treatment in Discussion of Cold Damage* (*shāng hán lùn zhèng zhì lèi quán*). Beijing: Science and Health Publishing House, 1959: 1–2

8 Wang Bing, op. cit., p.183

the same character, "寒 *hán*," does not bear the concept of a disease but rather the concept of a pathological factor, i.e. cold, because the same chapter also states that "when a person is attacked by cold, she or he will suffer from a febrile disease (人之傷於寒，則為病熱 *rén zhī shāng yú hán, zé wéi bìng rè*)."[9] Obviously, the character "寒 *hán*" in Chapter 31 does not only refer to the disease but can also refer to a pathological factor; therefore, as early as 1987, Fu You-Feng pointed out that the term "傷寒 *shāng hán*" was used as a concept for pathological factors, which is not limited to cold, in The Yellow Emperor's Inner Classic.[10] The concept of this term as a disease did not occur until it was discussed in Difficult Questions (難經 *nàn jīng*).

Shāng hán in a narrow sense

Externally contracted diseases due to invasion of wind-cold

It is correct that Zhang Ji had consulted The Yellow Emperor's Inner Classic and Difficult Questions, both of which are mentioned in the preface of his work. These classics are important for us to understand the content in Discussion of Cold Damage since they set up the basic theories for Zhang Ji's practice and writing. But his having mentioned the books is by no means an indication that Zhang Ji simply adapted these concepts without any modifications. The practical way to understand certain concepts, such as *shāng hán*, in his works (especially in Discussion of Cold Damage) is to explore how he applied such terms in the original text of this book and figure out whether or not he completely or partially adapted the concept of this term from The Yellow Emperor's Inner Classic and/or Difficult Questions. This is the only way that can provide concrete evidence of what this term really means in his work. By my calculations, the term "傷寒 *shāng hán*" appears 99 times in Discussion of Cold Damage: once in the title, once in the preface and 97 times in the text itself.

According to Zhang Ji's preface, two thirds of his family died within ten years, among whom seven of the ten people died from *shāng hán*. (It seems that this kind of *shāng hán* was contagious.) According to Li Han-Zhang and colleagues, Zhang Ji was good at medicine and saved many patients that suffered from contagious diseases when he worked

9 Ibid.

10 Fu You-Feng. "Textual research for the concept of shang han." *Helongjiang Journal of Traditional Chinese Medicine*, 1987 (2): 6–8

as commissioner in Changsha county at the end of the East Han Dynasty (c. 200 AD).[11] Also, based on studies from some scholars, yin yang yi disease, as recorded in Discussion of Cold Damage, is contagious;[12] therefore, it is probable that the term "傷寒 *shāng hán*" includes diseases that are contagious. As to the 97 occurrences of this term in Discussion of Cold Damage, they can be classified into two categories—either *shāng hán* is discussed alone or it is discussed compared with other conditions due to externally contracted pathological factors. The first category accounts for 93 occurrences and the second for 4 occurrences (lines 101, 119, 145 and 158). According to Zhang Zheng-Zhao, because the term "太陽 *tài yáng*" is put ahead of the term "傷寒 *shāng hán*" in line 119, this clearly demonstrates that the term "傷寒 *shāng hán*" in that line bears a narrow-sense meaning, which is that it is caused by invasion of cold.[13] Zhang's interpretation can be supported by the following facts from the original text of Discussion of Cold Damage: Zhang Ji has classified the exterior conditions in tai yang disease into two syndromes, shang han and zhong feng syndromes, at the very beginning of the first section of the chapter on tai yang disease. Both syndromes are caused by invasion of wind-cold. The difference between these two syndromes in terms of pathological factors is that the former is invaded by more cold while the latter is invaded by more wind, though they are both caused by wind-cold (see lines 2 and 3 for further details). Because Zhang Ji uses the term "太陽傷寒 *tài yáng shāng hán*" in line 119—but uses the term "太陽中風 *tài yáng zhòng fēng*" in lines 12, 38 and 152—Zhang Zheng-Zhao concludes that "when the names of three yin and three yang (tai yang, yang ming, shao yang, tai yin, shao yin and jue yin) are not put ahead of the term "傷寒 *shāng hán*," the term "傷寒 *shāng hán*" bears a broad sense, meaning it includes all externally contracted febrile diseases.[14] Zhang's statement is very instructive, but it cannot explain why this term is used differently in lines 101, 145 and 158, where the terms "傷寒 *shāng hán*" and "中風 *zhòng fēng*" are put together in lines 101 and 158, i.e. "傷寒中風 *shāng hán zhòng fēng*." The condition "傷寒 *shāng hán*" in

11 Li Han-Zhang et al. *History of Hunan Province* (*hú nán tōng zhì*). Changsha: Pavilion of Respect for Classics in Learning Palace, 1885: 2033

12 Cheng Wu-Ji. *Annotating and Explaining Discussion of Cold Damage* (*zhù jiě shāng hán lùn*). Beijing: People's Health Publishing House, 1978: 187

13 Zhang Zheng-Zhao. *Back to Truth for Discussion of Cold Damage* (*shāng hán lùn guī zhēn*). Changsha: Hunan Science and Technology Publishing House, 1993: 212

14 Ibid., pp.212, 213

women is discussed in line 145, where the condition "中風 *zhòng fēng*" in women is discussed in lines 143–144. Apparently, the term or condition "傷寒 *shāng hán*" in line 145 is paralleled or compared to the term or condition "中風 *zhòng fēng*" in lines 143 and 144. Of course, when the terms "傷寒 *shāng hán*" and "中風 *zhòng fēng*" are put together in one sentence in lines 101 and 158, they are paralleled too. As mentioned above, tai yang disease can be classified into two syndromes, shang han syndrome and zhong feng syndrome; therefore, there is no doubt that the term "傷寒 *shāng hán*" in lines 101, 145 and 158 bears a narrow sense, which refers to the syndrome as being due to wind-cold invasion, with cold being predominant. Interestingly, when the term "傷寒 *shāng hán*" appears with the term "中風 *zhòng fēng*" in the same sentence, it can also bear a broad sense, which refers to all externally contracted diseases (see line 96 for further details).

Based on the discussion above, we can see that the term "傷寒 *shāng hán*" in Discussion of Cold Damage has three meanings: first, it mostly refers to its broad sense, i.e. externally contracted diseases; second, it sometimes refers to its narrow sense, i.e. the syndrome is caused by invasion of wind-cold, especially with cold being predominant; third, it also refers to some contagious diseases. (Apparently, it does not include all diseases.)

Questions might be raised, such as the following: "According to your research, the term '傷寒 *shāng hán*' mostly refers to externally contracted diseases. Do you agree that the theories, treatment approaches and formulas in Discussion of Cold Damage can be used to treat diseases which are due to internal disorders rather than those which are externally contracted?"

This question refers to two different concepts: the meaning of "傷寒 *shāng hán*," and the application of theories, treatment approaches and formulas, as recorded in Discussion of Cold Damage, in clinical practice. The answer is yes, the concept of "傷寒 *shāng hán*" mostly refers to externally contracted diseases; however, the diseases which Discussion of Cold Damage discusses are not limited to externally contracted diseases. For example, in lines 53 and 54 there is mention of a sweating disorder, due to disharmony between the nutritive qi and the defensive qi in internal disorders, which is still treated by Cinnamon Twig Decoction (*guì zhī tāng*); in lines 16 and 267 there are deteriorated syndromes, which do not belong to three yin and three yang diseases; in lines 129 and 130 there is visceral bind disorder (yang deficiency and cold accumulation in the organs), which is similar to the chest-binding syndromes; in lines 338 and 340, respectively, there is cold located in the urinary bladder and the conception vessel (CV 4), or in various organs.

Many lines and formulas in Discussion of Cold Damage have been recorded in Essentials and Formula Discussions from the Golden Cabinet (金匱要略方論 *jīn gùi yào lüè fāng lùn*), a companion book written by Zhang Ji, and there is no doubt that the theories, treatment approaches and formulas in Discussion of Cold Damage can be applied for other internal disorders and women's disorders. In the 1900 years since the book was written, many scholars have in fact employed these theories, treatment approaches and formulas to treat various internal disorders and women's disorders, as well as skin problems. However, this just means that over the centuries, these tools have been applied with the same flexibility that Zhang Ji probably applied to them. In other words, it does not mean that "傷寒 *shāng hán*" encompasses all the disorders for which Discussion of Cold Damage was primarily designed.

2

BRIEF INTRODUCTION TO ZHANG JI AND HIS WORKS

Unlike Hua Tuo (a famous physician who lived c. 208 AD), very little information is available on Zhang Ji and his works; this information was not recorded in historical books such as History of the Later Han Dynasty (後漢書 *hòu hàn shū*), which was written by Fan Ye during the Northern and Southern Dynasties and recorded details about historical events and historical figures in the Eastern Han Dynasty when Zhang Ji was alive. During the past two decades, many scholars have made great effort to explore information about Zhang Ji and his works. The information given in this chapter represents general agreement from contemporary scholars.

Zhang Ji 張機, whose honorific name was Zhang Zhong-Jing 張仲景, was born in Nanyang county, Henan province, c. 150 AD and died c. 219 AD. Zhang Ji was very interested in studying the doctrine of Confucius when he was about 15 years old, and he became a government official later. According to "Preface for Version of Discussion of Cold Damage in Song Dynasty," written by Lin Yi and colleagues in 1065 AD, Zhang Ji was selected as an official due to his exemplary behavior in the regard of filial duty and honesty, and he was also appointed as a commissioner in Changsha county. He first learned Chinese medicine from Zhang Bo-Zu, a local physician. People at that time commented that Zhang Ji's incisive knowledge was better than that of his mentors. Later, he became a very skillful physician. Besides many legendary stories told locally, a very interesting case study was recorded by Huang Fu-Mi (also known as Huang Xuan-Yan, 215–282 AD) in the preface of his book, Acupuncture Jia and Yi Classic (針灸甲乙經 *zhēn jiǔ jiǎ yǐ jīng*) published c. 256 AD (see Chapter 3 for further details). Being a well-known physician, Zhang Ji had a lot of apprentices, among whom Wei Xun and Du Du would become quite famous for their medical practice and academic writings.

According to the preface by Zhang Ji, his classic book was originally titled *Discussion of Cold Damage and Miscellaneous Diseases*

(傷寒雜病論 *shāng hán zá bìng lùn*), which in total accounted for 16 volumes and covered various diseases such as externally contracted diseases, internal disorders, women's health and skin diseases. Based on Zhang Ji's preface, it is believed that this book was finished between 210 and 219 AD. The book was damaged due to the war during the Three Kingdoms period (220–265 AD). Fortunately, Wang Xi (also known as Wang Shu-He, 201–280 AD), a chief officer who was in charge of medical affairs in Wei Kingdom (220–265 AD) and the early stage of the Jin Dynasty (265–420 AD), found and collected the damaged fragments of the book. He reconstructed Zhang's work as 15 volumes between 220 and 235 AD and named it "Formulas by Zhang Zhong-Jing (張仲景方 *zhāng zhòng-Jǐng fāng*)." From 420 AD (Northern and Southern Dynasties) to 1065 AD (Northern Song Dynasty), there were many handwritten versions that bore different names related to this work. The official version of the book was not published until Lin Yi and colleagues did textual research for it. Based on Lin and colleagues' textual research on the previous versions of this work, two of which had already been presented—one related to externally contracted diseases and the other related to internal disorders, women's health, and skin diseases—the government in the Song Dynasty published Discussion of Cold Damage (傷寒論 *shāng hán lùn*), The Classic of the Golden Coffer and Jade Sheath (金匱玉函經 *jīn gùi yù hán jīng*) and Essentials and Formula Discussions from the Golden Cabinet (金匱要略方論 *jīn gùi yào lüè fāng lùn*) in 1065, 1066 and 1067 AD, respectively. The former two books are relevant to externally contracted diseases, while the latter one focuses on internal disorders, women's health, skin diseases and dietary contraindications. The Classic of the Golden Coffer and Jade Sheath (金匱玉函經 *jīn gùi yù hán jīng*) is just another ancient version of Discussion of Cold Damage, though it is not as popular. Based on the version of Discussion of Cold Damage published in 1065 AD, Cheng Wu-Ji annotated and explained the book and then published his own book, Annotating and Explaining Discussion of Cold Damage (註解傷寒論 *zhù jiě shāng hǎn lùn*), in 1144 AD. Both books are still popular and important.

Figure 2.1 gives a brief summary of the history of Zhang Ji's works.

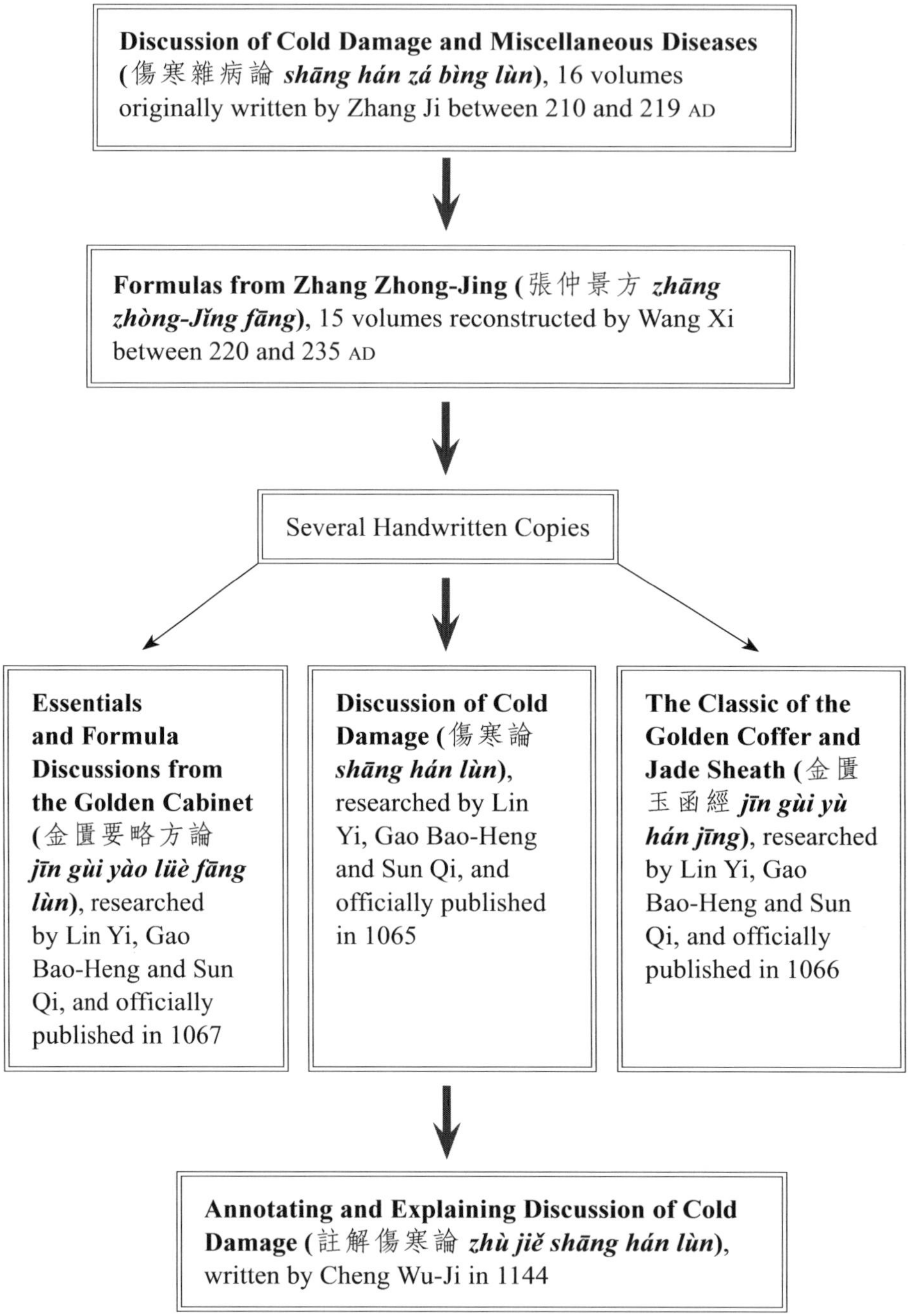

FIGURE 2.1 BRIEF INTRODUCTION TO ZHANG JI'S WORKS

3

EXPLORATION OF THE CULTURAL LANDSCAPE FOR WRITING DISCUSSION OF COLD DAMAGE

Medicine is a product of human society, and Chinese medicine is deeply rooted in traditional Chinese culture in regard to basic theory, academic contexts, and way of thinking. In the past 200 years, and especially in the past 50 years, scholars have published many articles and book chapters which discuss the cultural landscape, particularly the social and economic conditions, against which Zhang Ji wrote Discussion of Cold Damage. However, none of them have systematically explored this cultural landscape. As we know, Zhang Ji summed up the medical achievements gained before and during the Han Dynasty (206 BC to 220 AD) and developed new and practical differentiation and treatment systems for various kinds of diseases, systems which later had a tremendous influence on the theory and practice of Chinese medicine. Therefore, in order to thoroughly understand the theories and treatment approaches in Discussion of Cold Damage, one must study the cultural landscape on which the theories and treatment approaches of this classic were created and developed.

Culture is a fruit produced by the activity of human society. It basically stems from philosophical thinking. In the early stages of medical practice in China, Chinese medicine was based on sporadic accumulation of experience, though the knowledge of medicine was continually evolving. However, the medical knowledge of the time was superficial and scattered. When scholars and practitioners started to use both ancient and contemporary philosophy to view and guide medical practice, Chinese medicine gradually began to develop into a systematic, practical and effective discipline. During the Qin Dynasty (221–206 BC) and early Han Dynasty, the theory of qi, the theory of yin and yang, and the theory of five elements were blended into Chinese medicine, and several important books such as The Yellow Emperor's Inner Classic (黃帝內經 *huáng dì nèi jīng*), Materia Medica by Shen Nong (神農本草經 *shén nóng běn cǎo jīng*) and Difficult Questions (難經 *nàn jīng*), were produced. But what did the cultural landscape look like when Zhang Ji started to write Discussion of Cold Damage?

Cultural landscape when Zhang Ji wrote Discussion of Cold Damage

In Chinese history, the Spring and Autumn period (770–476 BC) and the Warring States period (476–221 BC) are the two eras when philosophers, such as Confucius, Lao Zi, Zhuang Zi, Xun Zi and others, abounded like stars in the galaxy. Of course, their doctrines—particularly those of Confucius and Lao Zi—have played an important role in the development of Chinese culture and Chinese medicine, especially since the Han Dynasty.

At the beginning of the Western Han Dynasty (206 BC to 24 AD), the economy was very bad and people were very poor as a result of one war after another due to peasant uprisings and the warlords fighting to control the country. In order to let peasants have a peaceful life for the recovery of the economy, the emperors and central government adopted the theory of Daoism, especially the statement, "when nothing is done, nothing is left undone," which appears in Chapter 48 of Morals Classic (道德經 *dào dé jīng*),[1] and this granted more freedom for local government and people. Daoism flourished at the beginning of the Western Han Dynasty. This flourishing is documented in the Historical Book for the Han Dynasty (漢書 *hàn shū*) written by Ban Gu (also known as Ban Meng-Jian, 32–92 AD), an historian of the early Eastern Han Dynasty (24–220 AD).[2] According to Zhang Heng-Liu and colleagues, in the section "Record of Art and Culture" (藝文志 *yì wén zhì*) of that book, which contains a list of books published c. 88 AD, Daoism held a prominent place in the literature of that era.[3]

1 Jia-Fu Feng and Jane English. *Tao Te Ching*. New York: Vintage Books, 1972: 57

2 Although the "Han Dynasty" is referred to in the title, Historical Book for the Han Dynasty only covers the Western Han Dynasty. The book is considered to be written by Ban Gu, but he did not finish the book before he died so it was completed by his sister, Ban Zhao, and another scholar, Ma Xu.

3 Zhang Heng-Liu et al. *Explanation and Clinical Application for Discussion of Cold Damage* (*shāng hán lùn jiě dú yǔ lín chuáng yìng yòng*). Shanghai: Publishing House of Shanghai University of Traditional Chinese Medicine, 2006: 2

Liu Che (140–87 BC), who was the seventh emperor and "Brave Emperor of the Han Dynasty," noticed that too much freedom for the people, especially for the local government controlled by royal family members, had compromised the power of the central government while the economy had begun to improve. Liu accepted the idea from Dong Zhong-Shu (179–104 BC) in 134 BC to "turn down all doctrines but respect the doctrine of Confucius," though in fact Dong's idea of Confucius' teachings was not based on the original doctrine of Confucius but rather was a "doctrine" that Dong himself had established, one that was based mainly on the doctrine of Confucius but had been combined with other doctrines as well—a new branch of Confucianism, as it were. According to this branch, everything had been put in its natural order, such as emperor and government ministers, father and sons, husband and wife. It was believed that the emperor was carrying out orders from gods in heaven and had the legal right to govern the country. This idea fitted very well with the intention of Liu Che to strengthen his power to control the country as a unified domain. However, this "unified domain" was broken apart by wars between warlords and peasant uprisings at the end of the Eastern Han Dynasty, and the country fell into chaos again. At that time, other philosophies (especially Daoism) were revived.

There is general agreement that Zhang Ji lived at the end of the Eastern Han Dynasty, and this was the social and cultural landscape in which he wrote Discussion of Cold Damage. How did this landscape influence Zhang Ji's writing? This question is answered in the next section.

Influence of Confucianism and Daoism on Zhang Ji

Evidence that Zhang Ji was influenced by Confucianism and Daoism is that he applied the concept of harmony, which was put forward by both (see Chapter 7 for further details). In Discussion of Cold Damage, there are many lines related to disharmony in the body and to the treatments to recover harmony. For example, Zhang Ji held the disharmony between the nutritive qi and the defensive qi responsible for spontaneous sweating (see lines 53, 54 and 95).

Compared with Hua Tuo, who lived at the same time as Zhang Ji, Zhang Ji was much less famous in his lifetime, though there are many legendary stories about him today. Among these stories, the story recorded in Book Reviewed by the Emperor of the Tai Ping Era (太平御覽 *tài píng yù lán*), published in 983 AD, demonstrates that Zhang Ji was very fond of Confucianism. Chapter 722, "Supplementary Biography for Mr. He Yong" (何顒別傳 *hé yóng bié zhuàn*), states:

> A fellow called Zhang Zhong-Jing, who was about 15 years old and came from the same town, paid a visit to Mr. He Yong (c. 168 AD) and wanted to learn from him. Mr. He told him, "You have a thoughtful mind, but it is not so charming. You can become a famous doctor."[4]

Given that He Yong served as a scholar and official in the highest institute and was quite famous for studying Confucianism, and because the country still functioned very well under Confucius' doctrine, when Zhang Ji was a teenager he was obviously very interested in studying Confucius' doctrine and becoming an official.

It was a tradition for authors who wrote books related to Chinese medicine during the Qin Dynasty and the Han Dynasty to absorb the essence of ancient Chinese philosophers. For example, Bamboo Slips in the Han Dynasty Dug from Zhang Jia-Shan (張家山漢簡 *zhāng jiā shān hàn jiǎn*), which is believed to have been written before The Yellow Emperor's Inner Classic, states: "To preserve health for the body, one must follow the principle of heaven and earth and act as a bellows. The shape changes but not the form. The more it moves, the more it yields."[5] This sentence is almost the same as the second part of Chapter 5 of Morals Classic (道德經 *dào dé jīng*), which states: "The space between heaven and earth is like a bellows. The shape changes but not the form. The more it moves, the more it yields."[6]

In the preface of Discussion of Cold Damage, Zhang Ji cites the following sentence from Confucius:

> Confucius says: "Those who know naturally from birth are greatest; those who understand by study are second to them; those who understand by broadly listening and memorizing are inferior." I have been respecting remedial arts for a long time and would like to follow this advice in my practice.

Zhang Ji also advocated the medical ethic that reflects benevolence and filial piety and duty, which is one of the fundamental concepts of

4 Li Fang et al. *Book Review by Emperor in Tai Ping era* (*tài píng yù lán*). Beijing: Chinese Publishing House, 1960: 3197

5 Gao Da-Lun. *Study on Qi Cultivation: Book on Bamboo Slips Dug from Tombs in Han Dynasty at Zhang Jia Mountain* (*zhāng jiā shān hàn jián yǐn shū yán jiū*). Chengdu: Bashu Publishing House, 1995: 63

6 Jia-Fu Feng and Jane English, op. cit., p.10

Confucianism. For example, in the preface of Discussion of Cold Damage, he encourages medical practitioners in the following way:

> Pay attention to medicine and proficiently study the remedial arts to treat the illnesses of emperors and parents above, then relieve the suffering of the poor and the lowly below, and finally, take care of one's own health as the center for preserving life.

In this context, the words "above" and "below" are literal translations of the characters "上 *shàng*" and "下 *xià*," respectively, which reflect another basic concept of Confucianism in the regard of classifying people according to their age, education level, economic status and political position in society. Craig Mitchell and colleagues wrote that "in Confucian philosophy, above, below and center describe social levels relative to the individual: above the individual are the sovereign and the individual's parents; below the individual are those less fortunate; the center is the individual himself."[7]

Additional concrete evidence that Zhang Ji studied Confucius is that he wrote in the preface of Discussion of Cold Damage, "If readers follow what I have written in this book, they will understand most of medicine." The words "they will understand most of medicine" share the exact structure of a sentence from the second section of the fourth appendix of the Book of Changes (周易 *zhōu yì*), which says that "if the wise look at this summary for one hexagram, he or she will understand most hexagrams,"[8] and there is general agreement that the whole appendix of the Book of Changes was written by Confucius and his followers.

In contrast to Confucianism, Daoism is not directly mentioned or cited by Zhang Ji. However, after carefully reviewing the literature that explores the sources for the formulas in his work, all contents of Discussion of Cold Damage, and related stories, one finds that Zhang Ji indeed applied Daoist doctrines, in his practice and his book, in the treatments for various kinds of diseases.

Indirect evidence to support that Zhang Ji was influenced by Daoism is a story in the preface of Acupuncture Jia and Yi Classic (針灸甲乙經 *zhēn jiǔ jiǎ yǐ jīng*) published c. 256 AD. In that story, a very interesting case study is recorded as the following:

7 Craig Mitchell et al. *Shāng Hán Lùn on Cold Damage*. Brookline: Paradigm Publications, 1999: 31

8 Li Wen-Bo. *General Explanation for the Book of Changes* (*yì jīng tōng jiě*). Beijing: China Publishing House of Contributing to Public, 2008: 326

> [Zhang] Zhong-Jing visited Wang Can, who was an official next to the prime minister and was about 20 years old. He told Mr. Wang, "You have suffered from the disease which can make eyebrows fall out at the age of 40, and you will die a half year after the falling out of the eyebrows. However, you can avoid this consequence if you take Five Stones Decoction." Mr. Wang was very annoyed by Zhang's words and did not take the decoction, though Mr. Wang did receive the prescription. Three days later, [Zhang] Zhong-Jing visited Mr. Wang and asked, "Have you taken the decoction?" Mr. Wang replied, "I did." [Zhang] Zhong-Jing said, "The color and expression on your face tell me that you have not taken the decoction. Why did you not take good care of your life?" Mr. Wang did not reply. Sure enough, Mr. Wang's eyebrows fell out 20 years later, which was exactly what [Zhang] Zhong-Jing had predicted, and Mr. Wang died 187 days after the falling out of his eyebrows.[9]

Jiang You-Li agrees about the influence of Daoism on Zhang Ji:

> Alchemy was very popular in the Western Han and Eastern Han Dynasty because of the close relationship between medicine and Daoism. The famous physicians and their books must have been affected by this relationship and stamped with this practice. Zhang Ji could not have been any exception to this influence...Five Stones Decoction consisted of five stones, although we do not know what exactly these five stones were. But it must have been relevant to five-stone powder (also called cold-stone powder) and five-miracle pills, which was very popular during that time.[10]

In the preface of Discussion of Cold Damage, little is revealed about where Zhang Ji learned to make his 113 formulas, though the books that might be related to Chinese herbs in this preface are called "胎臚藥錄 *tāi lú yào lù*." It is believed that these two books, which were written before Zhang Ji was born, are related to herbs used to treat women's disorders.[11]

---

9 Huang Fu-Mi. *Acupuncture Jia and Yi Classic* (*zhēn jiǔ jiǎ yǐ jīng*). Shanghai: Business Publishing House, 1955: 1

10 Jiang You-Li. *Taoist Culture and Chinese Medicine* (*dào jiā wén huà yǔ zhōng yī xué*). Fuzhou: Fu Jian Science and Technology Publishing House, 1997: 213

11 Guo Zhong-Guo. "Preliminary exploration of the meaning of Tai Lu and Yao Lu." *Forum for Doctors to Practice Chinese Medicine*, 2001 (1): 52

Fortunately, Huang Fu-Mi, who lived very close to the time when Zhang Ji lived,[12] has offered valuable information about the origin of Zhang Ji's formulas. In the preface of his book, Acupuncture Jia and Yi Classic published c. 256 AD, he wrote that "[Zhang] Zhong-Jing has studied and developed the formulas from Classical Methods to Make Formulas (湯液經法 *tāng yè jīng fǎ*),[13] and has written a book that has more than thirty chapters. The formulas recorded in his work are often effective in clinical practice."[14]

According to Liu Yong-Min's study, the three-chapter version of Classical Methods to Make Formulas, which Zhang Ji used as an important reference book, was written by some Daoist alchemists;[15] therefore, it is reasonable to deduct that Zhang Ji's writing was influenced by Daoism. Although Classical Methods to Make Formulas was available to readers during the Han Dynasty (206 BC to 220 AD) and the Northern and Southern Dynasties (420–589 AD), it seems that this book completely disappeared after the Song Dynasty (960–1279 AD), making it impossible to precisely know how Daoism influenced Zhang Ji's writing and practice, especially in regard to creating his formulas. Fortunately, the Rhymed Formula for Keys to Employ Herbs According to Zang-fu Organs (輔行訣臟腑用藥法要 *fǔ xíng jué zàng fǔ yòng yào fǎ yào*), which contains a lot of important information (especially formulas from Classical Methods to Make Formulas), was rediscovered by Zhang Guang-Rong, a veterinarian, in 1918.

12 According to Du Yu-Mao, Zhang Ji was born c. 151 AD and died c. 220 AD. See Du Yu-Mao, "Exploration of several issues related to Zhang Ji's life." *Journal of Shanxi College of Traditional Chinese Medicine*, 1982 (2): 38

13 There is general agreement that Classical Methods to Make Formulas (*tāng yè jīng fǎ*) was written by Yi Yin, a famous minister of the early Shang Dynasty (c. 1600 BC). According to Liu Yong-Min (see footnote 15), however, Classical Methods to Make Formulas (*tāng yè jīng fǎ*), which had 32 chapters as recorded in Record of Art and Culture of the Han Dynasty (*hàn shū yì wén zhì*), was not written by Yi Yin; instead, it has only three chapters and was written after the time when Materia Medica by Shen Nong (*shén nóng běn cǎo jīng*) was written but before Zhang Ji's work was written.

14 Huang Fu-Mi. *Acupuncture Jia and Yi Classic* (*zhēn jiǔ jiǎ yǐ jīng*). Shanghai: Business Publishing House, 1955: 1

15 Liu Yong-Min. "A study of Classical Methods to Make Formulas and Rhymed Formula for Keys to Employ Herbs According to Zang-fu Organs: Discussing the great influence of early Taoist culture on traditional Chinese medical science." *Dunhuang Research*, 2010 (3): 60

According to Wang Shi-Min, Rhymed Formula for Keys to Employ Herbs According to Zang-fu Organs was written by Tao Hong-Jing (also known as Tao Tong-Ming, 456–536 AD) and his followers, all of whom were Daoists,[16] between the Northern and Southern Dynasties and the Tang Dynasty (420–907 AD), and the formulas in it were adapted from Classical Methods to Make Formulas. In Rhymed Formula for Keys to Employ Herbs According to Zang-fu Organs, Tao Hong-Jing, a Daoist medical practitioner who lived a couple of hundred years after Zhang Ji, first proved what Huang Fu-Mi had said in the preface of Acupuncture Jia and Yi Classic—that Zhang Ji had followed Classical Methods to Make Formulas in developing his formulas. Tao wrote:

> During the Han Dynasty (206 BC to 220 AD) and Jin Dynasty (265–420 AD), all well-known physicians, such as Zhang Ji, Wei Si, Hua Yuan-Hua,[17] Wu Pu,[18] Huang Fu Xuan Yan,[19] Zhi Fa-Shi, Ge Zhi-Chuan,[20] Fang Jiang-Jun and others were all people of virtue, and all of them studied and followed Classical Methods to Make Formulas, diligently treating illness and benefiting mankind. They modified the formulas in this book and either specialized or found new applications for these formulas. Their practice seems not to have complied with the classic texts, but their objectives were in accordance with medical guidelines.[21]

But what did Zhang Ji actually learn from this book? Tao Hong-Jing answered as follows:

---

16 Wang Shi-Min. "Exploration of the relationship among Rhymed Formula for Keys to Employ Herbs According to Zang-fu Organs, Classical Methods to Make Formulas and Discussion of Cold Damage and Miscellaneous Diseases." *Journal of Traditional Chinese Medicine*, 1998 (11): 694

17 Hua Yuan-Hua was an honorific name for Hua Tuo.

18 Wu Pu was a student of Hua Tuo.

19 Huang Fu Xuan Yan was an alias for Huang Fu-Mi.

20 Ge Zhi-Chuan was a style name for Ge Hong (also known as Ge Ya-Chuan), a Taoist medical doctor who lived c. 284–364 AD.

21 Yi Zhi-Biao et al. *Study on Rhymed Formula for Keys to Employ Herbs According to Zang-fu Organs* (*fǔ xíng jué zàng fǔ yòng yào fǎ yào yán jiū*). Beijing: Learning Garden Publishing House, 2009: 16

> There are two dan formulas, six-gods[22] formulas, big and small formulas in Classical Methods to Make Formulas to treat externally contracted diseases and contagious diseases. In the past, Zhang Ji, who was from Nanyang county, adapted these formulas and wrote Discussion of Cold Damage. Since his book offers detailed treatment approaches, it has been well respected and followed by subsequent scholars and practitioners.[23]

What is the relationship between the two dan formulas, six-gods formulas and the major and minor formulas in Classical Methods to Make Formulas and the formulas in Discussion of Cold Damage? Wang Shi-Min states the following in his study on this question:

> There are 56 formulas recorded in Rhymed Formula for Keys to Employ Herbs According to Zang-fu Organs, among which...two dan formulas include five formulas (major, minor, yin and yang dan, and right yang dan decoctions), six-gods included 12 formulas [two types for each] (six gods: bluegreen dragon, white tiger, red bird, black warrior, hook old, flying snake)...Minor Yang Dan Decoction in Rhymed Formula for Keys to Employ Herbs According to Zang-fu Organs is identical to Cinnamon Twig Decoction (*guì zhī tāng*) in Discussion of Cold Damage...[24]

Table 3.1 provides a comparison (with slight adjustments) among the formulas in Rhymed Formula for Keys to Employ Herbs According to Zang-fu Organs and Discussion of Cold Damage.

22 According to Wang Xue-Tai, a scholar who was in charge of reconstructing this book in the early 1970s, "there are only four classic formulas recorded in this book. The six-gods formula appears to have been mistaken for the four-gods formula." See Wang Xue-Tai, *Textual Research, Commentary and Annotation for Rhymed Formula for Keys to Employ Herbs According to Zang-fu Organs* (*fǔ xíng jué zàng fǔ yòng yào fǎ yào jiào zhù*). Beijing: People's Military Medical Press, 2008: 28

23 Yi Zhi-Biao et al., op. cit., p.20

24 Wang Shi-Min, op. cit., p.694

Table 3.1 Comparison among formulas in Rhymed Formula for Keys to Employ Herbs According to Zang-fu Organs and Discussion of Cold Damage

R^x: Rhymed Formula for Keys to Employ Herbs According to Zang-fu Organs

D^x: Discussion of Cold Damage

Classification	Same	Similar
Decoctions contain Cinnamomi Ramulus (*guì zhī*)	Minor Yang Dan Decoction (*xiǎo yáng dàn tāng*) in R^x is the same as Cinnamon Twig Decoction (*guì zhī tāng*) in D^x.	Major Yang Dan Decoction (*dà yáng dàn tāng*) in R^x is Newly Augmented Cinnamon Twig Decoction with the Addition of One Liang Each of Peony and Fresh Ginger and Three Liang of Ginseng (*guì zhī jiā sháo yào shēng jiāng gè yì liǎng rén shēn sān liǎng xīn jiā tāng*) in D^x plus Astragalus.
Decoctions contain Scutellariae Radix (*huáng qín*) and/or Coptidis Rhizoma (*huáng lián*)	Minor Red Bird Decoction (*xiǎo zhū què tāng*) in R^x is the same as Coptis and Ass-Hide Gelatin Decoction (*huáng lián ē jiāo tāng*) in D^x.	Minor Yin Dan Decoction (*xiǎo yīn dàn tāng*) in R^x is Scutellaria Decoction (*huáng qín tāng*) in D^x plus Zingiberis Rhizoma Recens (*shēng jiāng*).
		Major Red Bird Decoction (*dà zhū què tāng*) in R^x is Coptis and Ass-Hide Gelatin Decoction in D^x plus Ginseng Radix (*rén shēn*) and Zingiberis Rhizoma (*gān jiāng*).
Decoction contains Bupleuri Radix (*chái hú*)		Major Yin Dan Decoction (*dà yīn dàn tāng*) in R^x is Minor Bupleurum Decoction (*xiǎo chái hú tāng*) in D^x plus Paeoniae Radix Alba (*bái sháo*).
Decoctions contain Ephedrae Herba (*má huáng*)	Minor Bluegreen Dragon Decoction (*xiǎo qīng lóng tāng*) in R^x is the same as Ephedra Decoction (*má huáng tāng*) in D^x.	
	Major Bluegreen Dragon Decoction (*dà qīng lóng tāng*) in R^x is the same as Minor Bluegreen Dragon Decoction (*xiǎo qīng lóng tāng*) in D^x.	

Decoctions contain Gypsum fibrosum (*shí gāo*)	Minor White Tiger Decoction (*xiǎo bái hǔ tāng*) in R^x is the same as White Tiger Decoction (*bái hǔ tāng*) in D^x.	Major White Tiger Decoction (*dà bái hǔ tāng*) in R^x is Lophatherum and Gypsum Decoction (*zhú yè shí gāo tāng*) in D^x minus Ginseng Radix (*rén shēn*) plus Zingiberis Rhizoma Recens (*shēng jiāng*).
Decoctions contain Aconiti Radix Lateralis (*fù zǐ*)		Major Black Warrior Decoction (*dà xuán wǔ tāng*) in R^x is True Warrior Decoction (*zhēn wǔ tāng*) in D^x plus Ginseng Radix (*rén shēn*) and Glycyrrhizae Radix (*gān cǎo*).
		Minor Black Warrior Decoction (*xiǎo xuán wǔ tāng*) in R^x is True Warrior Decoction (*zhēn wǔ tāng*) in D^x minus Zingiberis Rhizoma Recens (*shēng jiāng*) plus Zingiberis Rhizoma (*gan jiāng*).
Decoctions contain Pinelliae Rhizoma (*bàn xià*)	Minor Hook Old Decoction (*xiǎo gōu chén tāng*) in R^x is the same as Decoction to Drain the Epigastrium (*xiè xīn tāng*) in D^x.	
	Major Hook Old Decoction (*dà gōu chén tāng*) in R^x is the same as Pinellia Decoction to Drain the Epigastrium (*bàn xià xiè xīn tāng*) in D^x.	
Decoctions contain Natrii Sulfas (*máng xiāo*)		Minor Flying Snake Decoction (*xiǎo téng shé tāng*) in R^x is Major Order Qi Decoction (*dà chéng qì tāng*) in D^x minus Rhei Radix et Rhizoma (*dà huáng*) plus Glycyrrhizae Radix (*gān cǎo*).
		Major Flying Snake Decoction (*dà téng shé tāng*) in R^x is Major Order Qi Decoction (*dà chéng qì tāng*) in D^x plus Lepidii/Descurainiae Semen (*tíng lì zǐ*) and Zingiberis Rhizoma Recens (*shēng jiāng*).

Based on Table 3.1 and the discussion above, it is clear that most important formulas in Discussion of Cold Damage, such as Cinnamon Twig Decoction (*guì zhī tāng*), White Tiger Decoction (*bái hǔ tāng*), Ephedra Decoction (*má huáng tāng*), Decoction to Drain the Epigastrium (*xiè xīn tāng*), Major Bluegreen Dragon Decoction (*dà qīng lóng tāng*), Minor Bluegreen Dragon Decoction (*xiǎo qīng lóng tāng*), Coptis and Ass-Hide Gelatin Decoction (*huáng lián ē jiāo tāng*), Scutellaria Decoction (*huáng qín tāng*), Minor Bupleurum Decoction (*xiǎo chái hú tāng*) and True Warrior Decoction (*zhēn wǔ tāng*), are indeed very similar to their counterparts in Classical Methods to Make Formulas. Since both Huang Fu-Mi and Tao Hong-Jing mentioned that Zhang Ji developed his formulas based on Classical Methods to Make Formulas (湯液經法 *tāng yè jīng fǎ*), which was written earlier than Discussion of Cold Damage, and there are so many similarities among the formulas in these two books, the conclusion can be made that the formulas in Discussion of Cold Damage stemmed from Classical Methods to Make Formulas, i.e. Classical Methods to Make Formulas is the major source for formulas in Discussion of Cold Damage. What is more, this relationship has demonstrated that Zhang Ji was indeed influenced by Daoism, as bluegreen dragon, white tiger, red bird and black warrior are four gods worshiped by Daoists.

What is the difference between Black Warrior Decoction in Classical Methods to Make Formulas and True Warrior Decoction in Discussion of Cold Damage? In fact, they are similar in terms of meaning and their ingredients. One of the differences between them is the name has something to do with the taboo of using the personal names of emperors in Chinese history (see line 82 in section two of Discussion of Cold Damage for further details). If one reads Discussion of Cold Damage carefully, one should notice that Zhang Ji mostly used the names of herbs for naming the formulas. But why did he have such practice in the regard of naming the formulas? Tao Hong-Jing first offered a relatively reasonable answer to this question. He wrote that "Zhang Ji avoided using the Daoist name when writing Discussion of Cold Damage. Therefore, the formula he recorded did not bear the original Daoist name; rather, he named it after herbs, using chief herbs to name formulas."[26] It was a tradition to use chief herbs to name formulas between the Qin and Han Dynasties. For example, the authors who wrote The Yellow Emperor's Inner Classic had methods to name formulas such as Pinellia Decoction in Chapter 71 of Spiritual Pivot. In the case studies from Chun Yu-Yi, a well-known physician early in the Western Han Dynasty, there were formulas named after herbs such as "Pinellia Pill" and "Scrophlaria Decoction."[25] Therefore, it was reasonable for Zhang Ji to follow this tradition and name a formula after the chief herb in the formula. However, Zhang Ji did not completely give up all four-god decoctions in Daoism that are in charge of wind, dryness, fire and water. He used three of them for naming the formula, i.e. Bluegreen Dragon Decoction for wind, White Tiger Decoction for dryness and Black Warrior Decoction, which is changed to True Warrior Decoction in the later version of this book, for water, but he did not use Red Bird Decoction for fire, though there is Ass-Hide Gelatin Decoction (*huáng lián ē jāo tāng*) for fire. Apparently, Zhang Ji was hesitant to completely follow Classical Methods to Make Formulas and use Daoist names for naming all these formulas related to the four gods in Daoism.

Why did Zhang Ji struggle with this issue? In order to answer this question, one must review the cultural landscape in which Zhang Ji lived when he started to write Discussion of Cold Damage. As mentioned above, the doctrine of Confucianism had become the ruling ideology since 134 BC and the influence of Daoism was much less in various aspects. Zhang Ji grew up in this situation and became fond of Confucianism when he was a teenager. But this does not mean that Daoism disappeared from his mind, his practice and his writing. In fact, Daoism was revived at the end of the Eastern Han Dynasty when Zhang Ji started to learn Chinese medicine from the books that contain the profound philosophy of Daoism such as The Yellow Emperor's Inner Classic and Classical Methods to Make Formulas. At the end of the Eastern Han Dynasty, especially in 184 AD, there was a famous peasant uprising which was organized by a network of Daoists. Therefore, on one hand, as a commissioner of Changsha county, an official of government who was supposed to follow Confucius' doctrine, Zhang Ji had to deal carefully with something that was relevant to Daoism, and on the other hand, he did believe that ideas from Daoism were good for preserving the people's heath, because in the statement in the preface of his work he put forward that to study and practice medicine is to "take care of one's health as the center for preserving life," which reflects some ideas from Daoism. This is probably why he did not use all Daoist names from Classical Methods to Make Formulas to name

25 Han Zhao-Qi. *Commentary on Historical Records* (*shǐ jì pǐng zhù běn*). Changsha: Yue Lu Press, 2004: 1415–1416

formulas in Discussion of Cold Damage and did not mention that book as one of his references in the preface of his work.

Like discussing the influence of Confucianism, the impact on Zhang Ji's writing by Daoism can also be found in the text of Discussion of Cold Damage. One of the most important schools of thought in Morals Classic (道德經 *dào dé jīng*) is to follow the principles of nature. In Chapter 25 of Morals Classic (道德經 *dào dé jīng*), Lao Zi (also known as Li Er or Li Dan, c. 471 BC) pointed out that "man follows the earth. The earth follows heaven. Heaven follows the Tao. Tao follows what is natural."[26] Following Lao Zi's thought, Zhang Ji attached great importance to the natural healing ability of the human body when treating various kinds of diseases. In Discussion of Cold Damage, there are as many as 11 lines devoted to "automatic recovery," which demonstrates that Zhang Ji had noticed the potential ability of the human body to heal itself. He had not only noticed this self-healing ability but also observed that the human body is capable of finding natural ways to get rid of pathological factors, which are the promotion of sweating, promotion of vomiting, promotion of urination, purging and bleeding. In his book, Zhang Ji has 25 lines that use the characters "愈 *yù*" or "解 *jiě*," which mean "recovery," from the natural approach to eliminate pathological factors, for which there are ten lines related to promotion of sweating, seven lines related to purging and one line related to the promotion of urination. Of course, if one does not count on these characters in place of the formulas he recommended and one analyzes these treatment approaches, all 113 formulas can be viewed as following the body trend or natural way to eliminate pathological factors. Moreover, recognizing such potential healing ability in the human body, Zhang Ji discusses how to predict when a disease is about to resolve in 25 lines of his book.

Besides the thought to follow the principles of nature, reverse thought in Morals Classic (道德經 *dào dé jīng*) is another one to influence Zhang Ji's differentiation of disease in Discussion of Cold Damage. Reverse thought stresses mutual dependence and mutual transformation in two things that are opposed to each other. It requires one to view an objective from the opposite angle, which might be completely opposite to the direction of the movement of this objective, and to verify one thing through disapproving another thing. Lao Zi discusses this kind of thought

26 Jia-Fu Feng and Jane English, op. cit., p.50

in many chapters of Morals Classic (道德經 *dào dé jīng*). For example, in Chapter 2, he points out:

> Under heaven all can see beauty as beauty only because there is ugliness. All can know good as good only because there is evil. Therefore, having and not having arise together. Difficulty and easy complement each other. Long and short contrast each other, high and low rest upon each other; voice and sound harmonize each other; front and back follow one another.[27]

In Chapter 58, Lao Zi writes: "Happiness is rooted in misery. Misery lurks beneath happiness."[28] In Chapter 40, he writes: "Returning is the motion of the Tao."[29] In Chapter 78, he writes: "A positive word sounds like a negative word."[30]

Life is a process during which one disapproval comes after another disapproval. Because of this continual disapproval, one is born, grows, matures, gets old and dies. Likewise, the pathology of the disease process is the disapproval for normal physiology in the human body. In Chinese medicine, we often know the normal function of zang-fu organs through their clinical manifestations due to their dysfunctions, i.e. through their disapprovals. In fact, progression or regression of a disease is also the process of one disapproval coming after another disapproval. Carefully searching and studying a symptom or sign that disapproves of or disagrees with the previous one or other symptom and sign is a key to identifying this progression or regression in various kinds of diseases. Deeply understanding this philosophy stemming from Daoism, Zhang Ji created a special sentence which is called the sentence of showing manifestation that is opposite to the common condition and/or is unexpected according to regular thinking (反見證 *fǎn jiàn zhèng*). The way for him to present this reverse thought in his writing is to use the character "反 *fǎn*" or "復 *fù*," which can be translated as "but," "rather than," or "instead." For example, in line 287, Zhang Ji writes:

> In shao yin disease, there is a tight pulse. On the seventh or eighth day, there is automatically diarrhea, and the pulse suddenly becomes feeble, but the hands and feet become warm and the tight pulse is gone. This

27 Ibid., p.3

28 Ibid., p.105

29 Sha Shao-Hai and Xu Zi-Hong. *Complete Translation of Lao Zi* (*lǎo zǐ quán yì*). Guiyang: Guizhou People's Publishing House, 1989: 80

30 Ibid., p.158

> indicates that the disease is about to resolve. Although there is vexation and diarrhea, there will be automatic recovery.

In this line 287, Zhang Ji demonstrates what a key role the disapproval or disagreeable and unexpected symptom or sign plays in disease differentiation in his clinical practice. Yes, a feeble pulse indicates yang deficiency in shao yin deficiency, but it does occur after the tight pulse, which disapproves of or disagrees with the other symptoms and signs of yang deficiency and is unusual. Yes, the hands and feet should be cold as there is yang deficiency in shao yin disease, but the hands and feet become warm instead, which also disapproves of or disagrees with the combination of diarrhea and a feeble pulse or other symptoms and signs that might relate to yang deficiency, and the presentation of warm hands and feet is unusual. When analyzing these two symptoms and signs in combination, Zhang Ji would naturally know that yang qi is in the process of recovery. This is why he predicts that the disease is about to resolve though there is vexation and diarrhea. One must also learn that it is crucial to dynamically observe the change in symptoms, signs and pulses clinically for precise differentiation in time. According to my study, Zhang Ji deliberately used this special sentence in Discussion of Cold Damage to detect progression or regression of diseases. There are as many as 37 lines (more than 8% of the lines of this classic) devoted to this kind of thought: lines 11, 23, 24, 68, 89, 90, 104, 105, 110, 120–123, 126, 130, 136, 141, 182, 196, 215, 279, 287, 292, 301, 317, 322, 333–335, 341, 342, 347, 362, 363, 369, 377 and 384.

Knowing there is a possibility for such disapproval or disagreeable and unexpected symptoms or signs that present during the progression of a disease, Zhang Ji tried to exclude these symptoms or signs to determine whether or not a disease had progressed from one conformation to another. For example, in line 5, he writes that "neither yang ming syndrome nor shao yang syndrome is observed, though Cold Damage has been going on for two or three days. This indicates that there is no progression in tai yang disease." Such practices have been seen not only in disease differentiation but also in treatment approach. Zhang Ji used this thought to remind us of what treatment should be employed, what treatment should not be used, and what the consequence would be if the wrong treatment were applied. For example, in line 34, Zhang Ji states:

> A syndrome in tai yang disease that should be treated by Cinnamon Twig Decoction (*guì zhī tāng*) is purged instead. Consequently, incessant

> diarrhea ensues. If a cu pulse is felt, it indicates that the exterior syndrome has not been resolved; if there is panting and sweating, Pueraria, Scutellaria and Coptis Decoction (*gé gēn huáng qín huáng lián tāng*) should be prescribed.

Yes, wrong treatment should not be done in light of the theory of Chinese medicine. However, since there is always limitation for practitioners in the regard of their knowledge and skill, it is possible for them to make mistakes in differentiation and treatment when dealing with a disease. Knowing such possibilities (disapproval or disagreement with correct treatment) as much as possible, one cannot only avoid making the same mistakes but also learn what the consequences would be from this wrong treatment and get a clue as to what treatment would be appropriate for correcting these mistakes. Of course, our disease differentiation and treatment skills will be much improved by going through this process. In Chinese society, there is a famous proverb which states that "failure can be the mother of success." This is why Zhang Ji spent so much time and used so many lines to discuss deteriorated syndromes due to wrong treatment. Unfortunately, such wonderful skills in Discussion of Cold Damage stemming from reverse thoughts in Daoism have been largely ignored by contemporary scholars and practitioners. Now, the time has come to repay a visit to this insightful school of thought, that is, we must improve our study of Discussion of Cold Damage in order to make our treatment more effective in the clinic for various kinds of diseases.

Exploring the cultural landscape for writing Discussion of Cold Damage has been the only purpose of this chapter. Studying and understanding this cultural landscape, especially the philosophy that influenced Zhang Ji when he was writing this classic, is to open another window for readers to truly understand the content of Discussion of Cold Damage instead of only elaborating this classic according to contemporary theory in Chinese medicine. Understanding this can bring our knowledge to a deeper level and eventually improve our disease differentiation and treatment skills in our daily practice.

4

SCHOOL OF COLD DAMAGE AND SCHOOL OF STUDYING DISCUSSION OF COLD DAMAGE

In the history of Chinese medicine, nothing can compare with Discussion of Cold Damage in regard to its popularity. It is said that one cannot become a competent practitioner of Chinese medicine without studying Discussion of Cold Damage. According to Wen Chang-Lu and colleagues, there are as many as 600 versions of Discussion of Cold Damage since it was published and more than 10,000 books that study this classic have been published up to 2004.[1] In the past 100 years, there have been as many as 30,000 articles related to academic approaches to the study of this book and Zhang Ji's story.[2] Hao Wan-Shan has cited Liao Guo-Yu's article "Preliminarily Exploration for the Books that Study Theory from (Zhang) Zhong-Jing in the Past," which states that there are as many as 2763 books to study Discussion of Cold Damage among 3130 books related to the theories of Zhang Zhong-Jing.[3] Obviously, there is no doubt that all these figures demonstrate how important Discussion of Cold Damage is in Chinese medicine. Therefore, in order to be a skilled physician of Chinese medicine, one must study and understand this classic deeply. But questions are: What have these books and articles done for studying Discussion of Cold Damage? What kind of contribution have the authors who wrote these studies made to studying this classic or even to Chinese medicine? What can we learn from these books and

1 Wen Chang-Lu et al. *Collection of Studies for Works Written by Zhang Zhong-Jing* (*zhāng zhòng-jǐng yán jiū jí chéng*). Beijing: Chinese Medical Ancient Literature Publishing House, 2004: 2

2 Wen Chang-Lu. "Section one of review and commentary for theoretical study of Discussion of Cold Damage in recent hundred years." *Henan Journal of Traditional Chinese Medicine*, 2007 (3): 1

3 Hao Wan-Shan. "On establishing discipline of Discussion of Cold Damage and its content." *Journal of Beijing University of Traditional Chinese Medicine*, 1995 (11): 28

articles in terms of studying Discussion of Cold Damage and improving our clinical skills? Interestingly, systematic research for the books related to Discussion of Cold Damage and scholars who are dedicated to studying this classic did not appear until Zuo Ji-Yun (1891–1942) first discussed the classification for authors and their works related to studying Discussion of Cold Damage. In his book, Key Points to Study Discussion of Cold Damage (傷寒大要 *shāng hán dà yào*), written in 1937 but attached to his other work, Collections and References of Classified Formulas and Case Studies Related to Discussion of Cold Damage (傷寒論類方法案匯參 *shāng hǎn lùn lè fāng fǎ àn huì cān*) published in 2000, he first classified these scholars and their works into the following 12 schools:

1. one that compiles and annotates Discussion of Cold Damage
2. one that collects and records formulas from Discussion of Cold Damage
3. one that advocates warming and tonifying approach to treat Cold Damage due to internal injury
4. one that applies formulas in Discussion of Cold Damage according to geographic region
5. one that classifies the content of Discussion of Cold Damage according to the function of formulas
6. one that applies the theories in Discussion of Cold Damage based on movement of the five elements and six qi (五運六氣 *wǔ yùn liù qì*)
7. one that attaches great importance to tonifying yang
8. one that respects Discussion of Cold Damage as a classic without adding any personal opinion
9. one that pays special attention to the warming and clearing methods in Discussion of Cold Damage
10. one that corrects mistakes due to misplacement of bamboo slips or leaves questions unanswered
11. one that explains Discussion of Cold Damage by integrating both Chinese medicine and Western medicine

12. one that is skeptical of the existence of several chapters in Discussion of Cold Damage.[4]

As far I know, the term "school of Discussion of Cold Damage (傷寒學派 *shāng hán xué pài*)" was first introduced in the second version of the national textbook for Various Schools in Chinese Medicine (中醫各家學說 *zhōng yī gè jiā xué shuō*). Ren Ying-Qiu (1914–1984), a famous scholar from Sichuan who worked at Beijing University of Traditional Chinese Medicine, was a chief editor for the first three versions of this national textbook. He divided this school into three periods of time, i.e. authors and their books between the end of the Eastern Han Dynasty and Tang Dynasty, authors and their books in the Song Dynasty and authors and their books between the Ming Dynasty and the Republic of China. The greatest contribution he made for the school of studying Discussion of Cold Damage is that he classified the studies for this classic into three sub-schools. During the Ming Dynasty and Republic of China, there have been three sub-schools to study Discussion of Cold Damage. The first one comprises scholars who believed that the original text of Discussion of Cold Damage did not exist anymore and the versions of this classic we read had been edited and compiled by Wang Xi, Cheng Wu-Ji and other scholars. Therefore, one should do some research for these versions and recover the original presentation of Discussion of Cold Damage by changing the order of the lines in these versions. The second sub-school is completely opposite to the first one in that it is believed that Wang and Cheng made great contributions, respectively, to the passing down of this classic and the understanding of it. Therefore, it is not necessary to make any changes in the order of the lines for these versions. The third sub-school has attached great importance to the differentiation and treatment approaches according to various kinds of syndromes in Discussion of Cold Damage. Adherents to this sub-school believe that the most important thing in studying Discussion of Cold Damage is to gain benefit for clinical practice regardless of what is written by Zhang Ji and what is compiled or edited by Wang Xi and other scholars.[5]

4 Zuo Ji-Yun. *Collections and References of Classified Formulas and Case Studies Related to Discussion of Cold Damage* (*shāng hán lùn lè fāng fǎ àn huì cān*). Tianjin: Tianjin Scientific and Technological Publishing House, 2000: 560–564

5 Ren Ying-Qiu et al. *Various Schools in Chinese Medicine* (*zhōng yī gè jiā xué shuō*). Shanghai: Shanghai Scientific and Technological Publishing House, 1980: 91–107

Ren's approach had such a tremendous influence on the research for the schools of studying Discussion of Cold Damage that many scholars have followed his classification when discussing these schools. However, he confused two concepts when he wrote these textbooks—the school of Discussion of Cold Damage (傷寒學派 *shāng hán xué pài*) and the school of studying febrile diseases (傷寒學 *shāng hán xué*)—because he adapted citations from scholars who were dedicated to summarizing clinical experiences to treat exogenous febrile diseases due to pathological factors, which is not related to Discussion of Cold Damage. For example, he put Pang An-Shi (also known as Pang An-Chang, 1042–1099) as one of the scholars who specialized in the school of studying Discussion of Cold Damage. As a matter of fact, Pang An-Shi believed that the externally contracted diseases (the broad sense of the concept of *shāng hán*; see Chapter 1 of the present book for further details) are basically caused by cold-toxin, which does not agree with the content of Discussion of Cold Damage. Noticing this issue in Ren's classification, scholars have tried to demarcate these two concepts. Xi Zheng-Long has introduced the term "傷寒論學 *shāng hăn lùn xué*" (school of studying Discussion of Cold Damage) for clarifying the difference between these two concepts. He writes:

> What is called "傷寒學 *shāng hán xué*" refers to the discipline of treating acute febrile diseases in Chinese medicine. What is called "傷寒論學 *shāng hán lùn xué*" refers to the academic system formed by past scholars during their studying of Discussion of Cold Damage…it takes studying and explaining the principles and approaches of differentiation and treatment according to syndromes in Discussion of Cold Damage as its general goal. Its basic content is to elaborate the essence of six conformations, features of the theory, treatment methods and application of herbs in six conformations, and to annotate and comment on different versions of Discussion of Cold Damage.[6]

Wan Xiao-Gang points out that "strictly speaking, '傷寒學 *shāng hán xué*' is the discipline in Chinese medicine that takes the principles of the onset, progression, diagnoses and treatment approaches in febrile diseases

6 Xi Zheng-Long. "Section one of School of Studying Febrile Diseases and School of Studying Discussion of Cold Damage." *Shangdong Journal of Traditional Chinese Medicine*, 1991 (6): 22–23

as its study subject."[7] Because the contents of "傷寒學 *shāng hán xué*" (the school of studying febrile diseases) goes beyond Discussion of Cold Damage—though some of them are still helpful to understand theories, treatment approaches and formulas in Discussion of Cold Damage—I would focus on the literature that is specially dedicated to studying Discussion of Cold Damage alone and present what contribution scholars in this school in the past have made not only to Discussion of Cold Damage, the book itself, but also to Chinese medicine during their studying and clinically applying the theories, treatment approaches and formulas in Discussion of Cold Damage.

Generally, scholars and practitioners have made four contributions in studying Discussion of Cold Damage. These four contributions are: (a) arranging the order of the lines of the book; (b) completion of textual research; (c) annotation and explanation of the theories, treatment approaches, formulas and herbs; (d) discussion of the special topics and exploration of the application of the theories, treatment approaches and formulas. Since Discussion of Cold Damage has existed for more than 18 centuries, four periods of time have been classified by numerous scholars and practitioners for studying the book. These four periods are: early studies, intensive studies, introduction of new study approaches and multiple studies.

Early studies for Discussion of Cold Damage between the Jin Dynasty and Five Dynasties (265–960 AD)

The original book was written on bamboo slips between 210 and 219 AD. It contains 16 volumes, which covered Cold Damage, Miscellaneous Diseases and other disorders. The original book was lost long before it was finished due to political and social chaos either before or during the Three Kingdoms period (220–265 AD). The book was not intact when it was found as the string to connect the bamboo slips could be easily broken. However, information in the book must have been very insightful and had great value for excellent differentiation and treatment for various kinds of diseases, which made it so precious as to become top secret for some practitioners for quite a long period. No wonder Sun Si-Miao (581–682 AD),

7 Wan Xiao-Gang. "Brief History of School of Studying of Febrile Diseases and Its Development." In Xiong Man-Qi et al. (eds) *Discussion of Cold Damage in a Series of Advanced Books for Chinese Medicine* (*zhōng yī yào xué gāo jí cóng shū: shāng hán lùn*). Beijing: People's Health Publishing House, 2000: 972

a famous scholar and physician, sighed and stated that "practitioners south of the Yang Zi River hold key formulas from (Zhang) Zhong-Jing as top secret and have not passed them down"[8] even around the sixth century during the Tang Dynasty, 300 years after Discussion of Cold Damage was written. What most scholars and practitioners in that period did for this book was to reconstruct and copy it.

Among these scholars was Wang Xi (also known as Wang Shu-He, between 201 and 280 AD), a most brilliant figure in doing this kind of study. Wang Xi, a chief officer in charge of medical affairs in the Western Jin Dynasty (265–316 AD), collected those disconnected bamboos slips from various sources, reconstructed them (especially rearranged the order of the lines of the book) and named this reconstructed version "Formulas from Zhang Zhong-Jing (張仲景方 *zhāng zhòng-jǐng fāng*)." Besides this, he recorded most texts from Discussion of Cold Damage in his book, Pulse Classic (脈經 *mài jīng*) published c. 242 AD. In Pulse Classic, Wang Xi first classified the lines from Discussion of Cold Damage according to treatment approaches. It was a kind of studying process, which included figuring out the relationships among the lines in the regard of pathology and treatment. Based on the version of Discussion of Cold Damage published in 1065 AD (during the Song Dynasty), one can see that the order of the lines in three yin chapters and three yang chapters are not a random arrangement, and in each chapter they bear some meaning about onset, progression and prognosis of disease. It is very lucky for Chinese medicine that Wang Xi did exceptional work for the reconstruction of this classic. Without his hard work, the book probably would have been lost forever and there would be no Discussion of Cold Damage for guiding our practice in the clinic today. Without his thoughtful study and rearrangement of the lines of the book, which had been disorderly and unsystematic, what we would have now is a collection of experience-based formulas at most, and the book would not have become the milestone that it is for differentiation and treatment according to syndromes in Chinese medicine.

Besides Wang Xi, there were a few other scholars who did some useful study for Discussion of Cold Damage. Table 4.1 summarizes the contributions made by scholars and practitioners of that period.

---

8 Sun Si-Miao. *Thousand Ducat Formulas for Emergent Cases* (*bèi jí qiān jīn yào fāng*). Beijing: People's Health Publishing House, 1982: 187

Table 4.1 Major events in early studies for Discussion of Cold Damage

Author and date	Book and publication year	Contribution to study for Discussion of Cold Damage	Scholars influenced later
Wang Xi (201–280 AD)	Formulas from Zhang Zhong-Jing and Pulse Classic (c. 242 AD)	Collected bamboo slips, rearranged the order of the lines of the book. Classified the lines according to treatment approaches	Sun Si-Miao Qian Huang You Yi
Tao Hong-Jing (c. 456–536 AD)	Rhymed Formula for Keys to Employ Herbs According to Zang-fu Organs (date unknown)	Pointed out that Classical Methods to Make Formulas was the book from which Zhang Ji adapted formulas	Feng Shi-Lun
Sun Si-Miao (581–682 AD)	Thousand Ducat Formulas for Emergent Cases (652 AD) and Supplement to Thousand Ducat Formulas (682 AD)	Followed Wang Xi and classified the lines according to treatment approaches Classified the lines according to the relationship between syndromes and formulas, especially attaching great importance to Cinnamon Twig Decoction (*guì zhī tāng*), Ephedra Decoction (*má huáng tāng*) and Major Bluegreen Dragon Decoction (*dá qīng lóng tāng*) or Minor Bluegreen Dragon Decoction (*xiǎo qīng lóng tāng*)	Cheng Wu-Ji Fang You-Zhi Ke Qin Xu Da-Chun

Intensive studies for Discussion of Cold Damage between Song Dynasty and Qing Dynasty (960–1911)

Over a period of more than 1200 years, broad and deep studies for Discussion of Cold Damage have been done by many scholars. During the Song Dynasty and Yuan Dynasty, three important events related to studying Discussion of Cold Damage took place. The most important event for studying this classic during that period was that the official copy of Discussion of Cold Damage was published. In 1057, the government of the Song Dynasty set up the "Bureau of Textual Research and Correction for Medical Literature." The bureau invited many famous physicians and scholars and set up the schedule to collect, reconstruct and research important medical literature of the past. Among these scholars and physicians was Lin Yi, an unforgettable figure in the history of Chinese medicine, because he was in charge of doing textual research for different versions of Zhang Ji's works and left three precious versions of this work: Discussion of Cold Damage (published in 1065), The Classic of the Golden Coffer and Jade Sheath (which is another version of Discussion of Cold Damage published in 1066) and Essentials and Formula Discussions from the Golden Cabinet (published in 1067). It was Lin Yi's textual research that allowed the works of Zhang Ji, especially Discussion of Cold Damage, to be published, bringing an end to the 800 years of private copies and enabling this classic to be passed down. He provided us with the best version of Discussion of Cold Damage, and study for this book has flourished since then.

Zhu Gong (also known as Zhu Yi-Zhong, 1050–1125) first introduced the term "六經 *liù jīng*" for studying Discussion of Cold Damage in 1107 AD, though this term just means "six channels." He states:

> Scholars and practitioners in ancient times had a good method to study Discussion of Cold Damage since it is quite different from Miscellaneous Diseases in five aspects: It is treated according to six conformations (六經 *liù jīng*), onset and progression in yin channels, onset and progression in yang channels, the duration of the disease, as well as the warm and cold nature of the herbal formula, that should be prioritized accordingly.[9]

Nowadays, this concept has become the most important one to understand when studying Discussion of Cold Damage, though it was not the original one in the text and it does not bear the same meaning as Zhu's context (see Chapter 5 for further details). From the end of the Eastern Han Dynasty (220 AD) to the end of the Five Dynasties period (960 AD), what scholars have done for studying Discussion of Cold Damage is to focus on collecting disconnected bamboo slips, rearrange the order of

9 Zhu Gong. *The Book to Safeguard Life Based on Classifying Patterns* (*lèi zhèng huó rén shū*). In *Completed Medical Works of Zhu Gong and Pang An-Shi* (*zhū gōng páng ān-shí yī xué quán shū*) in *Collection of Works of Famous Physicians from the Tang, Song, Jin and Yuan dynasties* (*táng sòng jīn yuán míng yī quán shū dà chéng*). Beijing: China Chinese Medical Publishing House, 2006: 47

the lines and classify the lines. The first book to annotate Discussion of Cold Damage was not published until the work of Cheng Wu-Ji (1063–1156), Annotating and Explaining Discussion of Cold Damage (註解傷寒論 *zhù jiě shāng hán lùn*), went into print in 1144 AD. One of his methods of annotating this indispensable work was that he used theories from The Yellow Emperor's Inner Classic (黃帝內經 *huáng dì nèi jīng*) and Difficult Questions (難經 *nàn jīng*) as general guidelines to explain Discussion of Cold Damage. In his book, Cheng cites many statements from these two classics to elaborate the meaning of each line. Another of his methods was to elucidate the strategy for the 113 formulas (方論 *fāng lùn*), which included the principles of treatment and the combination of herbs as recorded in Discussion of Cold Damage. The former approach demonstrates the relationship between Discussion of Cold Damage and these two classics, and provides profound theoretical bases to deeply understand the original meaning of Discussion of Cold Damage, as these two classics were the texts to which Zhang Ji referred according to the preface of his works. The latter approach broke new ground in that the analysis of the formula had been absent in the studies done by previous scholars like Wang Xi and Sun Si-Miao.

In his book, Cheng first introduced some important terms for studying Discussion of Cold Damage such as "half interior and half exterior (半表半裡 *bàn biǎo bàn lǐ*)" for shao yang disease, "channel syndromes (經證 *jīng zhèng*)" and "fu syndromes (府證 *fǔ zhèng*)" for tai yang and yang ming disease, and the concept of "injury of the defensive qi by wind, injury of the nutritive qi by cold, injury of the defensive qi and nutritive qi by wind-cold." These terms and concepts have had a tremendous influence on the later study of Discussion of Cold Damage. Besides annotating and explaining this classic, Cheng provided another important work for us to study Discussion of Cold Damage, which is Understanding the Truth for Discussion of Cold Damage (傷寒明理論 *shāng hán míng lǐ lùn*) published c. 1142. In this book, Cheng first compared and differentiated 50 similar symptoms and signs, which is a prelude to the approach of differentiation of symptoms and signs in Chinese medicine. He also grouped the lines that contain the same symptom or sign and analyzed them for further exploring the way of thinking which Zhang Ji used for differentiation and treatment. In this book, he first explained the name of some formulas in Discussion of Cold Damage by applying his knowledge of ancient philosophy, astrology and geography. Yes, Lin Yi and colleagues made Discussion of Cold Damage available for the public. However, the book was written 1900 years ago. How to read and understand its content must be a big obstacle for scholars and practitioners. Of course, without a deep understanding of its theories, its application would be much limited. Obviously, Cheng's fruitful research on Discussion of Cold Damage made this book well received and led the school of studying Discussion of Cold Damage from early development to a flourishing time, and he played an indispensable role in terms of inheriting the past and ushering in the future.

As mentioned above, the school of studying Discussion of Cold Damage can be further classified into three sub-schools based on their attitude regarding the reliability of the text in the context of the various versions before the Song Dynasty, meaning (a) scholars who believe that the original book does not exist anymore and that the copy we have was edited and compiled by Wang Xi, Cheng Wu-Ji and other scholars; (b) scholars who are completely opposite to the first group, and believe that Wang and Cheng made great contributions to the passing down of the book and the understanding of it, respectively; and (c) scholars who have attached great importance to the differentiation and treatment according to various syndromes and ignore what was written by Zhang Ji and what was compiled or edited by Wang Xi and other scholars.

Among these scholars in the first sub-school, Fang You-Zhi (also known as Fang Zhong-Xing, 1523–1593) was the first to bring up disputes regarding the authenticity of the text of Discussion of Cold Damage, though Liu Wan-Su, Wang Lu and Huang Zhong-Li had already presented their questions about the reliability of the text according to the study by Guan Qing-Zeng and colleagues.[10] Having suffered the death of his two wives and five children from externally contracted diseases, Fang became determined to study Chinese medicine, he attached great importance to Discussion of Cold Damage, and spent much time on researching the order of the lines. After more than 20 years studying Discussion of Cold Damage, he wrote:

> Although the book is edited by (Wang) Shu-He (Wang Xi), it had been a long time since the book was written. Because time has changed and the book must have been eaten by worms and copied mistakenly by people, the book must not be the same as the original one. Scholars who annotated

10 Guan Qing-Zeng et al. *Ancient and Contemporary Study for Discussion of Cold Damage* (*shāng hán lùn gǔ jīn yán jiū*). Shenyang: Liaoning Scientific and Technological Publishing House, 1994: 36

> the book have largely ignored these facts and only given explanations according to the current copy of the book… It is clear that this practice has kept the mistakes made by previous scholars and continued to mislead people who read this book later… The reason I name this book by the term "條辨 *tiáo biàn*" is that I want to correct the mistakes made by (Wang) Shu-He (Wang Xi) and restore the original order of the lines as they should be.[11]

Fang strongly believed that the chapters "Normal Pulses," "Pulse Diagnosis" and "Precedent of Cold Damage" in Discussion of Cold Damage are not ones written by Zhang Ji, and that they were added by Wang Xi. Therefore, he deleted these three chapters in his book, Treatise on Discussion of Cold Damage (傷寒論條辨 *shāng hán lùn tiáo bìan*) published in 1592. Following Sun Si-Miao and Cheng Wu-Ji's approach to classify tai yang disease, Fang divided the content of the chapter on tai yang disease into three sections according to invasion of the defensive qi by wind, injury of the nutritive qi by cold and invasion of both the nutritive qi and defensive qi by wind-cold, and initially he introduced the concept of outline (提綱 *tí gāng*) for studying Discussion of Cold Damage. Fang's classification for tai yang disease is the prelude for what is called "the doctrine of three outlines that parallel each other like feet of an ancient vessel (三綱鼎立學說 *sān gāng dǐng lì xué shuō*)" in the history of the school of studying Discussion of Cold Damage. Like throwing a stone in a lake that stirs up thousands of waves, Fang's academic approach to studying Discussion of Cold Damage has been a hot topic debated by many subsequent scholars. Of course, some of them agreed with Fang, some of them blamed Fang's approach and some of them did not care about it. Apparently, Fang's study for Discussion of Cold Damage has livened up the academic atmosphere in studying this classic. Yu Chang (also known as Yu Jia-Yan, 1585–1644), a famous scholar and physician in the Ming Dynasty, greatly appreciated what Fang had done for Discussion of Cold Damage in regard to the rearrangment of the lines according to invasion of the defensive qi by wind, injury of the nutritive qi by cold and invasion of both the nutritive qi and defensive qi by wind-cold, though he held some reservations. He writes:

---

11 Fang You-Zhi. "Treatise on Discussion of Cold Damage" (*shāng hán lùn tiăo biàn*). In Business Publishing House (ed.) *Three Books on Discussion of Cold Damage* (*shāng hán lùn zhù sān zhǒng*). Beijing: Business Publishing House, 1957: 182

> In his book, Treatise on Discussion of Cold Damage (傷寒論條辨 *shāng hán lùn tiáo biàn*), Fang You-Zhi first deletes the chapter "Precedent of Cold Damage" added by (Wang) Shu-He, which has demonstrated great respect for the classic. However, there is the defect of being too extreme in this approach, and I would like to keep "Precedent of Cold Damage" and correct it. In this way, the correct and incorrect would be clear, and that is the contribution and mistakes Wang made. He made some changes to what (Wang) Shu-He did in the three chapters on tai yang disease, making the connection between wind-cold and the nutritive and defensive qi. This great approach transcended what his predecessors did for Discussion of Cold Damage.[12]

Yu rearranged the order of the lines of Discussion of Cold Damage not only based on the doctrine of three outlines that parallel each other like feet of a ancient vessel, but also according to different types of syndromes, diagnostic methods and treatment methods, which are the development from Fang's approach. For example, he assigned Cinnamon Twig Decoction (*guì zhī tāng*) for invasion of the defensive qi by wind, Ephedra Decoction (*má huáng tāng*) for the injury of the nutritive qi by cold, and Major Bluegreen Dragon Decoction (*dà qīng lóng tāng*) for invasion of both the defensive qi and nutritive qi by wind-cold. As a famous practitioner at that time, Yu attached great importance to the combination of theory and practice. He focused on the establishment of diagnostic and treatment methods and marked with the character "法 *fǎ* (method)" for each line and each chapter, which is helpful when distinguishing him from Fang You-Zhi. Besides this, Yu was probably the first scholar who annotated Discussion of Cold Damage while discussing the pathology of warm pathogen disease. He collected all lines that are relevant to warm pathogen disease in Discussion of Cold Damage and analyzed three pathological changes in warm pathogen disease, i.e. warm pathogen disease due to the attack of cold and lurking cold in winter, warm pathogen disease due to the failure of storing essence in winter and warm pathogen disease due to the attack of cold and the failure of storing essence in winter. However, some scholars have not agreed with Fang and Yu's attitude regarding what Wang Xi did and have given great credit to Wang Xi in the regard of reconstructing Discussion of Cold Damage. They

12 Yu Chang. *Writing on the Esteemed Discussion* (*shàng lùn piān*). In Yu Bo-Hai et al. (eds) *Collection of Famous Books on Discussion of Cold Damage, Essentials and Formula Discussions from the Golden Cabinet and Warm Disease* (*shāng hán jīn guì wēn bìng mīng zhù jí chéng*). Beijing: China Publishing House, 1997: 209

believe that Wang Xi did not make any mistakes in the rearrangement of the lines. He enabled this classic to be passed down and he is the person that has made the greatest contribution to Discussion of Cold Damage. In his book, Discussion of Cold Damage Annotated by Zhang Qing-Zi[13] (張卿子傷寒論 *zhāng qīng-zǐ shāng hán lùn*) published in 1644, Zhang Sui-Chen (also known as Zhang Qing-Zi, 1589–1668) followed the order of the lines as rearranged by Wang Xi. Zhang Zhi-Cong (also known as Zhang Yin-An, 1616–1674), one of his students and a famous scholar who annotated classics such as The Yellow Emperor's Inner Classic and Discussion of Cold Damage, stated:

> After carefully studying the art of composition to write a book, the lines are coherent to each other in good order. One can trust that these are not broken bamboo slips or residuals of chapters prior to the editing work done by (Wang) Shu-He.[14]

Chen Nian-Zu (also known as Chen Xiu-Yuan, c. 1753–1823), another well-known scholar who specialized in studying Discussion of Cold Damage, further pointed out:

> [Wang] Shu-He edited Discussion of Cold Damage and his great contribution will last forever. He added several chapters without putting his name on them, which was regretted by Wang An-Dao. However, all lines from "Differentiation and Treatment of Tai Yang Disease Based on Examining Both Pulses, Symptoms and Signs" to "Differentiation and Treatment for Yin Yang Yi Syndrome and Taxation Relapse Syndromes Based on Examining Both Pulses, Symptoms and Signs" are original texts written by (Zhang) Zhong-Jing.[15]

Overall, scholars in this sub-school believed that 397 lines in Discussion of Cold Damage are presented with the original sequence and are logical, though they realized that the three chapters, "Normal Pulses," "Pulse Diagnosis" and "Precedent of Discussion of Cold Damage," were added by Wang Xi.

---

13 Zhang Qing-Zi is the honorific name for Zhang Sui-Chen.

14 Zhang Zhi-Cong. *Ancestor Stamp for Discussion of Cold Damage* (*shāng hán lùn zōng yìn*). In Zheng Lin et al. (eds) *Complete Medical Works by Zhang Zhi-Cong* (*zhāng zhì-cōng yī xué quán shū*). Beijing: China Publishing House of Traditional Chinese Medicine, 2005: 756

15 Chen Nian-Zu. *Section Two of New Annotation and Collation for Books by Chen Xiu-Yuan* (*xīn jiào zhù chén xiū-yuán yī shū dì èr jí*). Fuzhou: Fujian Scientific and Technological Publishing House, 2003: 11

The doctrine of three outlines that parallel each other like feet of an ancient vessel and their treatments put forward by Fang You-Zhi and Yu Chang were not well received by most scholars, though there were still a few scholars, such as Qian Huang (also known as Qian Tian-Lai, c. 1707), who publicized and developed their ideas. For example, in his book, Connecting Pearls for Cold Damage (傷寒貫珠集 *shāng hán guàn zhū jí*) published in 1729, You Yi (also known as You Zai-Jing, 1650–1749), a famous scholar to study works written by Zhang Ji, made the following argument:

> Mild cold only injures the defensive qi, while severe wind can affect the nutritive qi. It would be difficult to eliminate wind when the defensive qi is in excess (stagnant). It would be impossible to prevent cold when the defensive qi is weak…Scholars should pay attention to whether or not there is sweating for determining application of Ephedra Decoction (*má huáng tāng*) and Cinnamon Twig Decoction (*guì zhī tāng*). And it is not necessary to differentiate injury by wind and injury by cold based on the excess or deficiency of the nutritive qi and defensive qi.[16]

In summary, the trend of this hot debate has pointed to keeping the 397 lines as they were in the version researched by Lin Yi and the version annotated by Cheng Wu-Ji, which leads to the presentation of this classic one read now. Concerning whether or not other chapters like "Normal Pulses," "Pulse Diagnosis" and "Precedent of Discussion of Cold Damage" were written by Zhang Ji or added by Wang Xi, we can continually debate but cannot arbitrarily state that they are useless, because they are at least the study done by Wang Xi for Discussion of Cold Damage, which can help us understand the book.

At the end of the Ming Dynasty (1368–1644) and during the Qing Dynasty (1644–1911), much more medical literature related to internal medicine, which address differentiation and treatment for various kinds of internal disorders, was published. This literature has made some scholars and practitioners in the school of studying Discussion of Cold Damage more practical and pay much attention to how to differentiate syndromes, especially classifying syndromes from various angles and giving treatments accordingly in six conformations, rather than try to figure out which chapter or line was originally written by Zhang Ji or added by Wang Xi. Scholars during that period classified syndromes in

16 You Yi. *Connecting Pearls for Discussion of Cold Damage* (*shāng hán guàn zhū jí*). Shanghai: Shanghai Science and Technology Publishing House, 1978: 7

Discussion of Cold Damage based on formulas, treatment approaches, qi transformations in six conformations, symptoms and signs, and causes.

Ke Qin (also known as Ke Yun-Bo, c. 1669), a quite fruitful scholar in studying Discussion of Cold Damage, made quite a few contributions to the school of studying Discussion of Cold Damage in his book, Surviving with Discussion of Cold Damage (傷寒來蘇集 *shāng hán lái sū jí*) published in 1669. The greatest contribution he made was that he rearranged the lines based on the relationship between the syndromes and formulas. Of course, as early as the seventh century, Sun Si-Miao had already classified the lines according to the relationship between syndromes and formulas, but this kind of classification done by Sun was just an embryonic form in which the concept of symptoms and signs (症 *zhèng*) and syndromes (證 *zhèng*) were not quite demarcated, and this is not practical in clinic settings. Ke's classification has the following two features:

- He highlighted the importance of syndromes, though he pointed out the conformation to which the syndromes belong, because syndrome is a very basic unit for diagnosis or differentiation and is also a base to set up the treatment approach, apply formulas and select herbs. Without clear differentiation of the syndrome, formulas and/or herbs would become sharp arrows that miss their targets. However, without formulas and herbs, the syndrome differentiated would not be resolved. In fact, knowing the mutually dependent relationship among syndromes, formulas and herbs, Zhang Ji stated "only if (the pathology of) the syndrome corresponds to (the function of) the formula can the formula be prescribed" in the footnote for the formula in line 317, and he used the formula's name to mark the syndrome such as the syndrome treated by Bupleurum Decoction (柴胡證 *chái hú zhèng*) in line 101.
- Learning from Zhang Ji and Sun Si-Miao, Ke systematically used the name of formulas to mark various syndromes. These not only included major formulas for each conformation in six conformations, such as the syndrome treated by Ephedra Decoction (麻黃湯證 *má huáng tāng zhèng*), the syndrome treated by Cinnamon Twig Decoction (桂枝湯證 *guì zhī tāng zhèng*) for tai yang disease, the syndrome treated by Bupleurum Decoction (柴胡湯證 *chái hú tāng zhèng*) and so on, but also cover the formulas

modified from them, such as the syndrome treated by Pueraria Decoction (葛根湯證 *gé gēn tāng zhèng*), the syndrome treated by Major Bluegreen Dragon Decoction (大青龍湯證 *dà qīng lóng tāng zhèng*).

This classification reflects the close relationship between the syndromes and formulas, and builds a bridge between the formulas and clinical situations, which makes it easier for practitioners to learn and apply the formulas. It is also quite helpful for practitioners to understand general pathology and individual development or special presentation for each syndrome and its treatment. For example, Ke Qin grouped 19 lines that contain the formulas modified from Cinnamon Twig Decoction (*guì zhī tāng*) under the syndrome treated by Cinnamon Twig Decoction (桂枝湯證 *guì zhī tāng zhèng*), which demonstrated the pathological development of the syndrome treated by Cinnamon Twig Decoction (*gui zhi tāng*) and special management of this formula, such as treating with this formula the disharmony between the nutritive qi and the defensive qi due to internal disorders. The classification of the lines in Discussion of Cold Damage done by Ke Qin according to the relationship between syndromes and formulas had a tremendous influence on ancient and contemporary scholars and practitioners in their studying and clinical practice related to Discussion of Cold Damage. For example, Xu Da-Chun (also known as Xu Ling-Tai, 1693–1771) duplicated the same classification approaches as Ke Qin and published his book, Classification of Formulas in Discussion of Cold Damage (傷寒論類方 *shāng hán lùn lèi fāng*) in 1759, Guo Zi-Guang and Feng Xian-Xun, professors from Chengdu University of Traditional Chinese Medicine, named their work in 1983 New Classification of Formulas and Syndromes in Discussion of Cold Damage (傷寒論湯證新編 *shāng hán lùn tāng zhèng xīn biān*). Although the research on the relationship between syndromes and formulas in Discussion of Cold Damage was done by Ke Qin and his followers, its theoretical and clinical significance is not limited to the understanding and application of the book and can be applied to all differentiation and treatment in Chinese medicine, because it has unveiled the logical relationship between the syndromes and formulas in the process of differentiation, treatment, formulas and herbs. Besides this lovely classification of the lines in Discussion of Cold Damage, Ke Qin first explained the book in the form of Discussion of Special Topic in Surviving with Cold Damage (傷寒來蘇集, 傷寒論翼 *shāng hán lái sū jí, shāng hán lùn yì*), such as "General View for the Whole

Book," "Correct Understanding of Six Conformations," and "Exploring the Significance of Dragging Over Diseases and Combinations of Diseases." In these special topics, he presents many of his own thoughtful, insightful and very valuable opinions to understand the content of this classic and its applications. For example, he points out:

> Six conformations differentiation created by (Zhang) Zhong-Jing was designed for hundreds of diseases rather than only externally contracted diseases. Externally contracted diseases and internal disorders should be treated by the same differentiation and treatment approach, which is six conformations differentiation.[17]

This statement has inspired many scholars and practitioners and made them attach great importance to employing the theories, treatment approaches and formulas in Discussion of Cold Damage to deal with various kinds of diseases in their life-long medical practices. Another contribution Ke Qin made was to put forward the idea of "six anatomical systems (六經形層 *liù jīng xíng céng*)" to explore the meaning of the term "六經 *liù jīng*," the very basic and hotly debated term in studying Discussion of Cold Damage (see Chapter 5 for further details). Like his other contributions, Ke Qin's study in this regard has influenced subsequent scholars.

Unlike Ke Qin, Qian Huang focused on diagnostic and treatment methods to study Discussion of Cold Damage. In his book, Trace to Source for Discussion of Cold Damage (傷寒溯源集 *shāng hán sù yuán jí*), first published in 1707, he realized that "almost all content in six conformations are methods related to diagnosis and treatment, and there is no exception in any lines"[18] based on his study of the book. Therefore, he "elucidates the reason to set up the methods related to diagnosis and treatment and explains the significance of making a formula when discussing differentiation and treatment for normal progression and abnormal progression in three yin diseases and three yang diseases."[19] In his book, he not only discusses what treatment methods should be for syndromes but also points out what wrong treatment methods are, such as the mistaken use of the promotion of sweating, vomiting, purging and

17 Ke Qin. *Discussion of Special Topic in Surviving with Cold Damage* (*shāng hán lái sū jí, shāng hán lùn yì*). Shanghai: Shanghai Science and Technology Publishing House, 1978: 2

18 Qian Huang. *Trace to Source for Discussion of Cold Damage* (*shāng hán sù yuán jí*). Shanghai: Shanghai Health Publishing House, 1957: 374

19 Ibid., p.6

firing methods recorded by Zhang Ji in three yin diseases and three yang diseases. Obviously, his study has offered a remedy for the defect of Ke Qin's approach, which only addressed the relationship between syndromes and formulas and ignored the treatment method that is a crucial part to guide the selection of formulas for resolving the related syndrome.

Qian was the first scholar who classified the lines in Discussion of Cold Damage according to the diagnostic and treatment methods. Besides this, his having stressed that there are wrong treatments recorded in the book can remind scholars and practitioners of not making the same mistakes made by previous practitioners and to improve their clinical skills in treating diseases. Following Fang You-Zhi and Yu Chang, who discussed injury of the nutritive qi and/or the defensive qi by wind and/ or cold in tai yang disease, Qian expanded this theory, especially injury by wind or cold, for all three yin diseases and three yang diseases, which does not stand up well to Chinese medicine theory.

Enlightened by Qian's approach in stressing diagnostic and treatment methods, You Yi systematically discussed eight diagnostic or treatment methods used in Discussion of Cold Damage in his book, Connecting Pearls for Discussion of Cold Damage (傷寒貫珠集 *shāng hán guàn zhū jí*) published in 1729. In this book, he tried to use these eight diagnostic or treatment methods to classify all lines in Discussion of Cold Damage and strongly believed that these methods are so precious, like pearls that connect on a string in the hands (hence, the title of the book). These eight diagnostic or treatment methods are regular treatment method, adapting method, mediating method, recovering method, classifying disease method, clear differentiating method, unusual method and acupuncture method, among which clear differentiating method and classifying disease method are related to diagnostic methods, while the rest are related to treatment approaches. In this book, You attached great importance to these methods and used them to govern syndromes and formulas, i.e. syndromes follow methods and formulas follow syndromes like connected pearls. Compared with Qian's approach, You's study offers a more orderly, clear and practical presentation of differentiation and treatment in Discussion of Cold Damage. This is why Tang Li-Shan (also known as Tang Da-Lie, c. 1792), a famous scholar at the end of the eighteenth century, commented the following:

> [You Yi] has unprecedentedly figured out a regular treatment method, adapting method, mediating method, recovering method, classifying

disease method, clear differentiating method, unusual method and so on, which make the essences of (Zhang) Zhong-Jing's work so clear with one glance, like the shining of snow and the light of the moon.[20]

According to Xi Zheng-Long, Wu Ren-Ju (also known as Wu Ling-Ya, date unknown) did an even better job in classifying the lines based on treatment methods. In his book, Inherit the Past and Usher in the Future for Medicine (醫宗承啟 *yī zōng chéng qǐ*), first published in 1702 (five years earlier than the works done by Qian), he used the following ten treatment methods to classify the lines in Discussion of Cold Damage: release the exterior, promotion of urination, promotion of vomiting, purging, harmonizing, rescue the interior, clear heat, warm the interior, acupuncture and moxibustion.[21]

As mentioned above, Cheng Wu-Ji analyzed 50 symptoms and signs recorded in Discussion of Cold Damage, an approach that had not been addressed very much by scholars who specialized in studying this classic for 600 years, until Shen Jin-Ao (also known as Shen Qian-Lu, 1701–1775) paid attention to this research approach. In his book, Detailed Outlines for Discussion of Cold Damage (傷寒論綱目 *shāng hán lùn gāng mù*), first published in 1774, he selected more than 100 symptoms and signs from Discussion of Cold Damage such as fever, aversion to cold, cough and so on to classify the lines in the book and then compared and analyzed them. The advantage of this approach is that it can clearly elucidate the pathology behind these symptoms and signs, their clinical presentations and the appropriate treatments. Therefore, Shen's work can be viewed as the first book related to differentiation and diagnosis of symptoms and signs for Discussion of Cold Damage. Later, Lü Zhen-Ming (also known as Lü Jian-Xun, 1798–1852) followed in Shen's footsteps to classify the lines according to symptoms and signs in his book, Searching the Source for Discussion of Cold Damage (傷寒尋源 *shāng hán xún yuán*) published in 1850. In 1959, Ren Ying-Qiu classified all lines except line 7, which was considered as an outline for differentiation of three yin diseases and three yang diseases, according to the 36 symptoms and signs in his book, Complete Classification of Syndromes and Their Treatments

20 Tang Li-Shan. *Collection of Papers of Physicians from Wu Area* (*wú yī huì jiáng*). Shanghai: Shanghai Science and Technology Publishing House, 1983: 22

21 Xi Zheng-Long. "Section two of School of Studying Febrile Diseases and School of Studying Discussion of Cold Damage." *Shangdong Journal of Traditional Chinese Medicine*, 1992 (1): 20

in Discussion of Cold Damage (傷寒論證治類詮 *shāng hán lùn zhèng zhì lèi quán*), first published in 1959.

The introduction of Western medicine in China can be traced back to the Northern and Southern Dynasties period (420–589 AD). But interaction of these two different medicines did not take place until Wang Hong-Han (also known as Wang Hui-Yuan, c. 1600) published his book, Beginning and Source of Medicine (醫學原始 *yī xué yuán shǐ*) in 1688. The first scholar who clearly stated "the connection of Chinese medicine and Western medicine (中西匯通 *zhōng xī huì tōng*)" is Tang Zong-Hai (also known as Tang Rong-Chuan, 1846–1897). As advocator for the combination of these two medicines, Tang applied this philosophy in his study for Discussion of Cold Damage. In his two works, Comprehensive Explanation for Syndromes and Formulas in Six Conformations (六經方證通解 *liù jīng fāng zhèng tōng jiě*) and Correction for Preliminary Commentary for Discussion of Cold Damage (傷寒論淺注補正 *shāng hán lùn qiān zhù bǔ zhèng*), he tried to integrate the main concepts of Chinese medicine and Western medicine to explain qi transformation in six conformations. His explanations are quite helpful for readers who have knowledge of Western medicine to exercise their imagination based on substantial anatomical parts of the body and get a better understanding of the function of the organs and pathology of the diseases. However, this kind of approach often led him to draw the wrong conclusions by false analogy and made him unable to have any fundamental breakthroughs in this area, though the work influenced Yun Shu-Jue's (also known as Yun Tie-Qiao, 1878–1935) book, Comments on Editorial Elaboration for Discussion of Cold Damage (傷寒論輯義按 *shāng hán lùn jí yì àn*), and Lu Pen-Nian's (also known as Lu Yuan-Lei, 1894–1955) book, Current Explanation for Discussion of Cold Damage (傷寒論今釋 *shāng hán lùn jīn shì*). All of them are important figures in the sub-school of connection between Chinese medicine and Western medicine (中西匯通學派 *zhōng xī huì tōng xué pài*) for studying Discussion of Cold Damage.

During the Song Dynasty and Qing Dynasty (960–1911), a particular sub-school in studying Discussion of Cold Damage, the sub-school of qi transformation, emerged and developed. The scholars who created this sub-school and developed its theory were Lu Zu-Chang (c. 1160), Lu Zi-Yi (also known as Lu Zi-Yao, 1599–1664), Zhang Zhi-Cong (also known as Zhang Yin-An, 1616–1674), Zhang Xi-Ju (also known as Zhang Ling-Shao, c. 1644), Huang Yuan-Yu (also known as Huang Kun-Zai, 1705–1750), Chen Nian-Zu (also known as Chen Xiu-Yuan, 1753–1823) and

Tang Zong-Hai (also known as Tang Rong-Chuan, 1847–1897). Scholars in this sub-school strongly believed that diseases in six conformations were the disorders of qi transformation in six conformations. The greatest achievement made by the school of qi transformation is that it has highlighted the importance of qi transformation in six conformations among the studies for Discussion of Cold Damage. It has offered quite an insightful approach for studying the book, especially for addressing some difficult issues in studying and practicing its theories, which have gradually been understood and valued by more contemporary scholars and practitioners, and have become an indispensable part of studying six conformations in Discussion of Cold Damage (see Chapter 6 for further details).

In the history of studying Discussion of Cold Damage, circulation of the book abroad did not draw attention from scholars in China until Wang Ke-Qin published his article "Discussion of Cold Damage in Japan"[22] in 1985 and Cui Xin-Ren wrote his masters thesis, "Circulation of Discussion of Cold Damage and Its influences on Medicine in Korea" in 2003. Since the literature for Discussion of Cold Damage in Korea has not been translated into Chinese or English, I am unable to offer more information about their studies and practices in Korea, though the circulation of this classic might be traced back to as early as the Sui Dynasty (589–618).

Historically, there have been two versions of Discussion of Cold Damage circulated in Japan, which are called "Kōhei"[23] (hand-copied in 1060) and "Kōji"[24] (hand-copied in 1143). Generally, the study for Discussion of Cold Damage in Japan has been influenced by two schools, the "school of applying ancient formulas" and the "school of applying both ancient formulas and contemporary formulas." Many Japanese scholars have done a great job regarding research and annotation for Discussion of Cold Damage, and they have published many valuable books. These scholars are Todo Yoshimasu (1702–1773), Sozan Shirozu (1713–1784), Motohiro Tamba (also known as Motohiro Taki, 1755–1810), Motosugu Tamba (also known as Motosugu Taki, 1789–1827), Motokata Tamba (also known as Motokata Taki, 1795–1857) and Koso Kitamura (1804–1876). There are two features for scholars and practitioners to study Discussion of Cold Damage in Japan: they attach great importance to the clinical

22 Wang Ke-Qin, "Discussion of Cold Damage in Japan." *Heilongjiang Journal of Traditional Chinese Medicine*, 1985 (1): 53

23 Kōhei refers to the period from 1058–1065 AD.

24 Kōji refers to the period from 1142–1144 AD.

application of formulas and "diagnostic skill in abdominal palpation" in this classic. "Diagnostic skill in abdominal palpation" has had great value in clinical diagnosis and differentiation, and it has been spreading in Western countries as well as in China. Although these scholars who were specialized in Discussion of Cold Damage did not use terms such as "six conformations (六經 *liù jīng*)" and "differentiation and treatment according to syndromes (辨證論治 *biàn zhèng lùn zhì*)" in their studies, they did have their theories such as "all diseases are caused by toxicity" and "qi, blood and water" to explain symptoms and signs recorded in Discussion of Cold Damage. Overall, ancient medicine in Japan originally comes from China, in which Discussion of Cold Damage has played an important role in the development of ancient medicine and has had a great influence on traditional medicine (漢方 *hàn fāng*) in modern-day Japan.

Introducing new studying approaches for Discussion of Cold Damage (1911–1949)

The 39-year period from 1911 to 1949 is definitely a short one in the history of the school of studying Discussion of Cold Damage. During this period, the war against the invasion of the Japanese and the civil war between the communist party and Nationalist party brought big turmoil in China. However, there were scholars and practitioner who continued their studies and practices in the field of Discussion of Cold Damage. Besides the publication of Exploring Real Meaning for Discussion of Cold Damage (傷寒發微 *shāng hán fā wēi*), written by Cao Jia-Đa (also known as Cao Ying-Fu, 1866–1937) in 1931, and Key Points to Study Discussion of Cold Damage (傷寒大要 *shāng hán dà yào*), written by Zuo Ji-Yun (1891–1942) in 1937, which belong to traditional approaches such as textual research, addressing differentiation and treatment, two new studying approaches were developed in this period. They were the sub-school of fire spirit (火神派 *huǒ shén pài*) and the sub-school of studying Discussion of Cold Damage at Shaoxing area (紹派傷寒 *shào pài shāng hán*). The latter one put forward the combination of the theory from the school of Discussion of Cold Damage and the theory from the school of warm-pathogen diseases.

In the history of Chinese medicine, especially during the Qing Dynasty (1644–1911), there have been some practitioners and/or scholars who have not cared very much about the school of Discussion of Cold

Damage and the school of warm pathogen disease. They strongly hold their faith that the clinical effect is their primarily concern regardless of which school works for diseases. Therefore, they would learn theories and apply formulas from both schools in their daily practice. For example, Ye Gui (also known as Ye Tian-Shi, 1666–1745), who was one of pioneers in the school of warm pathogen disease, especially in creating four-level differentiation, often adapted formulas from Discussion of Cold Damage in his practice. Since the eighteenth century, several scholars and practitioners from the Jiangsu province and Zhejiang province have written books to discuss the advantage of combining approaches from both schools. For example, Yu Zhao-Yuan (also known as Yu Gen-Chu, 1734–1799) wrote Popular Guide to the Discussion of Cold Damage (通俗傷寒論 *tōng sú shāng hán lùn*) and Wu Zhen (also known as Wu Kun-An, c. 1796) published his book, Completely Understanding Cold Damage (傷寒指掌 *shāng hán zhǐ zhàng*), in 1807. Both books are dedicated to the combination of theory and formulas from both schools in clinical practice. What they wrote, especially in Popular Guide to the Discussion of Cold Damage, drew great attention from many scholars and practitioners. Because most scholars and practitioners who have such practice came from the Shaoxing area in Zhengjiang province, they called themselves the school of studying Discussion of Cold Damage at Shaoxing area. The theory and practice of this sub-school were initiated by Yu Zhao-Yuan, but it was not systemized and did not become a unique sub-school until He Xiu-Shan (c. 1800), He Bing-Yuan (also known as He Lian-Chen, 1861–1929), Cao Bing-Zhang (also known Cao Chi-Dian, 1878–1956) and Xu Rong-Zhai (also known as Xu Guo-Chun, 1911–1982) annotated Yu's book, Popular Guide to the Discussion of Cold Damage. This school advocates combining theory from the school of Discussion of Cold Damage and the school of warm pathogen disease for exploring differentiation and treatment for externally contracted diseases, a broad sense of the concept of *shāng hán*. Scholars from this sub-school have developed many practical approaches and created many effective formulas to deal with externally contracted diseases.

The school of fire spirit (火神派 *huǒ shén pài*) is also called the school of strengthening yang (扶陽派 *fú yáng pài*). This school refers to a group of scholars and practitioners who attach great importance to yang qi and strengthening yang qi, especially being good at applying Aconiti Radix Lateralis (*fù zǐ*), Dry Ginger (*gān jiāng*), Cinnamomi Ramalus (*guì zhī*), Cinnamon Cortex (*ròu guì*) and other herbs with acrid flavor and hot nature in their clinical practice. They respect Discussion of Cold Damage, are familiar with six conformations differentiation and stress applying Aconiti Radix Lateralis (*fù zǐ*) early and in large dosage for various diseases. Zheng Shou-Quan (also known Zheng Qin-An, 1824–1911), who came from the Chengdu area, is considered to be the first scholar to establish this school. In his book, Truth Teaching in Medicine (醫理真傳 *yī lǐ zhēn chuán*), first published in 1869, he points out:

> Trigram 坎 *kǎn* refers to water, yin and blood, yet there is true yang contained. The line in the middle of this trigram refers to the heavens. The heavens and number one produce water, which corresponds to the kidney in the human body. However, there is one spot of true yang contained in two yins. This yang locates the place where there is extreme yin; it is a root for life and is really a true seed, which is called true yang by many books.[25]

In his other book, Flexible Medical Methods (醫法圓通 *yī fǎ yuán tōng*), first published in 1874, Zheng realized that yang plays a controlling role over yin and he states that "when yang is strong ten percent, yin would be strong ten percent; when yang is weak ten percent, yin would be weak ten percent."[26] Based on this philosophy, Zheng paid much more attention to strengthening yang qi for elimination of yin pathological factors and recovery of essence, blood and body fluid. He employed a large dosage of Zingiberis Rhizoma (*gān jiāng*), Cinnamomi Cortex (*róu guì*) and Aconiti Radix Lateralis (*fù zǐ*) for curing many severe syndromes due to yang deficiency and earned the nickname "fire god Zheng" (鄭火神 *zhèng huǒ shén*).

Because of his unique approach in the regard of theory and choosing herbs, Zheng got a lot of followers all over China during the end of the nineteenth century and the beginning of the twentieth century. They were Lu Yu-Chen (also known as Lu Zhu-Zhi, 1876–1963) and Tang Bu-Qi (1917–2004) from Chengdu, Wu Zhong-Quan (also known Wu Pei-Heng, 1888–1971) from Yunnan province and Zhu Wei-Ju (also known as Ao Shuang Xuan Zhu, 1884–1951) from Shanghai. Lu was called "Fire God Lu" (盧火神 *lú huǒ shén*) as he favored using acrid and hot herbs, while Wu and Zhu got the nicknames "吳附子 *Wǔ Fù Zǐ*" and "祝附子 *Zhù Fù Zǐ*"—related to Aconiti Radix Lateralis (*fù zǐ*) as they liked to use Aconiti Radix Lateralis to treat diseases.

25 Wang Ke-Qin. "Discussion of Cold Damage in Japan." *Heilongjiang Journal of Traditional Chinese Medicine*, 1985 (1): 53

26 Ibid., p.440

Historically, many scholars who specialized in Discussion of Cold Damage published their case studies, but none of them used their case studies to elucidate the content of Discussion of Cold Damage except for Cao Jia-Da, who first did so in his books, Exploring Real Meaning for Discussion of Cold Damage (傷寒發微 *shāng hán fā wēi*), written in 1931, and Records for Clinical Application of Classic Formulas (經方實驗錄 *jīng fāng shí yàn lù*), first published in 1937. Cao held that "if clinical experience is absent, the discussion of disease would be useless, though it might make sense."[27] Therefore, he "placed great attention on clinical experience and sometimes attached one or two case studies"[28] for explaining and exploring the pathology in Discussion of Cold Damage, proving the value of the formulas of Zhang Ji and answering confounding questions. In Records for Clinical Application of Classic Formulas, he even collected 92 case studies. Because case studies are more practical, Cao's approach made his study of Discussion of Cold Damage well received by subsequent scholars and practitioners.

As mentioned above, scholars in Japan have done a great job in textual research and annotation for Discussion of Cold Damage. At the end of the Qing Dynasty and the beginning of the Republic of China, there were many students sent to Japan to study various subjects. They also brought some books, including books related to Discussion of Cold Damage, back to China. These books were translated and circulated in China, and got the attention of some Chinese scholars. They not only relied on the literature offered by ancient scholars at home but also paid attention to what had been done by Japanese scholars in annotating this classic. Yun Shu-Jue (also known as Yun Tie-Qiao, 1878–1935) first took Editorial Elaboration for Discussion of Cold Damage (傷寒論輯義 *shāng hán lùn jí yì*), written by Motohiro Tamba (also known as Motohiro Taki, 1755–1810), as the chief source and wrote his book, Comments on Editorial Elaboration for Discussion of Cold Damage (傷寒論輯義按 *shāng hán lùn jí yì àn*) in 1928. Lu Pen-Nian (also known as Lu Yuan-Lei, 1894–1955), Yun's student, followed in his mentor's footsteps and cited more than ten books written by Japanese scholars when he wrote his book, Current Explanation for Discussion of Cold Damage (傷寒論今釋 *shāng hán lùn jīn shì*) in 1930. Introducing and citing the studies

27 Cao Jia-Da. *The Combined Book of Exploring Real Meaning for Discussion of Cold Damage and Essentials and Formula Discussions from the Golden Cabinet* (*cáo shì shāng hán jīn guì fā wēi hé kān*). Shanghai: Shanghai Health Publishing House, 1956: 72

28 Ibid., p.72

done by Japanese scholars has opened a window to broaden our view for studying Discussion of Cold Damage, giving us the opportunity to learn from Japanese scholars in order to improve our study in this field.

Multiple studies of Discussion of Cold Damage (1949 to present)

Unlike the regime of the Republic of China, the subsequent government of the People's Republic of China not only legalized Chinese medicine but also supported its development, though there was social turmoil during the Cultural Revolution that had a tremendously negative impact on traditional culture and philosophy. Generally, the time for Chinese medicine, including studying Discussion of Cold Damage, to flourish again has returned. According to Hao Wan-Shan, there were at least 5000 articles for studying Discussion of Cold Damage published between 1950 and 1990.[29] During that period, the areas and the approaches to study the book were largely expanded: many new theories in contemporary science, such as Pavlov's higher nervous activity theory, cybernetics and theory of communication were adapted to study Discussion of Cold Damage. Among these studies, the most attractive ones were: (a) systematic and textual research, annotation and translation; and (b) the principle of disease differentiation and treatment.

Systematic and textual research, annotation and translation for Discussion of Cold Damage

As mentioned above, Discussion of Cold Damage was researched by Lin Yi and colleagues in 1065. It has been almost 900 years since the last official textual research for the book. In 1959, scholars from Nanjing College of Traditional Chinese Medicine conducted the textual research for the version Completed Book by Zhong-Jing (仲景全書 *zhòng-jǐng quán shū*), compiled by Zhao Kai-Mei in 1575, which contains Discussion of Cold Damage, translated it into contemporary Chinese and published the book, Translation and Explanation for Discussion of Cold Damage (傷寒論譯釋 *shāng hán lùn yì shì*). In 1983, scholars from Shanghai College of Traditional Chinese Medicine selected ten chapters, including

29 Hao Wan-Shan. "On establishing discipline of Discussion of Cold Damage and its content." *Journal of Beijing University of Traditional Chinese Medicine*, 1995 (11): 28

the chapters on tai yang disease, shao yang disease, yang ming disease, tai yin disease, shao yin disease, jue yin disease, huo luan disease, yin yang yi syndrome and taxation relapse syndromes, from Completed Book by Zhong-Jing compiled by Zhao Kai-Mei and published Discussion of Cold Damage. Since the version of Discussion of Cold Damage of the Song Dynasty is not available, and Zhao's book has exactly copied the version of the Song Dynasty, there is general agreement that Zhao's work is faithful to the version of the book of the Song Dynasty. Because scholars from Shanghai College of Traditional Chinese Medicine did not do textual research for all the contents in the version of the book of the Song Dynasty, in 1991, Liu Du-Zhou (1917–2003) and colleagues conducted the textual research for Discussion of Cold Damage as a research project ordered by the Health Department of the Chinese government. Based on their research, they published Textual Research and Annotation for Discussion of Cold Damage (傷寒論校注 *shāng hán lùn jiào zhù*). This book has not only kept the presentation of the version of the Song Dynasty done by Lin Yi and colleagues, but also adapted some research achievements from contemporary scholars in their study of this classic. This book and the books published by scholars from Nanjing College of Traditional Medicine and Shanghai College of Traditional Chinese Medicine are considered as the three best versions thus far for learning and studying Discussion of Cold Damage in Chinese. Historically, besides the official publication of Discussion of Cold Damage in 1065, there was another ancient hand-copied version of Discussion of Cold Damage, which was researched by Lin Yi and colleagues during the Song Dynasty and published with the name The Classic of the Golden Coffer and Jade Sheath (金匱玉函經 *jīn gùi yù hán jīng*). Similar to the official 1065 version, this version of Discussion of Cold Damage has not been researched and annotated for 900 years since Lin Yi and colleagues did so in 1066. In 2007, with help from Qian Chao-Chen, a professor who specializes in reconstructing ancient medical literature at Beijing University of Traditional Chinese Medicine, Wu Zhong-Wen tried to do textual research and annotate The Classic of the Golden Coffer and Jade Sheath based on studying more than ten versions of Discussion of Cold Damage and published his research as a book, Study for The Classic of the Golden Coffer and Jade Sheath (金匱玉函經研究 *jīn gùi yù hán jīng yán jiū*). The publication of his book has provided reliable and supplementary literature for us to learn and study Discussion of Cold Damage.

Based on the demands of teaching Discussion of Cold Damage in many colleges and universities, since 1958 the Chinese government has invited many scholars who specialize in studying the book to write a national textbook for Discussion of Cold Damage and its supplementary reading books. Among these textbooks, the second, fifth and sixth versions of the national textbook for Discussion of Cold Damage and Teaching Reference Books for Traditional Chinese Medical Colleges: Discussion of Cold Damage (高等中醫院校教學參考書:傷寒論 *gāo děng zhōng yī yuàn xiào jiāo xué cān kǎo shū: shāng hán lùn*) have been quite well received. One of the features of these textbooks and teaching reference books is that they classify the lines of Discussion of Cold Damage according to the quality of pathology, which is quite different from the classifications done by past scholars. To meet these demands in teaching, each college or university has set up a Teaching and Research Section for Discussion of Cold Damage in which teachers have become specialists in studying the book. However, this teaching model has stemmed from Western medicine, in which a single textbook, single academic idea or single teaching method has greatly affected the integration of different sub-schools or academic ideas for studying Discussion of Cold Damage, though the model has made teaching easily accepted by students. Moreover, this single teaching model alone, without integrating apprenticeship, which is a traditional teaching model in Chinese medicine for more than 2000 years, would not be good for academic development of studying Discussion of Cold Damage.

Since the language used by Zhang Ji to write Discussion of Cold Damage was in use 1800 years ago, it is difficult for beginners who live in modern society to read and understand it. This would affect the understanding and application of the theories, treatment approaches and formulas in the book. Noticing this fact, there have been quite a few scholars who have translated the ancient texts in this classic into contemporary Chinese. Ren Ying-Qiu tried this translation in his book, Translation for Discussion of Cold Damage (傷寒論語譯 *shāng hán lùn yǔ yì*), first published in 1957. In his book, he not only translated this classic into contemporary Chinese based on his textual research and annotation but also summarized each line and each chapter for better understanding. Following his approach, Liu Du-Zhou and colleagues did a second translation with contemporary Chinese for this classic based on their study knowledge, Textual Research and Annotation for Discussion of Cold Damage (傷寒論校注 *shāng hán lùn jiào zhù*), the best version for this classic so far. Later, Hao

Wan-Shan worked with many scholars around the nation and presented the third translation with contemporary Chinese in their book, Translation for Discussion of Cold Damage with Contemporary Chinese (白話傷寒論 *bái huà shāng hán lùn*). Both Liu's and Hao's versions not only translated 398 lines, which is considered to be the original text of Discussion of Cold Damage by most scholars, but also gave translation for all other chapters such as "Normal Pulses," "Pulse Diagnosis" and "Precedent of Discussion of Cold Damage," which are viewed as added-on material. Without any doubt, these translations have made this classic widely accessible for readers and have helped its circulation and application. Interestingly, it seems that Discussion of Cold Damage is no longer a classic solely for professionals in Chinese medicine; it has now been more exposed to the general public, since Hao Wan-Shan, a professor at Beijing University of Traditional Chinese Medicine, was invited to teach Discussion of Cold Damage at the "Forum for Hundreds of Scholars" on Chinese Central Television in 2006.

Since the publication of the version of Discussion of Cold Damage in the Song Dynasty, there have been many scholars publishing their works for elucidating this classic based on their understanding and clinical experiences. These works have definitely made a great contribution to the understanding and application of the theories, treatment approaches and formulas. But so many explanations have made subsequent readers confused about the interpretations of these scholars and what is recorded or the original meaning of the book. Li Ke-Shao, a professor from Shangdong University of Traditional Chinese Medicine, and his colleagues, in their book, Explanation of Confusing Points in Discussion of Cold Damage (傷寒解惑論 *sháng háng jiě huò lùn*), first published in 1978, stressed that one should remain loyal to the original text of Discussion of Cold Damage and seek truth from this text. For example, they write:

> Commentators on and readers of Discussion of Cold Damage are used to calling three yin and three yang "six conformations (六經 *liù jīng*)" because "six conformations" is easier to pronounce [in Chinese]. However, this nomenclature can mislead readers to interpret the character "經 *jīng*" in the term "six conformations" as "channels" in the term "channels and collaterals (經絡 *jīng luò*)"...Zhang Zhong-Jing only mentioned three yin and three yang and never talked about "six conformations."[30]

30 Li Ke-Shao. *Explanation of Confusing Points in Discussion of Cold Damage* (*shāng hán jiě huò lùn*). Shandong: Shandong Scientific and Technological Publishing House, 1978: 11

Based on this approach, Li and colleagues have offered a very insightful explanation for many terms in this classic that are hard to understand such as "經 *jīng*," "傳 *chuán*," "中風 *zhòng fēng*" and "中寒 *zhòng hán*."

The circulation of Discussion of Cold Damage has not taken place only in China and Japan but also in Western countries. Luo Xi-Wen first translated most parts of the book into English and published "Treatise on Febrile Diseases Caused by Cold" in 1986. Although some of his translations were not accurate due to lack of medical background, his work has made the book available to scholars and practitioners in the West. In 1999, Craig Mitchell, Feng Ye and Nigel Wiseman took the national textbook for Discussion of Cold Damage as a main source and wrote Shāng Hán Lùn on Cold Damage. Since this work was done by three scholars who have a good background in Chinese, the translation has been well received and has produced textbooks available in the West, though lack of personal input in the theory and clinical experience has compromised the application of this book. Noticing this lack, Greta Yung Jie De and Robin Marchment, scholars and practitioners who practice in Australia, published their book, Shāng Hán Lùn Explained (傷寒論講解與臨床心得 *shāng hán lùn jiǎng jiě yǔ lín chuáng xīn dé*), in 2009. In their book, they offer some of their personal studies and clinical experience as well as cite many case studies to explain this classic and demonstrate its clinical significance.

The principle of differentiation and treatment in Discussion of Cold Damage

There is general agreement that Discussion of Cold Damage is not only a book to discuss externally contracted disease but also a work to present how to differentiate and treat various kinds of diseases. Since 1949, there have been many scholars who specialized in Discussion of Cold Damage who have attached great importance to exploring the principle of differentiation and treatment in this classic. They are Hu Xi-Shu (also known as Hu Xi-Xu, 1898–1984), Chen Yi-Ren (1924–2004), Li Pei-Sheng (1914–2009), Liu Du-Zhou (1917–2003), Yu Chang-Rong (1919–2003), Guo Zi-Guang, Nie Hui-Min, and Xiong Man-Qi. For example, in Passing Down Truth for a Classic Formula (經方傳真 *jīng fāng chuán zhēn*), which introduces his study and clinical experience for Discussion of Cold Damage, Hu Xi-Shu (also known as Hu Xi-Xu, 1898–1984) states that "differentiation according to eight diagnostic parameters and six conformations consists of the principle of differentiation and treatment in Discussion of Cold Damage."[31] Hu's idea has been echoed by Chen Yi-Ren (1924–2004), a professor from Nanjing University of Traditional Chinese Medicine. In his book, Search the Truth for Discussion of Cold Damage (傷寒論求是 *shāng hán lùn qiú shì*) first published in 1987, he writes that "the differentiation system [in Discussion of Cold Damage] mainly includes eight diagnostic parameters and six conformations."[32] Liu Du-Zhou holds that "the idea of eight diagnostic parameters comes from six conformations…six conformations is the main structure while eight diagnostic parameters is its application."[33] Some scholars have given detailed information in this regard according to their understanding and clinical experience. For example, Li Pei-Sheng (1914–2009), a chief writer of the fifth version of the national textbook for Discussion of Cold Damage, discussed ten differentiation methods in this classic, i.e. differentiating yin and yang, the exterior and interior, upper part and lower part of the body, deficiency and excess, cold and heat, true manifestation and false manifestation, similar syndromes, main manifestation and associated manifestations, urgent and trivial conditions, and prognosis. Following Ke Qin's approach, quite a few scholars, such as Hu Xi-Shu, Liu Du-Zhou, Nie Hui-Min and Guo Zi-Guang, have focused on "方證 *fāng zhèng*," the relationship between formulas and syndromes, to explore the principle of differentiation and treatment in Discussion of Cold Damage. Hu Xi-Shu gave the definition for the term "方證 *fāng zhèng*" as the following: "The term '方證 *fāng zhèng*' refers to the syndromes that correspond to formulas." He further states that "the substantial steps of differentiation and treatment according syndrome reflect on the management of '方證 *fāng zhèng*'."[34]

As mentioned above, original text like "the syndrome treated by Bupleurum Decoction (柴胡證 *chái hú zhèng*)" in line 101 implies that Zhang Ji noticed the relationship between formulas and syndromes. Liu Du-Zhou highly appreciated classifying the line according to the relationship

31 Feng Shi-Lun et al. *Passing Down Truth for a Classic Formula* (*jīng fāng chuán zhēn*). Beijing: China Publishing House of Traditional Chinese Medicine, 1994: 2

32 Chen Yi-Ren. *Search for the Truth for Discussion of Cold Damage* (*shāng hán lùn qǐu shì*). Shanghai: Shanghai Science and Technology Publishing House, 2008: 7

33 Chen Ming et al. *Key Points of Clinical Practice for Cold Damage by Liu Du-Zhou* (*liú dù-zhōu shāng hán lín zhèng zhǐ yào*). Beijing: Learning Garden Publishing House, 1998: 22–23

34 Feng Shi-Lun et al. *Passing Down Truth for a Classic Formula* (*jīng fāng chuán zhēn*). Beijing: China Publishing House of Traditional Chinese Medicine, 1994: 5

between syndromes and formulas and pointed out that "formulas and syndromes are essential for Discussion of Cold Damage. They are the keys to open the door for Discussion of Cold Damage."[35] Noticing this important relationship, Guo Zi-Guang and Feng Xian-Xun named their book New Classification of Formulas and Syndromes in Discussion of Cold Damage (傷寒論湯證新編 *shāng hán lùn tāng zhèng xīn biān*).

According to her study, Nie Hui-Min found that the corresponding relationship between syndromes and formulas had already been recorded in the footnote for line 317, which states that "Only when (the pathology of) the syndrome corresponds to (the function of) the formula can the formula be prescribed." Nie attached great importance to this relationship and pointed out:

> One of the features to compose the formulas of [Zhang] Zhong-Jing is to pair formulas with their corresponding syndromes…It requires establishing treatment approaches based on differentiated syndromes and selecting formulas according to the treatment approaches. Therefore, formulas must correspond with their syndromes when composing formulas.[36]

In the process of differentiation and treatment, there are many steps such as observation, smelling, inquiry, palpation, diagnosis or differentiation, selection of treatment approaches, choosing formulas and modifying formulas according clinical conditions, employing herbs, instruction of administering the decoction made from herbal formulas and recuperations. Obviously, among these steps, the formulas and syndromes, especially their relationships, are so crucial that they can have tremendous impact on the result of the treatment, because there are two fundamental factors in the differentiation and treatment, i.e. without knowing the pathology of the syndrome, there would be no treatment including selection of formulas; without selection of formulas, the treatment goal could not be fulfilled. Therefore, paying attention to the formulas and their corresponding syndromes is an important step to guarantee clinical success. It is essential, not only for treating diseases in six conformations of Discussion of Cold Damage, but also for every disease.

35 Chen Ming et al., op. cit., p.53

36 Nie Hui-Min. *Study of Discussion of Cold Damage by Nie Hui-Min* (*niè shì shāng hán xué*). Beijing: Learning Garden Publishing House, 2005: 13

Deep discussion for special topics

In regard to literature research, it will take a few years or maybe even one's whole life to write a book. But it might take only a few weeks or months to complete an article on a special topic. Modern media, especially more than 40 Chinese medical journals, have provided a good platform to discuss and debate special topics. Most research works on Discussion of Cold Damage are presented with special topics in these journals. These special topics have ranged from Zhang Ji's life, versions of his classic, academic approaches from scholars who have commented on and/or practiced the theories in the book in different eras, important concepts to study this classic such as six conformations, outlines for each disease, a single line and some terms, the theory of qi transformation, teaching methods for the book, treatment approaches such as harmonizing in shao yang and adjusting the nutritive qi and defensive qi, principles to applying herbs, the time for diseases in six conformations to resolve and so on. Among these topics, six conformations, harmonizing in shao yang and adjusting the nutritive qi and defensive qi, outlines for each disease, the unification of the school of Discussion of Cold Damage and the school of warm pathogen disease, and the theory of qi transformation have been hotly debated. The following discussion focuses on the unification of the school of Discussion of Cold Damage and the school of warm pathogen disease.

As early as the end of the Ming Dynasty (1279–1644), Yu Chang cited lines in Discussion of Cold Damage to analyze three pathological changes in warm pathogen disease. Later, scholars in the Shaoxing area put the theories and formulas from these two schools into their daily practice. Wan You-Sheng (1917–2003), a scholar who wrote Key Points to Learn from Discussion of Cold Damage (傷寒知要 *shāng hán zhī yào*), was the first contemporary scholar to state that "the school of Discussion of Cold Damage and the school of warm pathogen diseases can be united."[37] In 1980, he further pointed out that "six conformations in Discussion of Cold Damage, four levels and three burners differentiations in warm pathogen disease have their own defect, but it can be perfect when they are united. Therefore, both schools should be and can be united."[38]

37 Wan You-Sheng. "Discussion on transverse view in Discussion of Cold Damage and vertical view in warm pathogen disease." *Chinese Medicine in Jiangxi*, 1957 (1): 52

38 Wan You-Sheng. "On unification of six conformations in Discussion of Cold Damage, four levels and three burners differentiations in warm pathogen diseases." *Chinese Medicine in Jiangxi*, 1980 (4): 7

A year later, Wan proposed that "both schools can be united by putting theories, treatment approaches, formulas and herbs into the theories of six pathological factors, eight diagnostic parameters, zang-fu organs and channels."[39] Wang's proposal has drawn much attention from many contemporary scholars and it has been echoed and well received by many well-known scholars in China such as Mei Guo-Qiang (1939–) from Hubei, Guo Zi-Guang (1932–) from Chengdu, Shi Zhen-Sheng (1930–1998) from Beijing and Jiang Chun-Hua (also known as Jiang Qiu-Shi, 1908–1992) from Shanghai. However, there has been debate about how to unite these two schools, and the discussion on this special topic has been very much limited to theoretic exploration, and it has failed to be supported by clinical practice.

Besides unifying the school of Discussion of Cold Damage and the school of warm pathogen disease, the theory of qi transformation has been debated by many scholars for more than three decades (see Chapter 6 for further details).

Since 2007, the school of fire spirit (火神派 *huǒ shén pài*) has drawn much attention all over China, scholars and practitioners in this sub-school have set up the Forum to Strengthening Yang (扶陽論壇 *fú yáng lùn tán*) and have held three conferences since 2007. Lu Cong-Han (a grandson of Lu Zhu-Zhi), Wu Rong-Zu (a son of Wu Pei-Hen) and Liu Li-Hong (a follower of Lu) are the scholars who initiated these conferences. Besides organizing conferences, they have published books that contain the speeches presented in these conferences. Also, Zhang Cun-Ti, a scholar from Liaoning province, has published more than ten articles, especially analyzing case studies, in various journals to introduce and study the theories and practices related to this sub-school.

The school of fire spirit has produced practitioners who further study Discussion of Cold Damage, and therefore, the development and prosperity of this school has improved the theory and practice related to the book. However, due to sectarian bias, some of the adherents have stressed the importance of yang qi so much that it makes them denounce any other theories and approaches in the book, which obviously goes too far and requires awareness and attention.

For 1800 years, Discussion of Cold Damage has been studied and explored by scholars and practitioners. The theories it contains have

39 Wan You-Sheng. "On unification of Discussion of Cold Damage and warm pathogen diseases." *Yunnan Journal of Traditional Chinese Medicine*, 1981 (1): 1

served as guidelines for us to differentiate various kinds of diseases, and its formulas have become ancestor remedies for thousands of formulas. There have been numerous articles and a few hundred books in various sub-schools in regard to research on the book. Many scholars have dedicated their whole life to studying the book and applying its theories, treatment approaches and formulas in their daily practice. Based on their academic beliefs, their studies and clinical experience, they have offered many insightful and valuable yet different comments on this classic. They have built up the school of studying Discussion of Cold Damage and its many sub-schools through their constant and assiduous studies.

There have been disagreements and debates based on the academic backgrounds and clinical experience of such scholars. Some terms or theories that they have used are not recorded in the original text of Discussion of Cold Damage. But it is these disagreements and debates that have broadened our view. It is the introduction of these terms and theories that have deepened our understanding of the physiology and pathology of the human body and the treatment for various kinds of diseases. For example, debating on six conformations and the theory of qi transformation has presented a good picture about the physiological function of the body and progression of diseases based on the network of zang-fu organs and their channels, though they are not recorded in Discussion of Cold Damage. Classification of the lines of the book according to the formulas or treatment methods has facilitated the proper application of the formulas. Addressing the corresponding relationship between formulas and syndromes has offered two crucial keys for us to apply the theories and formulas in regard to differentiation and treatment. Like a piece of jade just dug up, time is needed to polish it for the shine of the beautiful jade to appear. Scholars and practitioners in the school of studying Discussion of Cold Damage have been working very hard for over eighteen centuries and have brought to us the very instructive and valuable classic, Discussion of Cold Damage, with their comments and explanations. Whatever the book means, its meaning will never be outdated. Therefore, it is reasonable to believe that there are still many things we need to study and explore in Discussion of Cold Damage.

5

SIX CONFORMATIONS, SIX CONFORMATIONS DISEASES AND SIX CONFORMATIONS DISEASE DIFFERENTIATION

Brief introduction to six conformations and six conformation diseases

Six conformations, six conformations disease and six conformations differentiation are translations for the terms "六經 *liù jīng*," "六經病 *liù jīng bìng*" and "六經辨證 *liù jīng biàn zhèng*," respectively. These three terms are so important that everyone who has studied Discussion of Cold Damage must be familiar with them, and everyone who wants to study this classic must not miss them. Obviously, without understanding six conformations, one cannot comprehend six conformations diseases and six conformations differentiation as it is a base for the other two terms. Therefore, six conformations are key and must be understood first. Yun Shu-Jue (also known as Yun Tie-Qiao, 1878–1935), a famous scholar who studied Discussion of Cold Damage in the first half of the twentieth century, stated:

> The most important thing in Discussion of Cold Damage is six conformations. And the most difficult to understand in this book is also six conformations. Therefore, everyone who discusses Discussion of Cold Damage has spared no efforts to explore it. Every scholar who wants to make commentary for Discussion of Cold Damage has also spared no efforts to do research for it. Without understanding this term, what one gets is a foggy picture for the whole book. And then how can one study Chinese medicine?[1]

1 Yun Shu-Jue. "On six conformations in Discussion of Cold Damage." *Literatures for Chinese Medicine*, 1936 (1): 134

Guan Qing-Zeng and colleagues further pointed out:

> Discussion of Cold Damage has established a system of pattern differentiation and treatment based on applying six conformations for naming diseases and demarcating pattern. [Therefore] correctly understanding six conformations is the basis and key to studying Discussion of Cold Damage.[2]

As a matter of fact, the term "六經 *liù jīng*" is not originally recorded by Zhang Ji in Discussion of Cold Damage. This term was first introduced as an approach to study this classic by Zhu Gong (also known as Zhu Yi-Zhong, 1050–1125) in his book, The Book to Safeguard Life Based on Classifying Patterns (類證活人書 *lèi zhèng huó rén shū*), in 1108. In this book, Zhu wrote:

> Scholars and practitioners in ancient times had a good method to deal with Cold Damage since it is quite different from Miscellaneous disease in the five aspects: It is treated according to "六經 *liù jīng*," onset and progression in yin channels, onset and progression in yang channels, the duration of the disease and the warm and cold nature of the herbal formula, all of which should be prioritized accordingly.[3]

The term "六經 *liù jīng*" has become an indispensable tool for ancient and contemporary scholars and practitioners to study and apply the theory for Discussion of Cold Damage. Because different scholars and practitioners have different depth and breadth of knowledge and practice, understanding this concept is quite different since the almost 1000 years that Zhu Gong first introduced this term. For example, scholars from Guangzhou College of Traditional Chinese Medicine and China Academy of Traditional Chinese Medicine viewed it as "six differentiating outlines" and "six comprehensive syndromes" in 1979,[4] and Craig Mitchell and

2 Guan Qing-Zeng et al. *Ancient and Contemporary Study for Discussion of Cold Damage* (*shāng hán lùn gǔ jīn yán jiū*). Shenyang: Liaoning Scientific and Technological Publishing House, 1994: 96

3 Zhu Gong. *The Book to Safeguard Life Based on Classifying Patterns* (*lèi zhèng huó rén shū*). In *Completed Medical Works of Zhu Gong and Pang An-Shi* (*zhū gōng páng ān-shí yī xué quán shū*) in *Collection of Works of Famous Physicians from the Tang, Song, Jin and Yuan dynasties* (*táng sòng jīn yuán míng yī quán shū dà chéng*). Beijing: China Chinese Medical Publishing House, 2006: 47

4 Guangzhou College of Traditional Chinese Medicine and China Academy of Traditional Chinese Medicine. Dictionary for Chinese Medicine (*zhōng yī dà cí diǎn*). Beijing: People's Health Publishing House, 1979: 72

colleagues translated it as "six channels" in 1999.[5] According to Wang Qing-Guo and Wang Zhen, there have been 41 opinions about the concept of "六經 *liù jīng*."[6] It is reasonable to speculate that many more opinions about this term have been developed since then. I would classify them into two categories and choose ones that have more influence on this study and present as viewing 六經 *liù jīng* as a physiological term or a term to describe disease pattern differentiation.

"六經 *liù jīng*" as a physiological term

"六經 liù jīng" as six channels

Zhu Gong first implied that this term refers to six channels. He writes:

> One must study channels when studying Discussion of Cold Damage. Without knowing channels, it is just like walking on a road that has dim light. One often treats shao yin channel when the disease is located in tai yang channel or harmonizes shao yang channel when the syndrome is located in jue yin channel.[7]

Wang Hu (also known as Wang Ling-You, c. 1680), a well-known commentator for Discussion of Cold Damage, further developed this idea in his book, Commentary on Differentiation in Discussion of Cold Damage (傷寒論辨證廣注 *shāng hán lùn biàn zhèng guǎng zhù*), first published in 1680. He wrote that "as to channels in Discussion of Cold Damage, [Zhang] Zhong-Jing only differentiates 六經 *liù jīng* without mentioning hand and foot channels. In fact, both foot channels and hand channels are involved in a disease."[8] Noticing that Zhu's understanding was too narrow to convey the meaning of the term "六經 *liù jīng*," Fang You-Zhi, a famous scholar to study Discussion of Cold Damage in 1589, pointed out:

> "六經 *liù jīng*" includes everything in the human body…if one arbitrarily views the character "經 *jīng*" in "六經 *liù jīng*" as channels of the human

5 Craig Mitchell et al. *Shāng Hán Lùn On Cold Damage*. Brookline, MA: Paradigm Publications, 1999: 10

6 Wang Qing-Guo and Wang Zhen. "Forty-one opinions about study on six conformations for Discussion of Cold Damage." *Journal of Beijing University of Traditional Chinese Medicine*, 1997 (20): 23

7 Zhu Gong, op. cit., p.21

8 Wang Hu. *Commentary on Differentiation in Discussion of Cold Damage* (*shāng hán lùn biàn zhèng guáng zhù*). Shanghai: Shanghai Health Publishing House, 1958: 7

> body, it does not lay out its meaning completely and gives rise to so many misunderstandings.[9]

The character "經 *jīng*" can be understood and translated into "channel" in English and six channels is exactly the literal translation for the term "六經 *liù jīng*." And yes, Zhang Ji indeed used this character "經 *jīng*" in the text of Discussion of Cold Damage. However, according to Liu Shao-Wu's study, Zhang Ji used this character ten times in this work and none of them refers to any of these channels.[10]

"六經 liù jīng" as six anatomical systems

Fang You-Zhi wrote:

> The channel in six conformations ("六經 *liù jīng*") is different from channels in the body. Like six classics in Confucius' school, "六經 *liù jīng*" refers to six parts (in the body). No matter how big the universe and how many things in the universe, the six parts in the classics can cover them; likewise, no matter how many things in the human body, "六經 *liù jīng*" can cover them completely.[11]

Based on this idea, in studying Discussion of Cold Damage, he first connected the skin to tai yang, muscle to yang ming, and interspaces between outer part of the body and zang-fu organs to shao yang. Fang's interpretation was echoed and developed by Ke Qin (also known as Ke Yun-Bo, c.1669), a famous scholar who specialized in making commentaries for Discussion of Cold Damage. In his book, Discussion of Special Topic in Surviving with Cold Damage (傷寒來蘇集・傷寒論翼 *shāng hán lái sū jí, shāng hán lùn yì*), first published in 1674, Ke wrote:

> "六經 *liù jīng*" from [Zhang] Zhong-Jing's work is to divide the human body into six parts and it covers vast areas. It does not focus on channels and collaterals, though vessels are considered as channels and collaterals. Let me take geography as an example: "六經 *liù jīng*" is like a special district in the country. The areas above the waist belong to three yang,

9 Fang You-Zhi. "Treatise on Discussion of Cold Damage" (*shāng hán lùn tiǎo biàn*). In Business Publishing House (ed.) *Three Books on Discussion of Cold Damage* (*shāng hán lùn zhù sān zhǒng*). Beijing: Business Publishing House, 1957: 1

10 Liu Shao-Wu. "Informally exploring that six conformations should be viewed as six diseases." *New Chinese Medicine*, 1979 (4): 12

11 Fang You-Zhi, op. cit., p.1

> which predominates the external parts of the body yet connect to the inside of the body. The heart is a place where three yang meet. Tai yang covers the areas that are from the heart and chest to the top of the head. It reaches frontal head, shoulder, back and feet, and connects to the urinary bladder internally. It governs the nutritive qi and defensive qi and is responsible for the exterior syndrome on the body, which is like the district on the border of the country.
>
> Yang ming covers the area that is from the heart and chest to the stomach and intestines. It reaches the head, face, abdomen and feet. Shao yang covers the areas that are from the heart to the throat. It goes along the cheek and reaches the ears, eyes and the top of the head. It connects to the gall bladder through the hypochondriac region. It locates between tai yang and yang ming, which are like surrounding areas of the capital. The areas below the waist belong to three yin. Three yin predominate the interior and the abdomen is the place where three yin meet. Tai yin covers the areas that are from the abdomen to large intestines, small intestines and anus. Shao yin covers the areas that are from the abdomen to the kidney, the urinary bladder and the urethra, while jue yin covers the areas that are from the abdomen to the liver, the diaphragm, the heart, the lower abdomen and outer genital organ.[12]

Followed Fang's and Ke's idea, Yu Zhao-Yuan (also called Yu Gen-Chu, 1734–1799), a well-known scholar and physician who combined theories from the school of Discussion of Cold Damage and the school of warm pathogen disease, developed a quite complete anatomical system for Discussion of Cold Damage in 1776. He states:

> Tai yang channel predominates the skin and hairs; yang ming channel predominates the muscles; shao yang channel predominates the interstices between muscles and skin; tai yin channel predominates the limbs; shao yin channel predominates the blood vessels; and jue yin channel predominates the tendons and membrane. In the body, tai yang predominates the chest; shao yang predominates the diaphragm; yang ming predominates the epigastrium; tai yin predominates the upper abdomen; shao yin predominates the lower abdomen; jue yin predominates the right and left low quadrant of the abdomen.[13]

12 Ke Qin. *Discussion of Special Topic in Surviving with Cold Damage* (*shāng hán lái sū jí, shāng hán lùn yì*). Shanghai: Shanghai Science and Technology Publishing House, 1978: 5–6

13 Yu Zhao-Yuan. *Revised Popular Guide to the Discussion of Cold Damage* (*chóng dìng tōng sú shāng hán lùn*). Hangzhou: New Medicine Press, 1956: 2

These interpretations, especially that of Yu Zhao-Yuan, are quite useful as they have developed a network which can help practitioners to visualize "六經 *liù jīng*" in the human body and apply it in clinical practice.

"六經 liù jīng" as three yin and three yang

Many ancient and contemporary scholars have realized that the term "六經 *liù jīng*" refers to three yin and three yang. For example, what is called the school of qi transformation has implied that "六經 *liù jīng*" refers to three yin and three yang and has discussed the relationship between six qi and three yin and three yang (see Chapter 6 for further details). The representative figure of this school is Zhang Zhi-Cong (also known as Zhang Yin-An, 1616–1674). In his book, Collection of Commentaries for Discussion of Cold Damage (傷寒論集注 *shāng hán lùn jí zhù*), first published in 1683, Zhang Zhi-Cong wrote:

> In Discussion of Cold Damage, there are tai yang, yang ming, shao yang, which are called three yang; there are tai yin, shao yin and jue yin, which are called three yin. Three yin and three yang are called six qi (wind, cold, summer-heat, damp, dryness and fire). As there is six qi in the heavens, there is six qi in the human body. Six qi in the human body correspond to the ones in the heavens and circulates (normally) when illness is absent.[14]

In the late 1950s, scholars from the Teaching and Research Section for Discussion of Cold Damage at Jiangsu School of Traditional Chinese Medicine were the first to clearly state that "'六經 *liù jīng*' refers to three yang (tai yang, yang ming, shao yang) and three yin (tai yin, shao yin and jue yin)."[15] A question might be raised: Why do not ancient and contemporary scholars use three yin and three yang rather than the term "六經 *liù jīng*"? Li Ke-Shao (1910–1996) offered a good explanation: "Scholars and readers are accustomed to calling three yin and three

---

14 Zhang Zhi-Cong. *Collection of Commentaries for Discussion of Cold Damage* (*shāng hán lùn jí zhù*). In Zheng Lin et al. (eds) *Complete Medical Works by Zhang Zhi-Cong* (*zhāng zhì-cōng yī xué quán shū*). Beijing: China Publishing House of Traditional Chinese Medicine, 2005: 621

15 Teaching and Research Section for Discussion of Cold Damage, Jiangsu School of Traditional Chinese Medicine. *Explanation for Discussion of Cold Damage* (*shāng hán lùn shì yì*). Nanjing: Jiangsu People's Publishing House, 1958: 2

yang '六經 *liù jīng*,' because '六經 *liù jīng*' is easier to pronounce [in Chinese]."[16]

"六經 *liù jīng*" as a complexity of channels, three yin, three yang, zang-fu organs and qi transformations in the human body

Ancient scholars, in fact, noticed that the channels, three yin and three yang, zang-fu organs and qi transformation in the human body are related to each other when they discussed the meaning of "六經 *liù jīng*." The first person who clearly related this term to zang-fu organs is Guo Yong (also known as Guo Zi-He, 1106–1187). In his book, Replenishment for Discussion of Cold Damage (傷寒補亡論 *shāng hán bǔ wáng lùn*), first published in 1181, Guo Yong wrote:

> Question: To which zang or fu organ does '六經 *liù jīng*' belong? Answer: Foot tai yang is the channel of the urinary bladder, foot yang ming is the channel of the stomach, foot shao yang is the channel of the gall bladder. These three fu organs belong to yang. Foot tai yin is the channel of the spleen, foot shao yin is the channel of the kidney, foot jue yin is the channel of the liver. These three zang organs belong to yin.[17]

In 1596, Li Shi-Zhen (also known as Li Dong-Bi, 1518–1593) tried to use the theory of zang-fu organs to explain the function of the formulas in Discussion of Cold Damage in his book, Detailed Outline of the Materia Medica (本草綱目 *běn cǎo gāng mù*). He stated:

> Ephedrae Herba (*má huáng*) is an agent to exclusively deal with the disorders of the lung and its channels...Ephedra Decoction (*má huáng tāng*) is indeed a formula to disperse stagnant fire in the lung and its channels, though it is considered as a strong formula to promote sweating in tai yang disease...Cinnamon Twig Decoction (*guì zhī tāng*) is indeed a formula to adjust the spleen and lung, though it is a mild formula to relieve flesh in tai yang diseases.[18]

16 Li Ke-Shao. *Explanation of Confusing Points in Discussion of Cold Damage* (*shāng hán jiě huò lùn*). Shandong: Shandong Scientific and Technological Publishing House, 1978: 12

17 Guo Yong. *Replenishment for Discussion of Cold Damage* (*shāng hán bǔ wáng lùn*). Shanghai: Shanghai Science and Technology Publishing House, 1959: 18

18 Li Shi-Zhen. *Detailed Outline of the Materia Medica* (*běn cǎo gāng mù*). Beijing: People's Health Publishing House, 1981: 1009

Jiang Chun-Hua (also known as Jiang Qiu-shi, 1908–1992), a well-known scholar from Shanghai, first introduced the term "綜合體 *zōng hé tí* (complexity)" to study the meaning of the term "六經 *liù jīng*" as early as 1962. He wrote:

> "六經 *liù jīng*" in Discussion of Cold Damage was originally recorded in The Yellow Emperor's Inner Classic. However, its contents were no longer the same as that which means "channels" in that book. The author (Zhang Ji) has orchestrated all concepts of yin and yang in The Yellow Emperor's Inner Classic, which includes the exterior, the interior, cold, heat, deficiency, excess, channels, zang-fu organs, the nutritive qi and defensive qi, wax and wane between pathological factors and anti-pathogenic qi, to make the condensed complexity that contains various concepts.[19]

In 1964, scholars from Chengdu College of Traditional Chinese Medicine pointed out that "六經 *liù jīng*" refers to complexity of channels, zang-fu organs and qi transformations. They pointed out:

> "六經 *liù jīng*" connects to the entire five zang and six fu organs. Qi transformation is the manifestation of the functions of zang-fu organs and channels…therefore, zang-fu organs, channels and qi transformations are closely related to each other. One cannot stress one of them for explaining the meaning of "六經 *liù jīng*" and must combine them for studying the meaning of "六經 *liù jīng*."[20]

This interpretation for the term "六經 *liù jīng*" has been widely received and developed by many contemporary scholars. For example, Li Ke-Shao (1910–1996), a famous scholar from Shandong province, echoed this interpretation as the following:

> "六經 *liù jīng*" is indeed three yin and three yang…Three yin and three yang is not only related to six qi, zang-fu organs and channels in Chinese medicine. They are also used by Zhang Zhong-Jing to mark types of diseases… In Discussion of Cold Damage, the six classifications of diseases are much closer to six qi, zang-fu organs and channels.

19 Jiang Chun-Hua. "Discussion of several issues on six conformations in Discussion of Cold Damage." *Shanghai Journal of Traditional Chinese Medicine*, 1962 (8): 17

20 Chengdu College of Traditional Chinese Medicine. *Textbook for Discussion of Cold Damage* (*shāng hán lùn jiáng yì*). Shanghai: Shanghai Scientific and Technological Publishing House, 1964: 3

> Therefore, employing three yin and three yang to name diseases is most comprehensive and appropriate.[21]

Liu Du-Zhou (1917–2003) , a well-known scholar from Beijing University of Traditional Chinese Medicine who specialized in Discussion of Cold Damage, pointed out as early as 1980 that "六經 *liù jīng*" includes 12 channels of the hands and feet and belongs to zang-fu organs internally."[22] He Zhi-Xiong also stated:

> "六經 *liù jīng*" in Discussion of Cold Damage was created upon the request to differentiate externally contracted diseases. It is another type of summary of human function based on the theory of zang-fu organs. First, zang-fu organs are classified into two types of yin and yang, i.e. five zang organs belong to yin, while six fu organs belong to yang. Then, they are further classified into three yin and three yang, named as tai yang, yang ming, shao yang, tai yin, shao yin and jue yin, based on the functions of different organs and different distribution of their channels. This is "六經 *liù jīng*" in Discussion of Cold Damage.[23]

Xiong Man-Qi and colleagues offered a good summary for these interpretations for the term "六經 *liù jīng*." In their book, Discussion of Cold Damage in a Series of Advanced Books for Chinese Medicine (中醫藥學高級叢書傷寒論 *zhōng yī yào xué gāo jí cóng shū: shāng hán lùn*) published in 2000, they wrote:

> "六經 *liù jīng*" is the succinct summary for physiological structure and function, and their relationship, and the relationship between nature and the human body. Specifically, it is the complexity of zang-fu organs, channels and qi transformation. In this whole system, it is classified into six sub-systems, i.e. tai yang, yang ming, shao yang, tai yin, shao yin and jue yin, based on the features of human structure and function and their relationship.[24]

---

21 Li Ke-Shao, op. cit., pp.10–12

22 Liu Du-Zhou. "Discussion of several issues in Discussion of Cold Damage." *Journal of New Medicine*, 1978 (1): 18

23 He Zhi-Xiong. "Exploration of the essence of six conformations in Discussion of Cold Damage." *New Chinese Medicine*, 1983 (2): 6

24 Xiong Man-Qi et al. *Discussion of Cold Damage in a Series of Advanced Books for Chinese Medicine* (*zhōng yī yào xué gāo jí cóng shū: shāng hán lùn*). Beijing: People's Health Publishing House, 2000: 2

"六經 *liù jīng*" as a term for disease pattern differentiation

"六經 liù jīng" as channels for disease pattern differentiation

As mentioned above, Zhu Gong (also known as Zhu Yi-Zhong, 1050–1125), the scholar who first introduced "六經 *liù jīng*" to study Discussion of Cold Damage, believed this term not only refers to channels but can also be used as a tool to identify their corresponding diseases. For example, he wrote:

> The kidney and the urinary bladder connect to each other. Therefore, the urinary bladder channel of foot tai yang and the kidney channel of foot shao yin relate to each other internally and externally. The urinary bladder channel of foot tai yang starts from the inner canthus, goes up to the head and connects to Feng Fu (Du 16) where it is divided into four sub-channels. There are six channels, including main channels and sub-channels, that go along the back of the body. The channels of tai yang dominate qi for all yang channels. If it is attacked by cold, there must be fever and aversion to cold. Since the head, nape, low back and vertebral column are the place where the urinary bladder channel runs, when there is headache, ache on the nape, general ache, stiffness on the low back and vertebral column or a floating pulse on the distal and proximal positions, one should know that the urinary bladder channel has been attacked.[25]

Wang Hu (also known as Wang Ling-You, c. 1680) further developed this idea. He pointed out:

> If one wants to study Discussion of Cold Damage by [Zhang] Zhong-Jing, one must also remember the channels in The Yellow Emperor's Inner Classic. Without knowing the channels, the progression of the disease in "六經 *liù jīng*" cannot be understood.[26]

"六經 liù jīng" as a tool to identify the exterior and interior, yin and yang for diseases

Layers to locate disease

Based on Fang You-Zhi's and Ke Qin's idea that viewed "六經 *liù jīng*" as anatomical portions of the body, in his book, True Classification and Analysis for Lines in Discussion of Cold Damage and Supplementary

25 Zhu Gong, op. cit., p.22

26 Wang Hu, op. cit., p.21

After-Reading Discussion of Cold Damage (傷寒論後條辨・讀傷寒論贅餘 *shāng hán lùn hòu tiǎo biàn, dú shāng hán lùn zhuì yú*), first published in 1670, Cheng Ying-Mao (also known as Cheng Jiao-Qian, c. 1669) pointed out:

> The reason that the book, Discussion of Cold Damage, contains "六經 *liù jīng*" is no more than a method to identify the location of disease in the regard of depth and superficiality...the character "經 *jīng*" also means border. When the border is settled, the territory can be demarcated. The character "經 *jīng*" means regularity too. When the regularity is known, one can detect changes. Therefore, when "六經 *liù jīng*" is applied, the exterior and interior, yin and yang, can be differentiated.[27]

Obviously, Cheng denounced the idea that "六經 *liù jīng*" has something to do with channels and considered it as an indispensable tool to differentiate diseases. Yun Shu-Jue (also known as Yun Tie-Qiao, 1878–1935) further elucidated this idea from Cheng and stated:

> What is called "六經 *liù jīng*" is to demarcate and locate the diseases based upon the clinical presentation of the human body. Therefore, "六經 *liù jīng*" is applicable only when there is a disease. When a disease is absent, it does not exist at all.[28]

It is true that "六經 *liù jīng*" can be viewed as a tool for disease pattern differentiation. But without physical structure, how can and where do the clinical manifestations present? Knowing this, You Yi (also known as You Zai-Jing, 1650–1749), a well-known scholar in commentating on Zhang Ji's work, pointed out the importance of this physical structure in the body for the term "六經 *liù jīng*." In his book, Connecting Pearls for Discussion of Cold Damage (傷寒貫珠集 *shāng hán guàn zhū jí*), first published in 1729, he stated:

> The twelve channels in the human body originally connect to each other and have their own borders. Therefore, when pathological factors invade them, there must be corresponding symptoms, signs and pulses which can be observed or felt. [Zhang] Zhong-Jing first ascertains that the symptoms, signs and pulses for tai yang are a floating pulse, headache, ache and stiffness on the nape and aversion to cold, because tai yang

27 Cheng Ying-Mao. *True Classification and Analysis for Lines in Discussion of Cold Damage and Supplementary After-Reading Discussion of Cold Damage* (*shāng hán lùn hòu tiǎo biàn, dú shāng hán lùn zhuì yú*). Beijing: China Publishing House of Traditional Chinese Medicine, 2009: 31, 175, 183

28 Yun Shu-Jue, op. cit., p.134

> locates on the exterior of three yang and its channel goes up to the frontal head, reaches to the top of the head, enters the brain and further goes down along the nape. Therefore, it presents with such clinical manifestations at the beginning of the disease regardless of zhong feng syndrome or shang han syndrome.[29]

Guo Zi-Guang, a famous scholar from Chengdu University of Traditional Chinese Medicine, first used the term "層次 *céng cì* (layers)" to study the meaning of "六經 *liù jīng*." In the chapter "Exploring the Essence of '六經 *liù jīng*'" he wrote:

> As a matter of fact, diseases in three yin and three yang are reactions in six major pathological layers: Tai yang disease refers to disorders of yin and yang on the body surface; yang ming disease locates inside of the body and often involves the chest, stomach and large intestine; shao yang disease locates in the half exterior and half interior and often involves in the gall bladder and three burners; tai yin disease locates relatively deep in the body and often involves the spleen and stomach; shao yin disease locates more deep in the body and often involves the heart and kidney; jue yin disease often involves the liver channels. Among these six major pathological layers, many small pathological layers can be further classified.[30]

Stages to classify externally contracted diseases

Zhu Wei-Ju (1884–1951), a famous physician who was good at employing warm and hot herbs like Aconiti Radix Lateralis (*fù zǐ*), Cinnamomi Ramulus (*guì zhī*) and Ephedrae Herba (*má huáng*) in the Shanghai area, viewed "六經 *liù jīng*" "as five stages to classify the externally contracted diseases. In the chapter "Outline of Five Stages for Discussion of Cold Damage" in his book, Answers to Difficult Questions for Discussion of Cold Damage (傷寒質難 *shāng hán zhì nàn*), he wrote:

> When diseases attack, the reaction of the body would be no more than these five stages. What do these five stages mean? When tai yang is invaded by pathological factors, anti-pathogenic qi is properly and initially fighting against the pathological factors due to stimulation from them. Yang ming disease refers to the condition that anti-pathological qi overacts since source qi is strong and fiercely fighting against pathological factors.

29 You Yi. *Connecting Pearls for Discussion of Cold Damage* (*shāng hán guàn zhū jí*). Shanghai: Shanghai Science and Technology Publishing House, 1978: 2–3

30 Guo Zi-Guang. "Exploring the principle of differentiation and treatment in Discussion of Cold Damage." *Journal of Chengdu College of Traditional Chinese Medicine*, 1979 (1): 2

> Due to the failure of qi to persistently fight against pathological factors, pathological factors frequently progress and regress in shao yang disease. In tai yin and shao yin disease, anti-pathogenic qi is so weak that it is unable to fight against pathological factors locally or in the whole body. In jue yin disease, anti-pathogenic qi tries to fight against pathological factors for the last time, and it is a critical condition. All externally contracted diseases can be classified into these five stages according to the fighting between anti-pathogenic qi and pathological factors.[31]

Zhu was probably the first person to introduce the term "階段 *jiē duàn* (stage)" to study the meaning of "六經 *liù jīng*." His interpretation has been followed by many contemporary scholars. Huang Wen-Dong, another famous scholar from the Shanghai area, first pointed out that "'六經 *liù jīng*' in Discussion of Cold Damage is to discuss the progressing principle for Cold Damage. It classifies this disease into six stages and six types of sub-disease based on clinical manifestation."[32] This was the first time that the term "six stages" was recorded in Chinese medical literature.

"六經 liù jīng" as a group of syndromes or diseases

A group of syndromes

The first person to introduce this term for "六經 *liù jīng*" was Lu Pen-Nian (also known as Lu Yuan-Lei, 1894–1955), a well-known scholar in studying Discussion of Cold Damage. He wrote:

> "六經 *liù jīng*" such as tai yang, yang ming and so on originates from ancient times and its meaning changes with time. First, it refers to channels. It is classified into twelve hand and foot channels, which is followed by acupuncturists and is recorded in Spiritual Pivot (靈樞 *líng shū*), Acupuncture Jia and Yi Classic (針灸甲乙經 *zhēn jiǔ jiǎ yǐ jīng*), Basic Questions (素問 *sù wèn*) and so on. Second, it refers to qi transformation, i.e. cold and water in tai yang, dry and metal in yang ming and so on, which is put forward by scholars who study Five Celestial Movements and Six Qi and is included in Chapter 66 and other chapters in Basic Questions (素問 *sù wèn*) by Wang Bing (also known as Qi Xuan-Zi, 710–804 AD). Finally, it refers to a group of syndromes in

---

31 Zhu Wei-Ju. *Answers to Difficult Questions for Discussion of Cold Damage* (*shāng hán zhì nán*). Shanghai: People's Bookstores, 1950: 78

32 Huang Wen-Dong. "My ideas on six conformations differentiation and treatments in Discussion of Cold Damage." *Shanghai Journal of Traditional Chinese Medicine*, 1955 (11): 24

> febrile diseases and was used by practitioners who prescribed herbs and was recorded in Discussion of Cold Damage and Chapter 31 of Basic Questions (素問 *sù wèn*).[33]

Huang Wen-Dong elaborated as follows:

> What is called "六經 *liù jīng*" actually refers to tai yang, yang ming, shao yang, tai yin, shao yin and jue yin, six groups of syndromes. It differentiates disease according to different conformations and identifies the exterior, the interior, cold, heat, deficiency and excess in terms of severity of the disease and applies different treatment approaches such as the promotion of sweating, vomiting, purging, harmonizing, warming, clearing, tonifying and astringing, and acupuncture and moxibustion.[34]

Six diseases

Based on the idea that "六經 *liù jīng*" refers to a group of syndromes, some contemporary scholars have developed the idea that this term refers to "six diseases," which is employed to classify syndromes. He Yun-He first adapted the term "六病 *liù bìng* (six diseases)" for explaining "六經 *liù jīng*" in 1957. He stated that "since [Zhang] Zhong-Jing called three yin and three yang diseases, "六經 *liù jīng*" should be called "six diseases" in regard to a group of diseases in Discussion of Cold Damage."[35] Liu Shao-Wu further explained that "six diseases" should be used to explain "六經 *liù jīng*." He pointed out:

> The concrete evidence to support "six channels" is absent in the original text of Discussion of Cold Damage. The term "diseases" is found in 137 lines of the book, which clearly identifies "tai yang disease," "yang ming disease"…What is more, the title for each chapter is named "diseases" rather than "channels." Therefore, if the term "six diseases" is applied according to the source book, it would be clearer when studying this classic and more simple and convenient when applying its contents. This is a reason that we believe that "六經 *liù jīng*" should be "six diseases"… the term "six diseases" is a pathological concept and is a method to artificially classify syndromes. If illness were absent, there would be no "six diseases."[36]

---

33 Lu Pen-Nian. *Current Explanation for Discussion of Cold Damage* (*shāng hán lùn jīn shì*). Beijing: Learning Garden Publishing House, 2008: 6

34 Huang Wen-Dong, op. cit., p.24

35 He Yun-He. "Brief explanation for six conformations." *Fujian Journal of Traditional Chinese Medicine*, 1957 (1): 1

36 Liu Shao-Wu, op. cit., p.12

In 1980, Zhang Zhi-Ming echoed Liu's idea and stated:

> The term "六經 *liù jīng*" is absent in Discussion of Cold Damage. And there is a term "six diseases" such as "tai yang disease" and "yang ming disease" in Discussion of Cold Damage. Scholars at later stages have made a mistake and viewed "六經 *liù jīng*" as six channels to classify syndromes. It should be called "six diseases" to classify syndromes. The character "病 *bìng* (disease)" mainly refers to six diseases in Discussion of Cold Damage, i.e. classify the course of progression in febrile disease into six stages and types to find out the location, pathology and quality of each disease.[37]

Obliviously, interpreting "六經 *liù jīng*" as "six diseases" has attached great importance to classifying and diagnosing role of this term. However, this interpretation might mislead readers to ignore the physiological foundations, especially the relationship between the channels and organs in regard to physical function, for diseases, and to view these diseases as individual ones that are irrelevant to each other like the diseases in zang-fu organ differentiation. Therefore, it would be hard to explain, monitor and predict the progression of diseases based on this interpretation, without connecting them to the physiology of the human body.

Almost 1900 years have passed since Zhang Ji wrote Discussion of Cold Damage. During this time, especially during the past 1000 years, the term "六經 *liù jīng*" has been introduced and has become the most important concept for studying this classic, though it was not recorded in the original text of the book. So far, more than 41 interpretations have been offered by scholars, and each of these interpretations have explored the meaning of "六經 *liù jīng*" based on their understanding and clinical practices, some of which are quite insightful. There is general agreement that "六經 *liù jīng*" must be related to three yin and three yang, i.e. tai yang, yang ming, shao yang, tai yin, shao yin and jue yin. Three yin and three yang were originally recorded in The Yellow Emperor's Inner Classic and bear both physiological and pathological meanings (see Chapter 6 for further details), which refer to channels, zang-fu organs, qi transformation and syndromes. Having studied The Yellow Emperor's Inner Classic,

37 Zhang Zhi-Min. "Primary exploration of the features and significance of classifying syndromes according to six diseases in Discussion of Cold Damage." *Zhejiang Journal of Traditional Chinese Medicine*, 1980 (1): 21

Zhang Ji did adapt the concept of three yin and three yang in Discussion of Cold Damage, as evidenced by line 270. In that line, he writes:

> After suffering from Cold Damage for three days, the involvement of three yang should be finished and three yin should be attacked by pathological factors. If the patient is nevertheless able to eat and does not have vomiting, this indicates that three yin are not attacked by pathological factors.

From line 270, one can learn that three yin and three yang is not only related to organs (rebellion of qi in the stomach and disorder of the spleen) but is also used as a tool to monitor the progression of a disease. Therefore, neither the organs, channel theory, nor the concept of pattern differentiation alone would be enough to explain "六經 *liù jīng*," i.e. three yin and three yang in Discussion of Cold Damage, though each of them has elucidated some meaning of this term from a different angle. According to my understanding, "六經 *liù jīng*" has become a most complex term in studying Discussion of Cold Damage. It refers to three yin and three yang, which are not only related to zang-fu organs, channels and qi transformation, and the physical structure, function and activity of the human body, but also it has become a differentiating tool to diagnose disease as well as monitor and predict the progression of disease. This is just as scholars from Hubei College of Traditional Chinese Medicine have stated:

> "六經 *liù jīng*" in Discussion of Cold Damage encompasses physiological functions and pathological changes for zang-fu organs, channels, qi and blood. It also analyzes and summarizes various syndromes in the course of externally contracted diseases for exploring the location of disorders, feature of syndromes, organs involved, cold and heat, wax and wane between pathological factors and anti-pathogenic qi, treatment approaches and herbs based on the strength and ability of the human body to fight against disease, attribution of pathological factors, progression of disease, and order of urgency. Therefore, "六經 *liù jīng*" is a principle to apply treatment as well as an outline for pattern differentiation.[38]

Based on this understanding, six conformations diseases (六經病 *liù jīng bìng*) are diseases caused by disorders of three yin and three yang, which includes their corresponding organs, channels and qi transformation. Six

---

38 Hubei College of Traditional Chinese Medicine. *Selected Reading from Discussion of Cold Damage* (*shāng hán lùn xuǎn dú*). Shanghai: Shanghai Scientific and Technological Publishing House, 1979: 2

conformations differentiation (六經辨證 *liù jīng biàn zhèng*) is a unique method to differentiate diseases and monitor the progression of disease, especially externally contracted disease based on three yin and three yang theory.

Scholars from Hubei College of Traditional Chinese Medicine and other colleges of traditional Chinese medicine have summarized these debates about what "六經 *liù jīng*" is as the following:

> Both ancient and contemporary scholars and practitioners have studied the meaning of "六經 *liù jīng*" based on the theory of zang-fu organs, theory of channels, theory of qi transformation, the concept of anatomical system, and the concept of stages. Each of these studies has made its contribution to understanding the meaning of "六經 *liù jīng*," but each of them has their one-sidedness, because zang-fu organs are the center of human function and activity, and zang-fu's function can affect the function and activity of different parts of the whole body, and vice versa. Therefore, the diseases of zang-fu organs should be explored from various aspects. While channels originate from zang-fu organs, they are a network over the body where qi and blood circulate.
>
> Channels have the relationship to zang-fu organ function as well as their own function. Therefore, one cannot explore the role channels play at the onset of a disease without addressing qi, blood, zang-fu organs and other factors. What is called qi transformation is an outline of the function and activity of zang-fu organs and channels. Therefore, qi transformation in the body must change when a disease takes place. Yes, it is quite helpful for understanding the physical and pathological conditions based on the theory of qi transformation. But if one wants to explore the origin of qi transformation, the zang-fu and channels must be considered. Obviously, without the zang-fu and channels, there is no base for qi transformation; without qi transformation, the function and activity of the zang-fu and channels cannot be presented.
>
> As to the anatomical locations and stages, they have their own clinical features and are indispensable parts for differentiation. However, the locations and stages on the exterior are often presentations of the disorders in zang-fu organs, channels and qi transformation. Therefore, one must orchestrate various factors for searching the root of a disease.
>
> In summary, one must start from the reality of clinical practice and combine syndromes in six conformations with zang-fu organs, channels, qi transformation, and location of diseases to study "六經 *liù jīng*." In this way, one can correctly understand the significance of

> six conformations differentiation (六經辨證 *liù jīng biàn zhèng*) in Discussion of Cold Damage.[39]

Why did Zhang Ji not use the zang-fu organs and channels involved, or pathological factors to name diseases, as was as done in The Yellow Emperor's Inner Classic, rather than use tai yang, yang ming, shao yang, tai yin, shao yin and jue yin, i.e. three yin and three yang? Zhang Zheng-Zhao, a scholar who specialized in Discussion of Cold Damage in Gansu province, has offered a reasonable answer for this question:

> The reason for the author of Discussion of Cold Damage to use "three yin and three yang" to name diseases is probably to attach great importance to the fact that three yin and three yang bear various meanings, which can reflect various features such as the location of disease (zang-fu, channels), trend of disease (the feature of qi transformation), quality of disease (yin, yang), strength of anti-pathogenic qi, strength of the ability to fight against pathological factors (quantity of "yin qi and yang qi") and so on.[40]

Obviously, without understanding qi transformation, which is the manifestation among organs and channels in three yin and three yang, one cannot understand deeply "六經 *liù jīng*" (see Chapter 6).

The next section provides a brief introduction to the physiology in six conformations and the etiology, pathology and progress in six conformations diseases.

Brief introduction to six conformations diseases

Tai yang and tai yang disease

Structurally, tai yang consists of the urinary bladder and the small intestine with their channels. It has an external-internal relationship to shao yin—the heart and kidney, respectively. There is general agreement that tai yang is in charge of the surface of the body and serves as the fence to defend the body as it governs the nutritive qi and the defensive qi, especially the defensive qi. The qi of tai yang comprises the nutritive qi and the defensive qi. The nutritive qi is generated by blood, which comes mainly from the processing of food by the spleen and stomach and can

39 Ibid., p.9

40 Zhang Zheng-Zhao. *Back to Truth for Discussion of Cold Damage* (*shāng hán lùn guī zhēn*). Changsha: Hunan Science and Technology Publishing House, 1993: 9

be generated by the essence stored in the kidney. The defensive qi, the most important qi to defend the body, can be produced in the following three ways: initially generated by the kidney yang warming the water in the urinary bladder; generated by qi from the middle burner; or generated locally in channels through warming the blood by the defensive qi when the defensive qi enters a channel. There are four ways for the defensive qi to get distributed from zang-fu organs: through the channels connection between the body surface and tai yang fu organs—the urinary bladder and the small intestine; through the connection between the muscles and the earth organs—the spleen and stomach; through the connection between the skin and the lung; and through shao yang's pivotal function (see Chapters 7 and 8 for further details).

According to the theory of qi transformation, tai yang bears the strongest yang among the three yang and contains cold water and it is called "three yangs." It is this strongest yang that makes it able to contend with cold water in the urinary bladder. This strongest yang is generated by heat qi in shao yin, i.e. the fire in the heart and the fire in the life gate acting on the water in the kidney. It is this strong yang that makes water warm instead of cold, and it is this cold water that keeps this strong yang in check. From this discussion, the production of tai yang qi relies on steaming water in the urinary bladder and the transformation of water, which depends on the warming function of yang qi. Since qi in tai yang is supposed to defend the body surface and prevent the body from being attacked by pathological factors, the movement of tai yang qi is outward. In light of the theory of opening, closing and pivot, its function falls into the category of opening.

Because tai yang serves as the defense on the first layer of the body, it is very common to first see tai yang disease in externally contracted diseases. At the very beginning of tai yang disease, the pathology comprises disharmony between the nutritive qi and the defensive qi. This disharmony is mainly caused by invasion of exogenous pathological factors. However, it can also be caused by internal disorders in organs (which is discussed in line 54 of Discussion of Cold Damage). Since tai yang bears the strongest yang qi, and is governed by cold qi and related to shao yin, which bears heat qi, any disorder in tai yang can change the relationship between yang qi, cold qi in tai yang and heat qi in shao yin, according to the theory of qi transformation. Therefore, the presentation of tai yang disease can be either cold or heat (see Chapter 6 for further details).

Zhang Ji not only discusses the treatment related to cold or cold and yang deficiency (see lines 12, 14 and 21) but also the treatment related to heat (see lines 6, 26, 38, 63 and 176) in tai yang disease. According to the theory of opening, closing and pivot, if tai yang opens too much, excessive sweating will be produced; if tai yang fails to open, there will be absence of sweating. Therefore, Cinnamon Twig Decoction (*guì zhī tāng*) and Ephedra Decoction (*má huáng tāng*) are two basic formulas to treat sweating disorders due to invasion of wind-cold in tai yang disease. Other formulas, like a Combination of Half Cinnamon Twig Decoction and Half Ephedra Decoction (*guì zhī má huáng gè bàn tāng*), a Combination of Two Parts Cinnamon Twig Decoction and One Part Ephedra Decoction (*guì zhī èr má huáng yī tāng*), Cinnamon Twig Decoction plus Pueraria (*guì zhī jiā gé gēn tāng*), are just modifications of these two formulas according to the severity of the syndromes and associated conditions. If tai yang fails to open and the disease progresses to the inside of the body, transmuted syndromes like the chest-binding syndrome, pi syndromes, water-accumulation syndrome and blood-amassment syndrome could present, depending on the body's constitution and the location of the disease. Therefore, in the early stage of Cold Damage, proper management of Cinnamon Twig Decoction (*guì zhī tāng*) and Ephedra Decoction (*má huang tāng*) bears important clinical significance, as they can cure disease when it is located at a very superficial level in tai yang or reduce the possibility for the disease to progress to the inside of the body. Among these transmuted syndromes, urination problems and diarrhea are quite common to see in tai yang disease, because qi transformation in the urinary bladder and small intestine, the tai yang fu organs, are affected.

Since the generation of tai yang qi involves so many organs and burners, tai yang disease can progress from the chest to the lower abdomen, including the lung, heart, chest, diaphragm, spleen, stomach, small intestine, shao yang, urinary bladder, uterus, chong channel and kidney. Among these progressions, the ones from tai yang to shao yin (the kidney and the heart) are discussed in lines 61, 64, 91, 112, 117 and 118 based on the external-internal relationship between tai yang and shao yin. Cinnamomi Ramulus (*guì zhī*) and Aconiti Radix Lateralis (*fù zǐ*), the herbs to deal with yang deficiency in the heart and kidney, respectively, are frequently used in the related formulas.

Figure 5.1 gives a brief summary for the progressions in tai yang disease according to Discussion of Cold Damage.

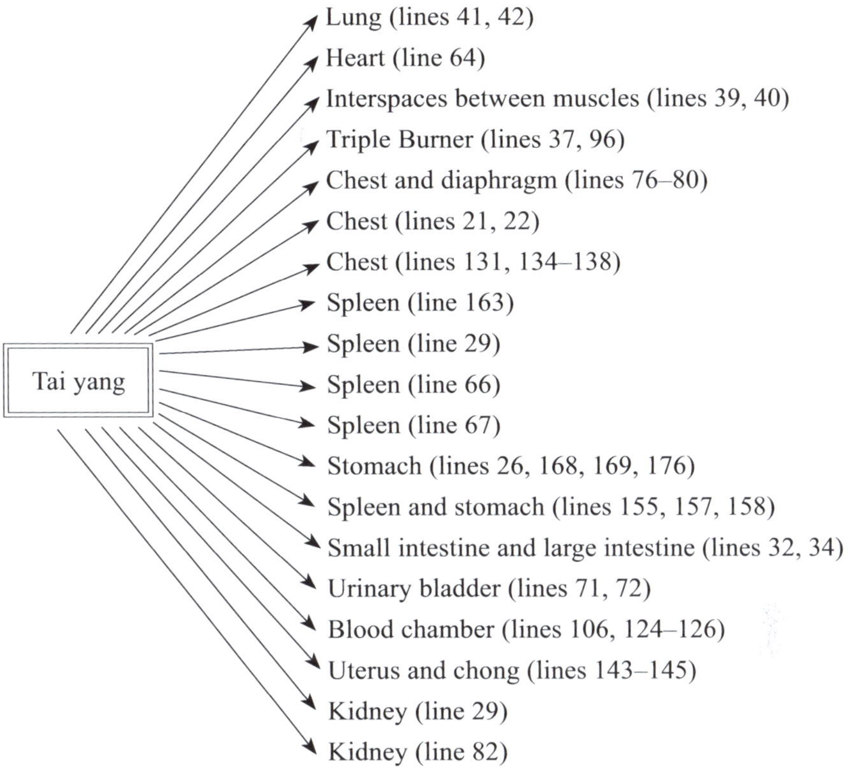
Tai yang
Lung (lines 41, 42)
Heart (line 64)
Interspaces between muscles (lines 39, 40)
Triple Burner (lines 37, 96)
Chest and diaphragm (lines 76–80)
Chest (lines 21, 22)
Chest (lines 131, 134–138)
Spleen (line 163)
Spleen (line 29)
Spleen (line 66)
Spleen (line 67)
Stomach (lines 26, 168, 169, 176)
Spleen and stomach (lines 155, 157, 158)
Small intestine and large intestine (lines 32, 34)
Urinary bladder (lines 71, 72)
Blood chamber (lines 106, 124–126)
Uterus and chong (lines 143–145)
Kidney (line 29)
Kidney (line 82)

FIGURE 5.1 BRIEF PROGRESSIONS FOR TAI YANG DISEASE

Yang ming and yang ming disease

Yang ming includes the large intestine and the stomach with their channels. It has an external-internal relationship to tai yin—the lung and the spleen, respectively. The stomach and large intestine are in charge of taking, ripening and transporting food and the discharge of waste, respectively. In Discussion of Cold Damage, Zhang Ji often uses the character "胃 *wèi*" to refer to these two organs. According to studies done by scholars for Discussion of Cold Damage, the exterior part of yang ming includes not only muscles and their channels but also the chest. As qi in yang ming is strong and very active, yang ming is called "two yangs." According to the theory of qi transformation, yang ming is governed by dryness qi. It is this dryness qi in yang ming that makes yang ming able to ripen, transport food and discharge waste. However, this dryness qi should be balanced by damp qi especially from the spleen. In other words, this strong and very active yang should be checked by tai yin, which bears the strongest yin in three yin. In this way, dryness qi in yang ming would be perfect in regard to its intensity and would not become excessively dry. With such balance of dryness qi and damp qi in yang ming and tai yin, the middle burner can function well in regard to descending and ascending, and taking charge of receiving, transforming and transporting food.

In light of the text of Discussion of Cold Damage, yang ming disease can progress from various sources: from tai yang, shao yang, tai yin, shao yin and jue yin, as well as being directly attacked by pathological factors. There is general agreement that pathological factors tend to turn into heat, leading to dry heat or the combination of dry heat and dry feces in yang ming because of its strong and active yang. The quality of yang ming disease is often interior excess heat. However, in light of the theory of qi transformation, the presentation of yang ming disease depends much on the interaction between dryness qi in yang ming and damp qi in tai yin. When yang qi, or dryness qi in yang ming, prevails, there is dry-heat presentations; when yang qi or dryness qi in yang ming is weak, damp qi prevails and cold is produced, and there is cold and deficiency in yang ming and yang ming disease progresses to tai yin disease. In Discussion of Cold Damage, Zhang Ji discusses these presentations and progressions in lines 187, 190, 191, 194, 195 and 259 after discussing dry-heat manifestations. In line 243, he even proposes the use of acrid and hot herbs in Evodia Decoction (*wú zhū yú tāng*) to deal with vomiting due to cold and yang deficiency in yang ming disease.

According to the theory of opening, closing and pivot, yang ming is in charge of inward qi movement and its function falls into the category of closing. If yang ming fails to close, i.e. the moving qi fails to move downward properly, there will be abdominal fullness, constipation, vomiting or diarrhea.

Shao yang and shao yang disease

Shao yang refers to the gall bladder and the three burners with their channels, and it has an external-internal relationship to jue yin—the liver and the pericardium. In regard to yang qi condition, shao yang bears the weakest yang qi among three yang and this is why it is called "one yang." However, shao yang is governed by ministerial fire and this fire should be facilitated by warm wind in jue yin according to the theory of qi transformation. In other words, yang qi and ministerial fire in shao yang would be healthy when they are supported by wind and wood in jue yin. The three burners is also a pathway for qi, blood, fire and water to circulate. The terms "half interior and half exterior" and "pivot" are two well-known concepts to describe the physical function for shao yang, they are the terms developed by scholars and commentators who study Discussion of Cold Damage. There are three ways to understand the term "half exterior and half interior":

1. It refers to the location of the shao yang channel among three yang channels, i.e. shao yang channel is located between the tai yang and yang ming channel.
2. It refers to the location of shao yang between three yang and three yin, i.e. shao yang is the place where qi moves from yang to yin in the body.
3. It refers to the term "pivot," which was introduced by the theory of opening, closing and pivot in The Yellow Emperor's Inner Classic. According to this theory, shao yang serves as the pivot to let qi in, out, up and down in the body (see Chapter 7 for further details).

Since shao yang governs fire and relates to jue yin, which belongs to wood—and wood can help fire—it is very common to see the presentation of the disorder of fire in the syndromes of shao yang. This is why all symptoms and signs, such as a bitter taste in the mouth, dry throat and dizziness, in the first line of the chapter on shao yang disease are the manifestation of flare-up fire from shao yang, especially from the gall bladder. However, when pathological factors affect the function of the three burners and/or the function of the pivot of shao yang, shao yang disease has its own special diversity, which ranges from qi stagnation, fire stagnation and water retention to the production of phlegm and damp. The organs it can affect range from the upper burner to the lower burner. Therefore, its location can be on the exterior as well as in the interior and its quality can be concurrently one of cold and heat. Since yang qi in shao yang is most weak among three yang and it locates between three yang and three yin, when tai yang disease or yang ming disease are not resolved, these diseases can progress to shao yang; when shao yang disease is not resolved, it can progress to three yin. While the yang qi is recovered in three yin diseases, the disease can regress to shao yang. Because shao yang serves as a pivot that lets qi in and out and/or up and down in the body, there is the chance to cure tai yang disease or yang ming disease through recovering the pivot function of shao yang, as discussed exquisitely in lines 37, 230 and 231.

Tai yin and tai yin disease

Theoretically, tai yin refers to the lung and spleen with their channels. It has an external-internal relationship to yang ming—the stomach and large intestine—although, in Discussion of Cold Damage, only the disorders of the spleen are discussed. Tai yin bears the strongest yin among three yin and is called "three yins." The spleen is supposed to transform what we eat into qi and blood and distribute them to the lung and other organs vertically and to the muscle on the body surface transversely. Tai yin is located on the most outer layer of three yin and can bring qi outward, its function falls into the category of opening in the theory of opening, closing and pivot. Also, according to the theory of qi transformation, tai yin is governed by damp qi. It is this damp qi which makes tai yin able to distribute qi and blood transformed from food ingested. However, this damp qi should be balanced by dryness qi in yang ming so as not to be too damp.

When pathological factors progress to tai yin, affect its transforming and opening functions that produce and distribute qi and blood to the lung and the body surface, the ingested food stays, ferments and makes damp qi in tai yin so strong that it goes beyond the control of dryness qi from yang ming. Also, since tai yin bears the strongest yin among the three yin, yang pathological factors tend to transform into yin pathological factors such as damp and cold. In this case, yang would be damaged and cold would be further produced and there would be diarrhea, abdominal fullness and/or pain in the abdomen.

According to the original text of Discussion of Cold Damage, there are three ways to suffer from tai yin disease: progression from tai yang disease due to wrong treatment such as improper application of promotion of sweating, purging and vomiting; direct attack of tai yin by cold; and progression from yang ming due to weakness of dryness qi in yang ming to balance damp qi in tai yin. Clinically, ingested cold and raw food is a common cause to make cold directly attack tai yin.

Generally, there are two progressions from tai yin disease when tai yin disease is not treated in time: it can progress to shao yin disease when yang qi in tai yin gets worse, or it can progress to yang ming disease when yang qi gets stronger and dryness qi in yang ming is able to balance damp qi in tai yin.

Shao yin and shao yin disease

Shao yin refers to the heart and kidney with their channels. It has an external-internal relationship to tai yang—the urinary bladder and the small intestine. Shao yin bears relatively strong yin among the three yin and is called "two yins." According to the theory of qi transformation, shao yin is governed by heat qi. As mentioned in tai yang and tai yang disease, tai yang is governed by cold water. It is this cold water in tai yang that keeps the heat qi of shao yin in check and makes it warm instead of hot in nature. While the kidney belongs to water and the heart belongs to fire in five elements theory, fire and water should communicate with each other for their balance, i.e. water in the kidney should go up to the heart for balancing fire in the heart and preventing hyperactive fire, while fire in the heart should descend to the kidney for warming the water in the kidney and preventing too much coldness in the water. On the way to warm the water in the kidney, fire in the heart can produce earth and help the function of the spleen (tai yin). Similarly, on the way to balance the fire in the heart, water in the kidney can nourish wood and help the function of the liver (jue yin). Shao yin is supposed to make this fire and water turn around and benefit tai yin and jue yin. Also, shao yin is located between tai yin and jue yin; therefore, shao yin is called the pivot for three yin.

In general, when a disease progresses to shao yin, there is deficiency of fire and water or deficiency in yin or yang. This is why the outline for shao yin consists of "thin and feeble pulse, only desire to sleep" in line 281 of Discussion of Cold Damage. Since there is a fire and water difference in shao yin, pathological factors can transform into heat when fire is relatively strong or transform into cold when water is relatively strong, leading to heat syndromes and cold syndromes, respectively.

In the text of Discussion of Cold Damage, there are two ways to suffer from shao yin disease. The first is through the progression from other diseases such as tai yang disease, shao yang diseases, and tai yin disease, among which tai yang disease is the one most discussed in the book because there is an external-internal relationship between tai yang and shao yin. The second way is direct attack of shao yin by cold. Since there is a close relationship between shao yin and tai yang, it is quite common to see concurrence of both tai yang disease and shao yin disease in Discussion of Cold Damage (for example, as discussed in line 301, fever can present in shao yin disease).

When shao yin disease is not treated in time, yang and/or yin in shao yin is further damaged and the condition in shao yin deteriorates, progressing to jue yin disease or leading to death. However, when yang qi is recovered, shao yin disease can progress to tai yang and yang ming, leading to heat in the urinary bladder and the clumping of dry heat and dry feces in the large intestine.

Jue yin and jue yin disease

Jue yin refers to the liver and pericardium and their channels. It has an external-internal relationship to the gall bladder and three burners, respectively. Jue yin bears the weakest yin among the three yin and is called "one yin." Jue yin is the end of yin in the cycle of qi circulation in yin and yang channels and locates between yin and yang. According to the theory of qi transformation, jue yin is governed by wind qi and closed to shao yang. On the one hand, like mild ventilation (wind) is warm and facilitates fire in the stove for cooking food, jue yin contains the fire, the liver contains the ministerial fire and the pericardium contains the fire of the heart, and can assist fire too; on the other hand, with help from fire in shao yang, qi in jue yin would be able to continually move from yin aspect to yang aspect, making yin and yang smoothly connected, and with help from fire in shao yang, wind qi in jue yin would be mild and warm, and wood in jue yin would not be frozen. Since the liver is supposed to store blood and contains the ministerial fire, and the pericardium contains the fire in the heart, it implies that qi in jue yin tends to move inward, jue yin falls into the category of closing in the theory of opening, closing and pivot. In this way, fire would not flare up, liver yang would not rise and qi and blood would circulate in the body like warm and mild wind move in spring.

Since jue yin locates between yin and yang, there would be an unsmooth connection between yin and yang when a disease progresses to jue yin. Consequently, the spread of cold feeling from the hands and feet to the limbs would ensue due to qi stagnation in jue yin. There are four pathological scenarios taking place in jue yin disease:

1. When qi is completely obstructed in yin aspect and fails to move to yang aspect, cold is produced, leading to the spread of cold feeling from the hands and feet to the limbs, or even death.

2. When qi is able to move in yin aspect but lacks momentum to continually move in yang aspect, there is qi stagnation in yang aspect and heat is produced. The more heat there is, the more qi stagnation there is, leading to the spread of cold feeling from the hands and feet to the limbs.

3. When qi is stagnated in both yin and yang aspect, there is concurrence of both heat and cold syndrome in various parts of the body, especially the upper part and lower part of the body.

4. When qi stagnation takes places more or less in yin or yang aspect, there is waxing and waning of heat and cold syndrome, which is a symbol for the movement of wind. However, since wind is yang in nature, jue yin encompass two fires—the ministerial fire in the gall bladder and king fire in the heart—and it is very common for jue yin to generate heat and present more heat syndrome clinically. This is probably why there is a "feeling of qi surging to the chest, pain and burning in the chest and hunger with no desire to eat," which demonstrates much more noticable heat than cold and is considered as the outline for jue yin disease.

According to Discussion of Cold Damage, there are two ways to suffer from jue yin disease: (a) progression from yang disease (such as shao yang and yang ming disease) or progression from yin disease (such as shao yin disease); or (b) direct attack by exogenous pathological factors.

The progression of jue yin disease depends much on the condition of anti-pathogenic qi. If anti-pathogenic qi is strong enough to overcome pathological factors and yang returns, the disease progresses to yang disease such as shao yang and yang ming disease. If yang collapses and/or exhaustion of yin occurs due to disconnection of yin and yang, death ensues.

6

THE THEORY OF QI TRANSFORMATION IN SIX CONFORMATIONS IN DISCUSSION OF COLD DAMAGE

Debate about qi transformation in Discussion of Cold Damage

Qi transformation is a literal translation for the term "氣化 *qì huà*" in Chinese medicine. According to Dictionary for Chinese Medicine (中醫大辭典 *zhōng yī dà cí diàn*) published in 1979, the term "氣化 *qì huà*" refers to "qi's movement and change."[1] As mentioned in Chapter 5, the school of qi transformation is one of the schools to study Discussion of Cold Damage. Historically, there has been much debating in studying Discussion of Cold Damage. However, nothing can compare to the school of qi transformation among those debating this classic. Therefore, it is impossible to avoid exploring the theory of qi transformation when studying Discussion of Cold Damage, unless one does not want to have serious study of this classic.

Historically, the debate about the theory of qi transformation can be classified into two groups: the group that strongly advocates it and the group that opposes it. In his book, Superficial Comments on Discussion of Cold Damage (傷寒論淺注 *shāng hán lùn qián zhù*) published in 1803, Chen Nian-Zu (also known as Chen Xiu-Yuan, 1753–1823), pointed out that "one cannot study Discussion of Cold Damage without understanding 本氣 *běn qì* (root qi), 標氣 *biāo qì* (branch qi) and 中氣 *zhōng qì* (middle

1 Guangzhou College of Traditional Chinese Medicine and China Academy of Traditional Chinese Medicine. *Dictionary for Chinese Medicine* (*zhōng yī dà cí diǎn*). Beijing: People's Health Publishing House, 1979: 58

qi)[2] in six qi."[3] Wan You-Sheng (1917–2003), a contemporary scholar from Jiangxi College of Traditional Chinese Medicine, stated:

> The theory of qi transformation can be considered as the spirit for Discussion of Cold Damage. Without it, Discussion of Cold Damage would become an inflexible doctrine. Therefore, one must attach great importance to it and further explore it. One cannot discuss the theory of three yin and three yang without the theory of qi transformation.[4]

The first person to oppose the theory of qi transformation was Zhang Bing-Lin (also known as Zhang Tai-Yan, 1869–1936), a famous scholar who studied ancient classics. In the preface for the book, Current Explanation for Discussion of Cold Damage (傷寒論今釋 *shāng hán lùn jīn shì*) written by Lu Pen-Nian, Zhang wrote:

> Zhang Zhi-Cong and Chen Xiu-Yuan[5] have made explanations for Discussion of Cold Damage in the name of the theory of the five constellation movement and six qi (五運六氣 *wǔ yùn liù qì*), drawn wrong conclusions by false analogy for the change of weather, and made unrealistic discussion of such a very practical book.[6]

Chen Yi-Ren (1924–2004), a well-known contemporary scholar from Nanjing University of Traditional Chinese Medicine who studied Discussion of Cold Damage, echoed Zhang's idea as the following:

> A common point from the school of the theory of qi transformation is that they have applied the "theory of 本氣 *běn qì* (root qi), 標氣 *biāo qì* (branch qi) and 中氣 *zhōng qì* (middle qi) in six qi" to all contents in Discussion of Cold Damage. Since they argue irrationally with difficult language, it is not helpful to study the theory of differentiation based on clinical manifestation in Discussion of Cold Damage. Rather, it can

2 Root qi, branch qi and middle qi (all discussed later in detail) are important in the theory of qi transformation.

3 Chen Nian-Zu. *Section Two of New Annotation and Collation for Books by Chen Xiu-Yuan (xīn jiào zhù chén xiū-yuán yī shū dì èr jí)*. Fuzhou: Fujian Scientific and Technological Publishing House, 2003: 14

4 Wan You-Sheng. "On the essence of three yin and three yang in Discussion of Cold Damage." *Jiangsu Journal of Traditional Chinese Medicine*, 1980 (4): 35

5 Zhang Zhi-Cong and Chen Xiu-Yuan were two scholars of the Qing Dynasty who made great contributions to the development of the theory of qi transformation.

6 Lu Pen-Nian. *Current Explanation for Discussion of Cold Damage* (*shāng hán lùn jīn shì*). Beijing: Learning Garden Publishing House, 2008: 1

> increase difficulty and compromise efficiency in studying Discussion of Cold Damage.[7]

In the late 1980s, Zhao En-Jian stated:

> Using the theory of six qi to explain six conformations is impractical. It has made six conformations differentiation based on pulses (clinical manifestation) become an unrealistic discussion. Because the theory of the five constellation movement and six qi (五運六氣 *wǔ yùn liù qì*) is not practical, it is not an ideal approach to use the theory of six qi to study six conformations.[8]

Naturally, a question must be raised in the reader's mind: Which idea is correct? To answer this question, one must know what qi transformation means in Chinese medicine, particularly in The Yellow Emperor's Inner Classic (黃帝內經 *huáng dì nèi jīng*), the book Zhang Ji mainly referred to when writing Discussion of Cold Damage.

Historical review for the theory of qi transformation in The Yellow Emperor's Inner Classic

The term "氣化 *qì huà* (qi transformation)" appears ten times in The Yellow Emperor's Inner Classic, particularly in Basic Questions (素問 *sù wèn*). This term is used nine times in the seven chapters (Chapters 66–71 and 74) of Basic Questions (素問 *sù wèn*) that discuss the five constellation movement and six qi (五運六氣 *wǔ yùn liù qì*), and one time this term is used (in Chapter 8) to elaborate the function of the urinary bladder. From this point of view, one can conclude that the term "氣化 *qì huà* (qi transformation)" was mostly used to discuss weather change in the universe in The Yellow Emperor's Inner Classic. There is general agreement that the theory of qi transformation in The Yellow Emperor's Inner Classic contains two aspects: distribution of 本氣 *běn qì* (root qi), 標氣 *biāo qì* (branch qi) and 中氣 *zhōng qì* (middle qi), and the transformation following the interaction among these three kinds of qi, while some scholars believe that the theory of opening, closing and pivot (開合樞理論 *kāi hé shū lǐ lùn*) also falls into the category of qi

7 Chen Yi-Ren. "Initial discussion for 'One cannot study Discussion of Cold Damage without understanding root qi, brand qi and middle qi in six qi'." *Jiangsu Journal of Traditional Chinese Medicine*, 1981 (5): 25

8 Zhao En-Jian. *Study on Discussion of Cold Damage* (*shāng hán lùn yán jiū*). Tianjin: Tianjin Science and Technology Publishing House, 1987: 47

transformation. According to cosmology and the macrocosm in The Yellow Emperor's Inner Classic, primordial qi in spacious sky is the foundation of the change in the universe and for the revolving of the celestial bodies, especially five constellations of wood, fire, earth, metal and water, and stars in the universe produce qi movement of the five elements (五運 *wǔ yùn*). The book states:

> The generation of all things depends on this qi (primordial qi) in the universe. As the nine stars illuminate above and the seven celestial bodies revolve regularly, qi of the five elements moves regularly in the universe, and it will distribute its refined qi and control the origin of all things on the earth. In this way, the distinction of yin and yang, and the different properties between firmness and softness, can be distinguished. Cold and summer-heat in the four seasons comes and goes regularly, presenting with generation, transformation and classification of all things in nature.[9]

Also, according to The Yellow Emperor's Inner Classic, the qi movement of the five elements (五運 *wǔ yùn*) generates six qi (六氣 *liù qì*) in the heavens. It states that "the qi of movement of five elements in the heavens determines the five orientations and produces cold, summer-heat, dryness, damp, wind [and fire]."[10] In this classic, the concept of yin and yang, and the concept of three yin and three yang, are used to study these six qi. The book states that "the cold, summer-heat, dryness, damp, wind and fire are yin and yang in the heavens; three yin and yang are used to correspond with them upward."[11] The descending of these six qi in the heavens produces different yin and different yang, and five elements on the earth. Figure 6.1 can be used to summarize the qi transformation in the heavens and on the earth according to The Yellow Emperor's Inner Classic.

9 Wang Bing. *Basic Questions of The Yellow Emperor's Inner Classic* (*huáng dì nèi jīng sù wèn*). Beijing: People's Health Publishing House, 1963: 364

10 Ibid., p.363

11 Ibid., p.366

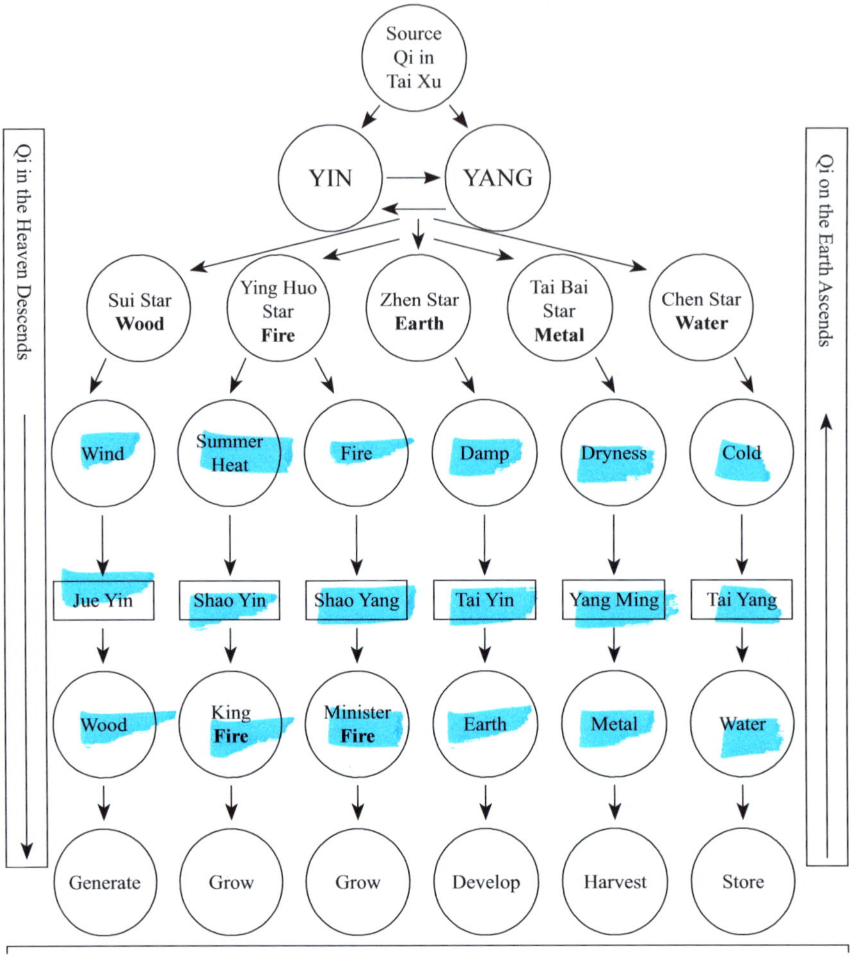

FIGURE 6.1 COSMOLOGY AND MACROCOSM IN THE YELLOW EMPEROR'S INNER CLASSIC

"The qi in the heaven and qi on the earth attract each other while the descending and ascending promote each other. Therefore change occurs." This figure is made based on Chapter 66, 67 and 68 of Basic Questions of The Yellow Emperor's Inner Classic (*huáng dì nèi jīng sù wèn*)

From Figure 6.1, one might deduce that wind, heat, fire, damp, dryness and cold are kinds of qi that circulate in the universe and have a relationship with three yin and three yang.

How do these relationships present in the universe? The authors of The Yellow Emperor's Inner Classic offer an explanation:

> In Chapter 68 of Basic Questions of The Yellow Emperor's Inner Classic, these relationships are discussed as the following:
>
> > shao yang is dominated by fire qi and jue yin is its 中氣 *zhōng qì*
> >
> > yang ming is dominated by dryness qi and tai yin is its 中氣 *zhōng qì*
> >
> > tai yang is dominated by cold qi and shao yin is its 中氣 *zhōng qì*
> >
> > jue yin is dominated by wind qi and shao yang is its 中氣 *zhōng qì*
> >
> > shao yin is dominated by heat qi and tai yang is its 中氣 *zhōng qì*
> >
> > tai yin is dominated by damp qi and yang ming is its 中氣 *zhōng qì*
> >
> > six qi is 本氣 *běn qì*, while what is located below the 本氣 *běn qì* is 中氣 *zhōng qì*
> >
> > what is located below the 中氣 *zhōng qì* is 標氣 *biāo qì*.[12]

The discussion can be summarized in Table 6.1.

Table 6.1 Summary of the relationship between 本氣 *běn qì*, 中氣 *zhōng qì* and 標氣 *biāo qì*, and three yin and three yang according to The Yellow Emperor's Inner Classic

本氣 ***běn qì***	中氣 ***zhōng qì***	標氣 ***biāo qì***
Wind qi	Shao yang (fire qi)	Jue yin
Heat qi	Tai yang (cold qi)	Shao yin
Fire qi	Jue yin (wind qi)	Shao yang
Damp qi	Yang ming (dryness qi)	Tai yin
Dryness qi	Tai yin (damp qi)	Yang ming
Cold qi	Shao yin (heat qi)	Tai yang

What do the characters "本 *běn*," "標 *biāo*" and "中 *zhōng*" mean? According to Origin of Chinese Characters (辭源 *cí yuán*), the character "本 *běn*" originally refers to the root of grass or trees but can be interpreted as "foundation," the character "標 *biāo*" originally refers to the branch of trees but can also be interpreted as "mark" and the character

12 Ibid., p.388

"中 *zhōng*" means "medium or middle."[13] Based on the observation of movement of constellations and weather change, ancient scholars and practitioners realized that the movements of six qi in the universe are the cause for the change of weather, while three yin and three yang come after these movements and changes. Therefore, they used the characters "本 *běn*," "標 *biāo*" and "中 *zhōng*" to reflect this root and branch, and the relationship between six qi and three yin and three yang. Each 標氣 *biāo qì* is used to mark and identify the quantity of yin and yang for its corresponding 本氣 *běn qì*. For example, shao yang, which is 標氣 *biāo qì*, is used to mark fire qi, its 本氣 *běn qì*, and indicates that yang is not strong in regards to quantity.

Questions might be raised, such as the following:

- It makes sense that tai yin is considered to be 標氣 *biāo qì* for damp qi as both tai yin and damp fall into the yin category according to the definition of yin and yang. However, why is tai yang, which is considered to be 標氣 *biāo qì*, used to mark cold qi, which is a type of yin qi, while tai yang is called "three yangs" (the strongest yang among three yang)?
- Why is jue yin, which is considered to be 標氣 *biāo qì*, used to mark wind qi, which is a type of yang qi, while jue yin is called "one yin"?
- Why is yang ming, which is considered to be 標氣 *biāo qì*, used to mark dryness qi, which is a type of yin qi, while yang ming is called "two yangs"?
- Why is shao yin, which is considered to be 標氣 *biāo qì*, used to mark heat qi, while shao yin is called "two yins"?
- Why is shao yang, which is considered to be 標氣 *biāo qì*, used to mark fire qi, which has strong yang, while shao yang is called "one yang"?

All of these questions that challenge the relationship between 標氣 *biāo qì* and本氣 *běn qì* have probably puzzled scholars and readers for a couple of thousand years, and have never been answered clearly when studying qi transformation. To answer these difficult questions, first we

13 Editorial Department of Business Publishing House. *Origin of Chinese Characters* (*cí yuán*). Beijing: Business Publishing House, 1980: 83, 1501, 1620, 1621

have to understand why the demarcation of three yin and three yang are introduced in The Yellow Emperor's Inner Classic. In Chapters 66 and 74, the conversation between the Yellow Emperor, Gui Yu-Qu and Qi Bo (the emperor's medical advisors), is recorded as the following:

> The Yellow Emperor asked, "Well, what does plenty and few for qi mean in the universe? Gui Yu-Qu replied, "There is differentiation for plenty and few for yin and yang; hence, there are distinctions between three yin and three yang."[14] The Yellow Emperor also asked, "I am told that there are three yin and three yang, and what is the reason? Qi Bo replied, "This is because the energies of yin and yang may be more or may be less in quantity."[15]

According to these differentiations, each qi in the universe can be viewed by the theory of yin and yang in terms of quantity; and yin and yang are divided into three yin and three yang following this thought; tai yang bears three yangs, yang ming bears two yangs, and shao yang bears one yang, while tai yin bears three yins, shao yin bears two yins, and jue yin bears one yin. We have to follow the method which ancient scholars used to observe the universe and figure out the principles in the universe. In Chapter 67 of Basic Questions of The Yellow Emperor's Inner Classic, this method is described as "starting to observe the change of weather can lead to understanding the principles in the universe. One must follow it."[16] According to my observations and study of weather change year-round, Table 6.2 suggests why three yin and three yang are used to mark six qi. For example, cold qi, which prevails in winter, must be counteracted by maximum yang, which is the strongest yang; otherwise, the impact of cold and freezing would last forever and there would be no spring. Ancient scholars might realize that there is extreme yang, tai yang, inside of cold qi, though it has not come to the surface for observation. They used tai yang to mark cold qi for reminding people that such cold qi is not pure cold, as there is the strongest yang balancing it.

Obviously, this table only demonstrates the relationships between six qi and three yin and three yang in the way 標氣 *biāo qì* marks for 本氣 *běn qì*, i.e. what three yin and three yang do for six qi, and fails to answer the following question: What does six qi do for three yin and three yang in the universe in detail? So our discussion must continue.

14 Wang Bing, op. cit., p.365

15 Ibid., pp.528–529

16 Ibid., p.371

Table 6.2 Relationship among the seasons, six qi, three yin and three yang

Seasons of lunar calendar	Spring (January to February)*	Spring (March to April)	Summer (May to June)	Summer and later summer (July to August)	Autumn (September to October)	Winter (November to December)
Six qi	Wind qi	Heat qi (king fire)	Fire qi (ministerial fire)	Damp qi	Dryness qi	Cold qi
Presentation of weather and vegetation	Warm wind blows; new buds of vegetation appear quietly.	Warm wind qi goes up and becomes heat qi. The leaves of greens open very fast.	Heat changes into fire, but this fire is only hot and has no flame to make things burn. Luxuriant flowers bloom everywhere.	Summer heat prevails, but it is compromised by damp qi.	Leaves on vegetation fall and dryness prevails.	Cold and frozen, but not frozen forever. There will be warmth again next spring.
Rationale	Yang starts to move. One yin starts to grow. Yang is relatively more active than yin.	Yang rises but does not make fire as there must be stronger yin to control it. This indicates yin has developed from one yin to two yins.	Like sunrise, the quantity of yang increases fast; like embers in the oven, it is hot but does not flare up and make food burn.	The most active yang must be controlled by extreme yin. Yin must develop from two yins to three yins to do this job.	Damp qi is the strongest yin, which needs stronger yang to counteract it; otherwise, the weather would stop changing and damp qi would last forever. Yang has moved from one yang to two yangs and become more active to make dryness qi in autumn.	Extreme cold must be counteracted by extreme yang, and extreme yang is able to open this cold and bring spring back. Yang has developed from two yangs to three yangs, the strongest yang.

Relationship between six qi, three yin and three yangs	Jue yin is one yin that cannot strongly control yang, making yang more active. The attributes of jue yin share some similarities with the yin that makes things change in nature during January and February, i.e. yang qi starts to move and becomes more active and generates wind qi. Therefore, Jue yin is used to mark wind qi.	Shao yin is two yins and can prevent yang from flaring up and moving in a reckless way. The attributes of shao yin share some similarities with the yin that makes things change in nature during March and April, i.e. yang becomes stronger and generates heat qi to speed up growth but not flare up because of control from stronger yin in shao yin. Therefore, Shao yin is used to mark heat qi.	Shao yang is one yang. It is hot but moderate and lacks flame. The attributes of shao yang share some similarities with the yang that makes things change in nature during May and June, i.e. yang generates fire qi that does not cause harm. Therefore, shao yang is used to mark fire qi.	Tai yin, which bears three yins and is extreme yin, can control most active yang. The attributes of tai yin share some similarities with the yin that makes things change in nature during July and August, i.e. there it is the strongest yin to check the fire qi, making qi movement in nature turn around. Therefore, tai yin is used to mark damp qi.	Yang ming is two yangs and has stronger yang that can check extreme yin to some degree. The attributes of yang ming share some similarities with the yang that makes things change in nature during September and October, i.e. there is stronger yang to check the strongest yin and make dryness qi in nature. Therefore, yang ming is used to mark dryness qi.	Tai yang is three yangs, which is the strongest yang. It can control the stronger yin, i.e. cold and open cold. The attributes of tai yang share some similarities with the yang that makes things change in nature during November and December, i.e. there is the strongest yang to check the stronger yin, making qi ready to turn around in nature. Therefore, tai yang is used to mark cold qi and is a reminder that the strongest yang opens yin, bringing spring back.

*According to the theory of qi movement of the five elements and qi transformation in six qi in the universe in Basic Questions of The Yellow Emperor's Inner Classic, all years are divided into six sections (六節 *liù jié*) or six steps (六部 *liù bù*). Each section or step counts for 60.875 days and comprises four periods (節氣 *jié qì*).

The reader might notice that there is interaction between yin and yang in either yin controlling yang or yang controlling yin in Table 6.2. This is key to answering this question. When we discuss three yin and three yang, it seems that three yin and three yang are pure yins or pure yangs, respectively. However, according to the conversation between the Yellow Emperor, Gui Yu-Qu and Qi Bo, each yin or each yang is the combination of yin and yang, and the only difference between three yin and three yang is that they bear more or less yin and yang. For example, the term "tai yin" only indicates that it bears much more yin than shao yin and jue yin. Otherwise, how can the lung and spleen, organs that corresponds to tai yin in the human body, activate and do their job in dispersing and descending or transforming and transporting, respectively, if they are pure yin. Likewise, each qi embraces yin and yang. According to cosmology and the macrocosm in The Yellow Emperor's Inner classic, six qi is the root while three yin and three yang are the branch. Chen Bo-Tan (also known as Chen Wen-Wei or Chen Ying-Qi, 1863–1938), a well-known physician who specialized in studying and practicing the theories in Discussion of Cold Damage, particularly qi transformation, in the Canton area, offered a concise yet insightful summary for this root-and-branch relationship. He pointed out that "six qi is the root for transformation while what are transformed are the branches of six qi."[17] In the universe, it is this interaction between yin and yang due to the different quantity of yin and yang that generates six qi. From the theory of yin and yang, it is the interaction between yin and yang due to the different quantity of yin and yang in six qi that generates three yin and three yang, and makes them have different movements. Observing and comprehending this production of different yins and different yangs generated by six qi, and the similarity between three yin and three yang and each qi in six qi, ancient scholars used tai yin, shao yin and jue yin, tai yang, yang ming and shao yang to mark six qi as well as classify three yin and three yang.

Furthermore, ancient scholars discovered that there is another interaction among these six qi based on mutual support and control, one of the principles in the universe. Based on this principle, they classified these six qi and three yin and three yang into three pairs of groups: (a) a pair of fire qi and wind qi, shao yang and jue yin; (b) a pair of dryness qi and damp qi, yang ming and tai yin; and (c) a pair of cold qi and heat qi, tai

17 Chen Bo-Tan. *I Have Read Discussion of Cold Damage* (*dù guò shāng hán lùn*). Beijing: People's Health Publishing House, 1954: 13

yang and shao yin. If each qi were to bear the complete balance of yin and yang without support or control from other qi, there would be no regular movement of qi in the universe, and regular change of weather would not take place. For example, if damp qi in late summer is not controlled by dryness qi, movement of qi in the universe will stop and the weather will be humid forever. Of course, in each pair of qi, one qi should be in charge in its season while its paired qi serves as a mediator to support or control it. For example, without support from fire qi, wind qi, which bears fewer yin, would not warm enough to bring initial growth for trees and crops in early spring; without support from wind qi, fire qi would not spread enough to make flowers bloom in early summer. In the first scenario, wind qi plays a major role while fire qi supports it; in the second scenario, fire qi is in charge of the related season while wind qi supports it. When these paired qi interact with each other, the qi they produce is called 標氣 *biāo qì*. Tai yang, yang ming, shao yang, tai yin, shao yin and jue yin are called 標氣 *biāo qì* generated by the corresponding interaction in six qi, and are also used to name and mark them based on the ratio of yin and yang in such qi for each season. The qi which plays a major role or is in charge of the related season is called 本氣 *běn qì*, and the qi which serves as a mediator to support and/or control 本氣 *běn qì* is called 中氣 *zhōng qì*, which means "medium qi." 中氣 *zhōng qì* is also one of six qi that serves as a mediator when it is not in charge of a season but acts as 本氣 *běn qì* when it governs a season. 標氣 *biāo qì* is different from 本氣 *běn qì* as well as 中氣 *zhōng qì*, because it is the qi produced by the interaction between 本氣 *běn qì* and 中氣 *zhōng qì*. Like 本氣 *běn qì* and 中氣 *zhōng qì*, 標氣 *biāo qì* is the combination of yin qi and yang qi, though these yin and yang might be variable in terms of quantity. Moreover, 標氣 *biāo qì* is not the same as its 本氣 *běn qì* and 中氣 *zhōng qì* anymore. Since the ratio between yin and yang in 本氣 *běn qì* and 中氣 *zhōng qì* cannot be seen with "half an eye," the terms "本氣 *běn qì*" and "中氣 *zhōng qì*" cannot be used to mark themselves in terms of yin and yang. Three yin and three yang, i.e. tai yang, yang ming, shao yang, tai yin, shao yin and jue yin can demonstrate the difference in terms of quantity of yin and yang and share some similarities with 本氣 *běn qì* are used to name and mark 標氣 *biāo qì*. In this process, 本氣 *běn qì* is a root and an internal cause, 中氣 *zhōng qì* is an external cause and 標氣 *biāo qì* is their product and a branch.

The next two sections relate to the interaction between 本氣 *běn qì* and 中氣 *zhōng qì*, and the process of the production of 標氣 *biāo qì* in regard to weather change. They are based on a summary of the thoughts mentioned above and insightful thoughts from Luo Mei, a famous scholar and practitioner in the late seventeenth century and early eighteenth century.[18]

Interaction between 本氣 *běn qì* and 中氣 *zhōng qì*

Yang in the universe wakes up and starts to present, leading to presentation of wind qi when spring is approaching. However, yang is still weak at the very beginning as the season has just turned from winter, and wind qi from such movement of yang can still be chilly, though it is time for the end of yin and generation of yang in the universe. In order to bring the initial growth of everything, fire qi is needed to make this wind qi warm since the flame from fire can generate warmer wind, which is critical for initial growth. During the interaction between wind qi and fire qi, wind qi is a main player while fire qi serves as a supporter. The production of qi from this interaction is not the same as either wind qi or fire qi, though the main part of this qi consists of wind qi. Obviously, this qi is warmer than wind qi but not as hot as fire qi as there are still fewer yins in it. Therefore, this kind of qi cannot be called wind qi or fire qi. One yin (jue yin), which means the end of yin and beginning of yang and can delineate the exact difference of this qi in the regard of quantity of yin and yang, is used to call and mark this qi. The term "one yin" (jue yin) is a reminder of where this qi comes from and what the composition of this qi would be in terms of yin and yang. In this process, wind qi is called 本氣 *běn qì*, fire qi is called 中氣 *zhōng qì* and one yin (jue yin) is called 標氣 *biāo qì*.

In late spring, heat qi in the universe continually grows. If heat qi in the universe grows too fast, there would not be enough time for full development of everything, and everything would become premature, which is not healthy growth. Therefore, cold qi is needed for pacing this growth. In this process, yang energy from heat qi would slowly but steadily climb and present like the king climbs the steps and shows up in front of his palace. Therefore, heat qi is also called king fire. During the interaction between heat qi and cold qi, heat qi is a main player while

18 Luo Mei. *Broad Discussion of The Yellow Emperor's Inner Classic* (*nèi jíng bó yì*). In Qiu Qing-Yuan (ed.) *Collection of Rare Chinese Medical Books* (*zhēn běn yī shū jí chéng*). Shanghai: Shanghai Science and Technology Publishing House, 1985: 6–7

cold qi serves as a mediator to control it. The production of qi from this interaction is not the same as either heat qi or cold qi, though the main part of this qi consists of heat qi. This qi is hot but not too hot since there is much yin from cold qi to control. Therefore, this kind of qi cannot be called heat qi or cold qi. Two yins (shao yin), which can perform this controlling while not compressing heat qi in this interaction, is used to call and mark this qi. The term "two yins" (shao yin) is a reminder of how this qi is produced and what the composition of this qi is with respect to yin and yang. In this process, heat qi is called 本氣 *běn qì*, cold qi is called 中氣 *zhōng qì* and shao yin is called 標氣 *biāo qì*.

Summer is the season when fire qi prevails. Unlike fire on the stove, this fire qi does not scorch everything in summer. Why? Because the fire qi is controlled and supported by chilly wind qi. On the one hand, wind qi can spread this fire qi evenly for full development; on the other hand, chilly wind qi will contain the hot nature of this fire qi. It is this interaction between fire qi and wind qi that makes the summer hot but not too hot to burn everything, and makes fire qi stay where it should and do as it should, like humble ministers in the government. Therefore, it is also called minister fire. During the interaction between fire qi and wind qi, fire qi is a main player while wind qi serves as a mediator to control and support it. The production of qi from his interaction is not the same as either fire qi or wind qi, though the main part of this qi consists of fire qi. Therefore, this kind of qi cannot be called fire qi or wind qi. And one yang (shao yang), which means activity of yang is modest enough not to harm anything, is used to call and mark this qi. The term "one yang" (shao yang) is a reminder of how this qi is produced and what the composition of this qi is with respect to yin and yang. In this process, fire qi is called 本氣 *běn qì*, wind qi is called 中氣 *zhōng qì* and one yang (shao yang) is called 標氣 *biāo qì*.

In the universe, one qi cannot continually stay. Otherwise, qi would go in one direction without return and the life cycle would end. Therefore, fire qi cannot exist forever and there must be something to make the upward and outward movement of fire qi turn around. Here comes damp qi, which brings autumn. It is damp qi that brings rain for containing fire qi and turning the movement of qi. However, if damp qi persistently exists without control, rain will continue and flooding will ensue. Therefore, dryness qi, a kind of yang qi in the universe, is needed to control damp qi, making some rain but not a continual downpour. In this interaction, damp qi is a main player while dryness qi serves as a mediator that makes humidity but not flooding. The production of qi from his interaction is not the same as either damp qi or dryness qi, though the main part of this qi consists of damp qi. Therefore, neither damp qi nor dryness qi would be appropriate for naming this kind of qi. One might notice that energy continually grows and ascends in the universe from the beginning of spring and reaches its climax in the middle of summer but turns around after the middle of summer. One cannot image how the universe makes the growing yang energy turn and descend in the middle of summer without the strongest yin. Only three yins (tai yin), which bear the strongest yin among three yin, must exist mainly in the qi produced by the interaction between damp qi and dryness qi for making this turn. Therefore, three yins (tai yin) are used to call and mark this qi from the interaction between damp qi and dryness qi. The term "three yins" (tai yin) is a reminder of how this qi is produced and how it embraces the strongest yin. In this process, damp qi is called 本氣 *běn qì*, dryness qi is called 中氣 *zhōng qì* and three yins (tai yin) are called 標氣 *biāo qì*.

In autumn, dryness qi that has been counteracting damp qi in late summer prevails. However, if there is only dryness qi, there will be no humidity contained in the soil for the growth next year, or no water in the rivers. Therefore, some damp qi is retained for controlling dryness qi. In the interaction of dryness qi and damp qi, dryness qi is a main player while damp qi is a mediator to control it. The qi produced from this interaction is no longer the same as damp qi or dryness qi. Therefore, neither damp qi nor dryness qi would be appropriate to name this kind of qi. Once this qi is produced by this interaction, the sky would not be so foggy or gray and would become clear and bright, and the sun would be shining again. Also, dryness qi, which can counteract damp qi and make it slow down in regard to descending, must bear relatively strong yang energy. Therefore, two yangs (yang ming, literally called "sun bright") is used to call and mark this kind of qi produced by the interaction between dryness qi and damp qi. The term "two yangs" (yang ming) is a reminder that it contains more yang than yin. In this process, dryness qi is called 本氣 *běn qì*, damp qi is called 中氣 *zhōng qì* and two yangs (yang ming) is called 標氣 *biāo qì*.

Winter is the season when cold qi prevails. One might get the impression that yang is absent in this season, because the water in the lakes and rivers, snow, and ice are cold to touch. Yang does not present on the surface of the lakes and rivers, but yang energy has astringed and hidden below frozen water, snow and ice. Of course, yang energy cannot hide forever; otherwise, spring would not come. This yang energy should be boosted. Heat qi is needed to enhance yang energy to break and melt this icy and frozen water. In the interaction between cold qi and heat qi, cold qi is a main player that keeps winter for a while to accumulate yang energy while heat qi serves as a mediator, which makes cold qi able to be dispersed by yang at the end of winter and the beginning of spring, on the one hand, and continually build up yang energy under this ice and frozen water, on the other hand. Therefore, qi produced by the interaction between cold qi and heat qi is not the same as cold qi and heat qi. It is not pure cold at all. Therefore, neither cold qi nor heat qi would be appropriate to name this kind of qi. Without strongest yang, how can this ice be broken and melted, how can this cold winter end and warm spring return? Only three yangs (tai yang) are capable of doing this job. Therefore, three yangs (tai yang) are used to call and mark the qi produced by the interaction between cold qi and heat qi. The term "three yangs" (tai yang) is a reminder that there is the strongest yang below this cold water and ice, and such cold water and ice will be broken soon by this yang and warm spring will be just around the corner. In this process, cold qi is called 本氣 *běn qì*, heat qi is called 中氣 *zhōng qì* and three yangs (tai yang) is called 標氣 *biāo qì*.

Process of production of 標氣 *biāo qì* in regard to weather change

As stated earlier, the observations of ancient scholars did not stop at six qi but also explored the relationship between the two qi in the three groups, which are wind qi and fire qi, damp qi and dryness qi, cold qi and heat qi. They discovered there is mutual control and/or support between these two qi, in which these two qi take turns serving as a main player or a mediator during this interaction based on observing the change of weather. Therefore, the terms "本氣 *běn qì*" and "中氣 *zhōng qì*" have been introduced to name and mark, respectively, these qi based on the roles they play in different seasons. The qi produced by such interaction bears differences and also similarities between its 本氣 *běn qì* and 中氣 *zhōng qì* in regard to the quantity of yin and yang. Therefore, the term "標氣 *biāo qì*" is used to name and mark this qi. The term "標氣 *biāo qì*" not only reveals the differences and similarities between itself and 本氣 *běn qì* in terms of quality and quantity of yin and yang but it also reveals the sequence of yin and yang during the process of weather change year-round.

The exploration of qi transformation in the universe by ancient scholars does not stop there. They also found that interaction does not only occur in those three groups in six qi but also takes place among 本氣 *běn qì*, 中氣 *zhōng qì* and 標氣 *biāo qì*. This is what is called qi transformation following the interaction among 本氣 *běn qì*, 中氣 *zhōng qì* and 標氣 *biāo qì*, and the second aspect of the theory of qi transformation.

The qi transformation following the interaction among 本氣 *běn qì*, 中氣 *zhōng qì* and 標氣 *biāo qì* was first discussed in Chapter 74 of Basic Questions of The Yellow Emperor's Inner Classic as the following:

> The Yellow Emperor said, "There are differences for the transformation following 本氣 *běn qì* and 標氣 *biāo qì* in six qi. What are they?" Qi Bo replied, "There is the transformation following 本氣 *běn qì*; there is the transformation following 標氣 *biāo qì*; there is the transformation that does not follow 本氣 *běn qì* and 標氣 *biāo qì*." The Yellow Emperor said, "I would like to learn it comprehensively." Qi Bo said, "The transformation for shao yang and tai yin follows their 本氣 *běn qì*; the transformation for shao yin and tai yang follows either their 本氣 *běn qì* or their 標氣 *biāo qì*; and the transformation for yang ming and jue yin does not follow either their 本氣 *běn qì* or their 標氣 *biāo qì* but 中氣 *zhōng qì*. The transformation following their本氣 *běn qì* means the change tends to move towards their 本氣 *běn qì*; the transformation following either their 標氣 *biāo qì* or their 本氣 *běn qì* is likely to move towards either their 標氣 *biāo qì* or their 本氣 *běn qì*; and the transformation following their 中氣 *zhōng qì* tends to move to their 中氣 *zhōng qì*."[19]

Wang Bing (also known as Qi Xuan-Zi, 710–804 AD), a famous scholar who specialized in Basic Questions (素問 *sù wèn*), first offered an explanation for why there is such different transformation in three yin and three yang. He stated:

> The 本氣 *běn qì* for shao yang is fire qi and the 本氣 *běn qì* for tai yin is damp qi. The 本氣 *běn qì* and 標氣 *biāo qì* share the same yin and yang property in shao yang and tai yin, respectively; therefore, the transformations for shao yang and tai yin tend to move towards their 本氣 *běn qì*. The 本氣 *běn qì* for shao yin is heat qi, while its 標氣 *biāo qì* falls into the yin category; the 本氣 *běn qì* for tai yang is cold qi, while

19 Wang Bing, op. cit., pp.532–533

> its 標氣 *biāo qì* belongs to the yang category. The 本氣 *běn qì* and 標氣 *biāo qì* are different in the regard of yin and yang for shao yin and tai yang, respectively; therefore, the transformations for shao yin and tai yang are likely to move towards either their 本氣 *běn qì* or their 標氣 *biāo qì*. Damp qi is 中氣 *zhōng qì* for yang ming and fire qi is 中氣 *zhōng qì* for jue yin. Since the 本氣 *běn qì* and 標氣 *biāo qì* are different from 中氣 *zhōng qì* in yang ming and jue yin, their transformations tend to move towards their 中氣 *zhōng qì*.[20]

This explanation has set up basic and useful methods to study the qi transformation among these three pairs of qi, and it especially attaches great importance to yin and yang property for qi transformation among 本氣 *běn qì*, 標氣 *biāo qì* and 中氣 *zhōng qì*. However, it is far from clear why and how these transformations take place.

Later, some scholars tried to explore the reason for such transformation based on the theory of five elements. For example, Zhang Jie-Bin (also known as Zhang Jing-Yue, 1563–1640), a famous scholar who specialized in studying The Yellow Emperor's Inner Classic, offered a better explanation for why the transformation of shao yang and tai yin tend to move towards their 本氣 *běn qì* while the transformation of yang ming and jue yin tend to move towards their 中氣 *zhōng qì* based on the five elements theory:

> Why does the transformation of shao yang and tai yin not move towards their 中氣 *zhōng qì* though they also have 中氣 *zhōng qì*? Because the 中氣 *zhōng qì* of shao yang is jue yin (wood). Wood and fire share the same energy and wood likes to turn to fire. Therefore, the transformation of shao yang does not move towards its 中氣 *zhōng qì*. The 中氣 *zhōng qì* of tai yin is yang ming (metal). The metal is produced by earth, and dryness qi is likely to transform into damp qi. Therefore, the transformation of tai yin does not move towards its 中氣 *zhōng qì*...
>
> The transformation of yang ming and jue yin move towards their 中氣 *zhōng qì* rather than 標氣 *biāo qì* and 本氣 *běn qì*, because the 中氣 *zhōng qì* of yang ming is tai yin (damp qi and earth), and the dryness qi tends to transform into damp qi. The 中氣 *zhōng qì* of jue yin is shao yang (fire), and wood is likely to transform into fire. Therefore, the transformation of yang ming and jue yin tends to move towards their 中氣 *zhōng qì* rather than 標氣 *biāo qì* and 本氣 *běn qì*.[21]

---

20 Ibid., p.533

21 Zhang Jie-Bin. *Illustration of the Classified Classic* (*lèi jīng tú yì*). Beijing: People's Health Publishing House, 1982: 140

Zhang first applied the theory of qi transformation to the network of zang-fu organs and created a diagram (Figure 6.2) of zang-fu organs corresponding to 本氣 *běn qì*, 中氣 *zhōng qì* and 標氣 *biāo qì* in the heavens.

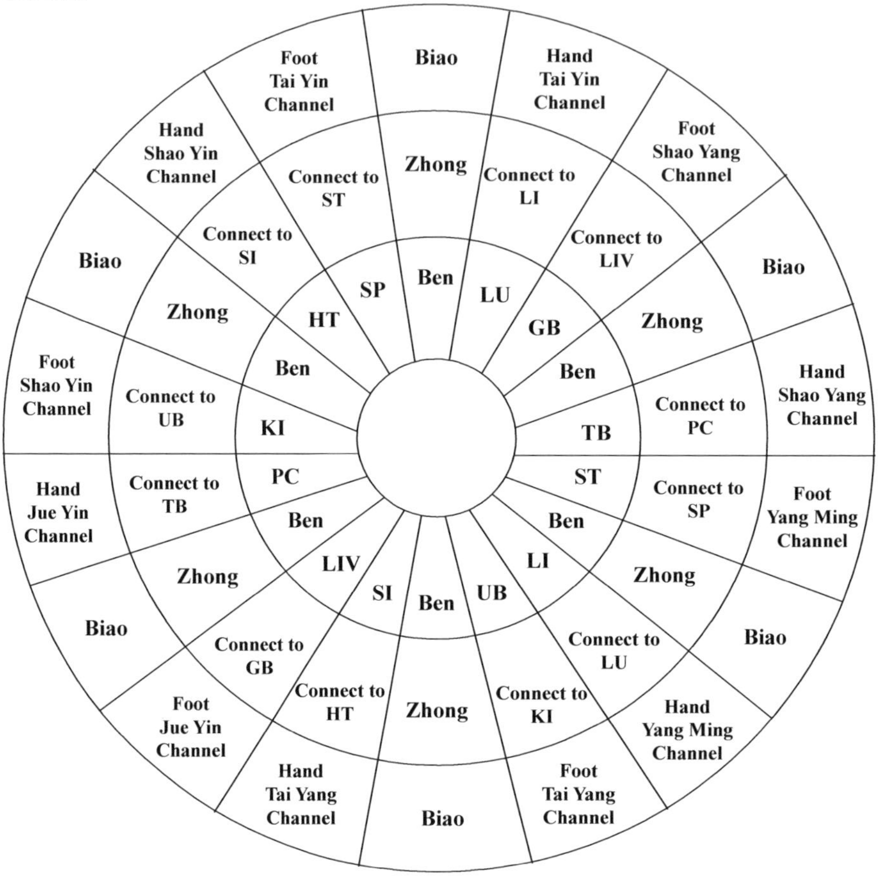

FIGURE 6.2 ZANG-FU ORGANS CORRESPONDING TO 標 BIĀO, 本 BĚN AND 中 ZHŌNG QÌ IN THE HEAVENS[22]

In the footnote for this diagram, Zhang wrote:

> Concerning 標氣 *biāo qì* and 本氣 *běn qì* in zang-fu organs, channels and collaterals, zang-fu organs are 本氣 *běn qì* as they locate in the interior of the body, while the twelve channels are 標氣 *biāo qì* as they locate on the body surface. What is connecting the exterior and interior is 中氣 *zhōng qì*, as it locates between the exterior and interior.[23]

22 Ibid., p.139

23 Ibid., p.139

In 1994, Hao Yin-Qing first applied both the theory of yin and yang and the theory of five elements to these transformations and offered an insightful explanation for these transformations based on researching results from past scholars.[24] Hao Ri-Jin, his son, followed up his father's study and wrote:

> Jue yin relates to wind qi in six qi and pertains to wood in five elements; shao yin relates to heat qi in six qi and pertains to king fire in five elements. Shao yang relates to fire qi in six qi and pertains to ministerial fire in five elements. Tai yin relates to damp qi in six qi and pertains to earth in the five elements. Yang ming relates to dryness qi in six qi and pertains to metal in the five elements. Tai yang relates to cold qi in six qi and pertains to water in the five elements. They are classified into three pairs, which correspond to each other. The following are the transformations among them:
>
> Fire qi is 本氣 *běn qì* for shao yang, which is ministerial fire and marked by yang. Its 中氣 *zhōng qì* is wind qi that relates to jue yin. Since its 本氣 *běn qì* and 標氣 *biāo qì* share the same energy (quality of yin and yang is the same), and its 中氣 *zhōng qì* is wind qi in six qi that relates to jue yin, wind qi transforms into fire. While jue yin belongs to wood according to the theory of five elements, wood can produce fire. Therefore, the transformation for shao yang must follow its 本氣 *běn qì* and turns to fire qi.
>
> Damp qi is 本氣 *běn qì* for tai yin that relates to earth and is marked by yin. Its 中氣 *zhōng qì* is dryness qi that relates to yang ming and metal. Its 本氣 *běn qì* and 標氣 *biāo qì* share the same energy, which is yin energy, and its 中氣 *zhōng qì* is dryness qi in six qi that relates to yang ming. The real change in weather is that dryness qi follows damp qi. According to the theory of five elements, dryness qi belongs to metal, earth is the mother of metal, and the transformation of the son should follow that of its mother. Therefore, the transformation for tai yin must follow its 本氣 *běn qì* and turns to damp qi. This is the reason why The Yellow Emperor's Inner Classic states that "the transformation for shao yang and tai yin follows their 本氣 *běn qì*."
>
> Cold qi is 本氣 *běn qì* for tai yang that relates to water and is marked by yang. Its 中氣 *zhōng qì* is heat qi (king fire) that relates shao yin. Its 本氣 *běn qì* and 標氣 *biāo qì* are different (opposing quality of yin and yang). While its 中氣 *zhōng qì* is heat qi in six qi that relates to shao yin, heat qi belongs to king fire according to the theory of five elements. Like

24 Hao Yin-Qing. "Searching for the root of the theory of qi transformation in six conformations of Discussion of Cold Damage." *Shanxi Journal of Traditional Chinese Medicine*, 1994 (4): 52

> tai yang, the 本氣 *běn qì* and 標氣 *biāo qì* for shao yin are different in terms of yin and yang. Both 本氣 *běn qì* and 標氣 *biāo qì* in tai yang and shao yin oppose each other as the cold and heat are supposed to control each other. There is a chance for tai yang to transform into either cold qi or heat qi.
>
> Heat qi is 本氣 *běn qì* for shao yin that relates to king fire and is marked by yin. Its 中氣 *zhōng qì* is cold qi that relates to tai yang and water. The mechanism for its transformation is the same as in tai yang. There is no necessity to give this in detail. This is the reason why The Yellow Emperor's Inner Classic states that "transformation for shao yin and tai yang follows either their 本氣 *běn qì* or their 標氣 *biāo qì*."
>
> Dryness qi is 本氣 *běn qì* for yang ming that relates to metal and is marked by yang. Its 中氣 *zhōng qì* is damp qi that relates to tai yin. Because dryness qi is qi in autumn and belongs to yin, its 本氣 *běn qì* and 標氣 *biāo qì* is different (in terms of yin and yang). Its 中氣 *zhōng qì* is damp qi in six qi. The change in weather is that dryness qi follows damp qi. Since earth can produce metal according to the theory of five elements, the transformation for yang ming must follow its 中氣 *zhōng qì*, damp qi.
>
> Wind qi is 本氣 *běn qì* for jue yin that relates to wood and is marked by yin. Its 中氣 *zhōng qì* is fire qi that relates to shao yang and ministerial fire. Like yang ming, the way 本氣 *běn qì* and 標氣 *biāo qì* relate to jue yin is different (with regard to yin and yang). Since its 中氣 *zhōng qì* is fire qi in six qi and the wind qi can follow fire qi for its transformation according to the theory of five elements, jue yin belongs to wood and wood can produce fire. Therefore, the transformation for jue yin must follow its 中氣 *zhōng qì*, fire qi.[25]

Hao's study has elaborated the mechanism for qi transformation in six qi and three yin and three yang. The great achievement this study made was that it was the first to point out that different qi transformations are brought about by the interaction among 本氣 *běn qì*, 標氣 *biāo qì* and 中氣 *zhōng qì* in regard to the quality of yin and yang. However, Hao's explanation is still not quite clear, particularly regarding the details of the mechanism. Enlightened by Hao's study, I offer Table 6.3 to explain qi transformation among 本氣 *běn qì*, 標氣 *biāo qì* and 中氣 *zhōng qì*, based on the waxing and waning of yin and yang.

---

25 Hao Ri-Jin. *Literature study for theoretical source and development of qi transformation in six conformations in Discussion of Cold Damage*. Wuhan: Hubei College of Traditional Chinese Medicine, 2008: 20–21

Table 6.3 Tendency of qi transformation among three yin and three yang according to the theory of 本氣 *běn qì*, 標氣 *biāo qì* and 中氣 *zhōng qì*

Three yin and three yang	標氣 *biāo qì*	中氣 *zhōng qì*	本氣 *běn qì*	Interactions	Tendency of qi transformation
Jue yin	One yin	Shao yang	Wind qi	Wind qi and shao yang are yang while jue yin is yin. 標氣 *biāo qì*, i.e. jue yin (yin), is different from its 本氣 *běn qì*, i.e. wind qi (yang). Among these three factors, there are two yangs and one yin, which make their movement more likely towards yang. Therefore, the transformation for jue yin tends to move towards its 中氣 *zhōng qì*, shao yang, i.e. it changes into fire.	Toward its 中氣 *zhōng qì*
Yang ming	Two yangs	Tai yin	Dryness qi	Dryness and tai yin are yin while yang ming is yang. 標氣 *biāo qì*, i.e. yang ming (yang), is different from its 本氣 *běn qì*, i.e. dryness qi (yin). Among these three factors, there are two yins and one yang, which make their movement more likely towards yin. Therefore, the transformation for yang ming tends to move towards its 中氣 *zhōng qì*, tai yin, i.e. it changes into damp qi.	Towards its 中氣 *zhōng qì*
Tai yang	Three yangs	Shao yin	Cold qi	Like jue yin and yang ming, there are differences between 標氣 *biāo qì* and 本氣 *běn qì* (tai yang and cold) in regard to yin and yang. The tendency of the movement between them depends on the results from the interaction between yang in tai yang and cold with the mediation of 中氣 *zhōng qì*, shao yin (heat qi). With strong heat qi from shao yin, yang in tai yang overcomes cold and the transformation of tai yang moves towards heat qi; otherwise, the transformation moves towards cold qi.	Towards qi either 標氣 *biāo qì* or 本氣 *běn qì*

Three yin and three yang	標氣 ***biāo qì***	中氣 ***zhōng qì***	本氣 ***běn qì***	Interactions	Tendency of qi transformation
Shao yin	Two yins	Tai yang	Heat qi	Like jue yin and yang ming, there are differences between 標氣 *biāo qì* and 本氣 *běn qì* (shao yin and heat qi) in terms of yin and yang. The tendency of the movement between them depends on the results from the interaction between yin in shao yin and heat qi with the mediation of 中氣 *zhōng qì*, tai yang (cold qi). With cold qi from tai yang, yin in shao yin overcomes heat qi and the transformation of shao yin moves towards cold qi; otherwise, the transformation moves towards heat qi.	Towards either 標氣 *biāo qì* or 本氣 *běn qì*
Tai yin	Three yins	Yang ming	Damp qi	Damp qi and tai yin are yin while yang ming is yang. 本氣 *běn qì*, i.e. damp qi (yin), shares the same energy with tai yin (yin). Among these three factors, there are two yins and one yang, which make their movement more likely towards yin. Also, tai yin and its 本氣 *běn qì*, damp qi, share the same energy, yin, and are quite compatible with each other. Therefore, tai yin tends to move towards yin, i.e. its 本氣 *běn qì*, damp qi.	Towards 本氣 *běn qì*
Shao yang	One yang	Jue yin	Fire qi	Fire qi and shao yang are yang while jue yin is yin. 本氣 *běn qì*, i.e. fire qi shares the same energy with shao yang (yang). Among these three factors, there are two yangs and one yin, which make their movement more likely towards yang. Also, shao yang and its 本氣 *běn qì*, fire qi, share the same energy, yang, and are quite compatible with each other. Therefore, shao yang tends to move towards yang, i.e. its 本氣 *běn qì*, fire qi.	Towards 本氣 *běn qì*

According to The Yellow Emperor's Inner Classic, the role that three yin and three yang play in the human body is variable. This is related to what is called the theory of opening, closing and pivot for three yin and three yang (Table 6.4) recorded in Chapter 5 of Spiritual Pivot and Chapter 6 of Basic Questions in The Yellow Emperor's Inner Classic. Their functions are described as the following: "Tai yang is supposed to open, yang ming to close, while shao yang serves as a pivot. Tai yin is supposed to open, jue yin to close, while shao yin serves as a pivot."[26]

Table 6.4 Opening, closing and pivot function for three yin and three yang

Opening	Closing	Pivot
Tai yang (three yangs)	Yang ming (two yangs)	Shao yang (one yang)
Tai yin (three yins)	Jue yin (one yin)	Shao yin (two yins)

Why are there the opening, closing and pivot in three yin and three yang and what do they mean? Two scholars who specialized in studying The Yellow Emperor's Inner Classic offered insightful interpretations for them. Wang Bing (also known as Qi Xuan-Zi, 710–804 AD) stated:

> The reason to discuss opening, closing and pivot for three yin and three yang is because qi in three yin and three yang are different in terms of quantity, activity and function. The opening refers to the beginning of qi movement, closing refers to the power to control and the pivot is in charge of turning of qi elegantly.[27]

Wu Kun (also known as Wu Shan-Fu, 1551–1620), the third scholar who made commentary for Basic Questions of The Yellow Emperor's Inner Classic, wrote:

> Tai yang locates on the exterior of the body and is supposed to distribute yang qi. Therefore, its function is called opening. Yang ming locates in the interior of the body and is supposed to receive and bring yang qi in. Therefore, its function is called closing. Shao yang locates between the exterior and the interior is supposed to turn and transport yang qi like a door hinge. Therefore, its function is called pivot…
>
> Tai yin locates in the middle part of the body and is supposed to distribute yin qi. Therefore, its function is called opening. Jue yin is the end of yin and is supposed to receive and bring yin qi in. Therefore, its

26 Wang Bing, op. cit., pp.50–51

27 Ibid., p.50

> function is called closing. Shao yin refers to the kidney and is full of essence and qi. The spleen is in charge of opening and the liver governs closing. If qi in the kidney is not full, the normal function of the opening and closing would be affected. Therefore, the function of shao yin is called pivot.[28]

Following Wu's thought, Zhang Jie-Bin (also known as Zhang Jing-Yue, 1563–1640) further explained:

> The opening of tai yang refers to the externally distribution of yang qi, and tai yang locates on the exterior in three yang. The closing of yang ming refers to internal accumulation of yang qi, and yang ming locates in the interior in three yang. The pivot of shao yang refers to the movement of qi between the exterior and interior and it can let qi move in and out like a door hinge. The opening of tai yin means that tai yin locates on the exterior in three yin. The closing of jue yin means that jue yin locates in the interior in three yin. The pivot of shao yin means that shao yin locates in the middle in three yin. The opening is in charge of outward movement of qi, the closing governs the inward movement of qi and the pivot controls in and out of qi movement.[29]

Since there are differences among three yin and three yang in terms of quantity of qi and function of qi, each yin and yang bears a different function. In order to make qi circulate continually and smoothly in the body, each yin and yang must play a role that makes qi in the body move in, out, upward and down; hence the terms for opening, closing and pivot for three yin and three yang have been adapted for the theory of qi transformation. In his doctoral dissertation, Li Hang-Zhou offers a very interesting opinion for the opening and closing function for tai yang and tai yin, and yang ming and jue yin, which is quite helpful for one to have deep understanding these concepts:

> The opening implies the meaning of communication between yin and yang. Qi in tai yin starts to open, leading to the communication and transformation between yin and yang, resulting in changing from yang to yin, i.e. moving to tai yin through the closing function of yang ming. And the trend of qi transformation is receiving, descending and hiding.

28 Wu Kun. *Commentary by Mr. Wu on Basic Questions of The Yellow Emperor's Inner Classic* (*huáng dì nèi jīng sù wèn wú zhù*). In Cheng Shi-De et al. *Selected Explanations for Basic Questions* (*sù wèn zhù shì huì cuì*). Beijing: People's Health Publishing House, 1982: 113, 115

29 Zhang Jie-Bin. *Classified Classic* (*lèi jīng*). Beijing: People's Health Publishing House, 1980: 286–287

> Tai yin belongs to three yins and has a good capacity of yin since it can accept yang qi accumulated and descended from yang ming. Therefore, tai yin is supposed to open and it is a gate for three yin. It is crucial for qi transformation for shao yin and jue yin, because it not only opens the gate to receive qi accumulated and descended from yang ming, but also can foster source yang with its high virtue to take charge of an important thing, and make qi transformation continue in jue yin.
>
> The closing function of yang ming and jue yin refers to the process from closing, to accumulating and transforming. They are turning points for ascending and descending of qi and qi transformation. The closing of yang ming refers to the process from tai yang to yang ming, during which yang has gradually changed from its peak to yin, and descends. The significance of jue yin to close is to connect shao yin to shao yang. If yin qi only lifts and disperses, it can easily be exhausted. After going through the process of closing from jue yin, yin qi accumulates and becomes stable. Just like yang ming can make yang transform to yin, jue yin can make yin transform to yang. It can receive qi from tai yin and mix this qi with qi in shao yin and finally deliver qi to shao yang.[30]

We have reviewed the theory of qi transformation in The Yellow Emperor's Inner Classic in great detail. Liang Hua Long has offered a good summary for the significance of this theory:

> The significance for the theory of the opening, closing and pivot are that it not only elaborates the process for transformation of yin and yang from yang to yin, from yin to yang, from the beginning to the climax, from the climax to the declining and from the declining to the flourishing again, but also this process as a whole should be viewed as a dynamic system—if there is opening, there should be closing; if there is closing, there should be opening; both opening and closing must be related to the pivot to make qi turn around. Therefore, the opening, closing and pivot are three movements for one thing. They cannot be separated from each other, though each plays a special role in the movement of qi.[31]

However, one should know that originally the concept of those three yin and three yang in Chapter 5 of Spiritual Pivot and Chapter 6 of Basic Questions of The Yellow Emperor's Inner Classic is somewhat different

30 Li Hang-Zhou. *Exploration for Balanced View of Qi Transformation Reflected by Resolving Time for Diseases in Six Conformation in Discussion of Cold Damage* (*shāng hán lùn liù jīng bìng yù jiě shí suǒ àn hán qì huà píng héng guān tān jiū*). Beijing: Beijing University of Chinese Medicine, 2011: 67

31 Liang Hua-Long. "Origin and application of the theory of opening, closing and pivot in six conformations." *Henan Journal of Traditional Chinese Medicine*, 1998 (2): 5

from the concept of three yin and three yang in Chapters 66–70 and 74 of Basic Questions. The former chapters only refer to 12 channels, i.e. analyzing yin and yang in nature for 12 channels in the human body and classifying them into three yin and three yang, while the latter chapters refer to the six qi in the universe. In other words, classifying three yin and three yang and their opening, closing and pivotal function, respectively, in Chapter 5 of Spiritual Pivot and Chapter 6 of Basic Questions is only based on qi and blood circulation in those channels and distribution of those channels. They have nothing to do with the six qi in the heavens and the function of zang-fu organs originally. This is probably why some scholars do not consider the theory of opening, closing and pivot for three yin and three yang as the content of the theory of qi transformation in The Yellow Emperor's Inner Classic. However, from my point of view, it is probably this difference that demonstrates that scholars and practitioners in ancient times already applied this theory to the physiological function of the human body as well as the six qi in the universe.

Based on the discussion above, what is called qi transformation in six qi was originally used to study the interactions among 本氣 *běn qì*, 標氣 *biāo qì* and 中氣 *zhōng qì* in the light of observing the change in weather. Also, the theory of qi transformation in The Yellow Emperor's Inner Classic (黃帝內經 *huáng dì nèi jīng*) not only refers to what happens in the universe but also can be applied for understanding physiological function of the human body. However, how has the qi transformation in the universe been applied to analyze the pathological changes in the human body, especially externally contracted diseases?

The theory of qi transformation for Discussion of Cold Damage, presented below, was based on the application of the theory by many ancient and contemporary scholars over a period of a few hundred years, of qi transformation in The Yellow Emperor's Inner Classic to the study of Discussion of Cold Damage.

Development of the school of qi transformation in six conformations in Discussion of Cold Damage

The main stream of studying Discussion of Cold Damage has been focused on six conformations, especially three yin and three yang, based on the theory of channels and collaterals, and the theory of zang-fu organs, from the twelfth to the sixteenth centuries. At the end of the sixteenth century, some scholars found that these two theories could not be explained completely in terms of what happens for three yin diseases and three yang diseases in Discussion of Cold Damage. Some scholars tried to apply the theory of qi transformation in six qi recorded in The Yellow Emperor's Inner Classic to the disorders of three yin diseases and three yang diseases in Discussion of Cold Damage for a more satisfying explanation, and a new school to study Discussion of Cold Damage was gradually established.

The early explorer for this school was Lu Zu-Chang who lived c. 1160 in Zhejiang province. He tried to use the theory of qi transformation to explain the pathology of shao yang disease. He wrote that "tai yang belongs to cold and water. Shao yang belongs to ministerial fire. When diseases in tai yang progress to shao yang, there will be a fight between fire and water, leading to alternating fever and chills."[32] Lu Zi-Yi (also known as Lu Zi-Yao, 1599–1664), who also lived in Zhejiang province, further applied the theory of qi transformation, especially 本氣 *běn qì* and 標氣 *biāo qì*, for an explanation of symptoms and signs for three yin diseases and three yang diseases in Discussion of Cold Damage. For example, he wrote that "aversion to cold indicates that patients dislike cold transformations from 標氣 *biāo qì* (tai yang)...fever is a yang presentation from 標氣 *biāo qì*."[33] Another contribution made by Lu was that he first adapted the theory of opening, closing and pivot from The Yellow Emperor's Inner Classic to explain the pathology and treatment for three yin diseases and three yang diseases in Discussion of Cold Damage. For example, he stated:

> Tai yang is supposed to open. When there is a disorder of this opening in tai yang, qi will be closed inside of the body. This formula [Cinnamon Twig Decoction (*guì zhī tāng*)] with acrid and sweet flavor can make the muscle layer open, dispersing wind that invades externally. In this way, the function of opening and closing will be normalized.[34]

Lu further stated:

---

32 Lu's statement was recorded in 1445 and was published in 1957 by Jin Li-Meng, a Korean scholar; see Jin Li-Meng et al. *Section Two of Collection of Medical Formulas According to Their Different Types* (*yī fāng lèi jù dì èr fēn cè*). Beijing: People's Health Publishing House, 1957: 203

33 Lu Zi-Yi. *Copy and Comment That Can Help in Deeply Understanding Discussion of Cold Damage by Zhong-Jing* (*zhòng-jǐng shāng hán lùn shū chāo jīn pī*). In Nie Hui-Ming et al. (eds) *Collection of Explanations on Discussion of Cold Damage* (*shāng hán lùn jí jiě*). Beijing: Learning Garden Publishing House, 2001: 204

34 Ibid., p.208

> Tai yin is supposed to open. Tai yin is unable to open when it is diseased, and it will affect the function of closing [for yang ming], leading to failure of tai yin and yang ming in taking food in, processing food, supporting the body and separating the clear from the turbid, resulting in progressively severe diarrhea.[35]

Following Lu's studying approach to Discussion of Cold Damage, there came one of the brilliant figures in the development of the theory of qi transformation for Discussion of Cold Damage, Zhang Zhi-Cong (also known as Zhang Yin-An, 1616–1674). His book, Collection of Commentaries for Cold Damage (傷寒論集注 *shāng hán lùn jí zhù*), was published c. 1683. What Zhang put forward in his book was based on the philosophy of "as above, as below" discussed in The Yellow Emperor's Inner Classic. He wrote:

> Six qi in the heavens is rooted and located above, while three yin and three yang in the human body are branches that corresponds to six qi in the heavens. This is called "there is six qi in the heavens and there is six qi in the human body."[36]

How do six qi in the heavens and six qi in the human body (three yin and three yang) interact with each other? Zhang explained it as follows:

> In the original text of Discussion of Cold Damage, tai yang, yang ming and shao yang are three yang while tai yin, shao yin and jue yin are three yin. Three yin and three yang are called six qi (in the human body). Since there are six qi in the heavens, there are six qi in the human body. Six qi in the human body circulate normally and correspond to six qi in the heavens when diseases are absent. When wind-cold invades the human body, it indicates that six qi in the heavens have turned into evil qi (pathological factors) and damaged anti-pathogenic qi.
>
> The evil qi interferes with the circulation of six qi in the body at the very beginning and then progresses to the channels due to the disorder of qi circulation. Practitioners nowadays do not understand the theory of qi transformation. They only think of the urinary bladder when discussing tai yang; only think of the stomach when discussing yang ming; only think of the gall bladder when discussing shao yang. They have been focusing on substantial things (channels and organs) and have forgotten non-substantial

35 Ibid., p.768

36 Zhang Zhi-Cong. *Collection of Commentaries for Discussion of Cold Damage* (*shāng hán lùn jí zhù*). In Zheng Lin et al. (eds) *Complete Medical Works by Zhang Zhi-Cong* (*zhāng zhì-cōng yī xué quán shū*). Beijing: China Publishing House of Traditional Chinese Medicine, 2005: 750

> things (six qi), addressing the least important things and ignoring the most important things. This is not the way to study Discussion of Cold Damage.[37]

Based on his observations, Zhang reminds us:

> What is called Cold Damage in six conformations refers to diseases that are related to the disorders of six qi and reflects on the pulses. The chance for Cold Damage to affect qi transformation and invade the body through the points of channel is 20–30%. This is the most important part, which must be realized by readers in studying Discussion of Cold Damage.[38]

According to his study, Zhang concluded:

> The essence of the theory of six qi (qi transformation) does not originate from Lu Zi-Yi [also known as Lu Zi-Yao, 1599–1664] and it has been discussed in detail in The Yellow Emperor's Inner Classic. In this classic, it states that 'wind, cold, summer-heat, damp, dryness and fire is six qi in the heavens; three yin and three yang correspond to them upward.' What is called three yin and three yang refers to six qi in the human body, because yin and yang in the human body correspond to yin and yang in the heavens through qi. Therefore, with qi moving in and out between the exterior and interior, the progression of disease between the interior and exterior is not limited.
>
> If one explores this circulation and progression based on only substantial channels, it will be very difficult to understand what is going on with them. Since channels are substantial while qi is non-substantial, six qi can encompass six channels, whereas six channels cannot cover six qi.[39]

Zhang also addressed the importance of the theory of opening, closing and pivot for six conformations in Discussion of Cold Damage. In the article "Comprehensively Studying the Relationship Between Discussion of Cold Damage and Six Qi," he wrote:

> The classic states that "yin and yang bear names but do not have a fixed shape." Therefore, three yin and three yang have movements such as in, out, combination and separation. Without thoroughly understanding the principle of the change in yin and yang, one cannot study Discussion of Cold Damage.[40]

37 Ibid., p.621

38 Ibid., p.750

39 Ibid., p.670

40 Ibid., p.750

Huang Yuan-Yu (also known as Huang Kun-Zai, 1705–1750) is another important figure who made a great contribution to the development of the theory of qi transformation in studying Discussion of Cold Damage. In his work, Explanation for Difficult Questions in Discussion of Cold Damage (傷寒懸解 *shāng hán xúan jiě*) published in 1748, he tried to use the theory of qi transformation in The Yellow Emperor's Inner Classic to explain six conformations and their pathologies. He wrote:

> There are twelve channels in the human body. The reason that [Zhang] Zhong-Jing only established six conformations is because they relate to six qi. In shao yin, shao yang and yang ming, hand channels are in charge of qi and the qi transformation in foot channels follow ones in hand channels, while in jue yin, tai yin and tai yang, foot channels are in charge of qi and the qi transformation of hand channels follow ones in foot channels. However, foot channels rather than hand channels are addressed in six conformations in Discussion of Cold Damage. This is because foot channels distribute over the body and they cover larger areas, while hand channels only go along two hands and cover smaller areas. In fact, when there is a disease, both hand and food channels are involved as they share the same qi…
>
> The urinary bladder of foot tai yang is in charge of cold and water, and the fire from the small intestine of hand tai yang follows the urinary bladder of foot tai yang and transforms into cold. The large intestine of hand yang ming is in charge of dryness qi and metal, and the earth from the stomach of foot yang ming follows the large intestine of hand yang ming and transforms into dryness. The three burners of hand shao yang is in charge of ministerial fire, and the wood from the gall bladder of foot shao yang follows the three burners of hand shao yang, and transforms into fire. The spleen of foot tai yin is in charge of damp and earth, and the metal from the lung of hand tai yin follows the spleen of foot tai yin, and transforms into damp. The heart of hand shao yin is in charge of king fire, and the water from the kidney of foot shao yin follows the heart of hand shao yin, and transforms into fire. The liver of foot jue yin is in charge of wind and wood, and the fire from the pericardium of hand jue yin follows the liver of foot jue yin, and transforms into wind. These are normal qi transformations in six conformations. When they are attacked by pathological factors, the presentation of tai yang is cold, the presentation of yang ming is dryness, the presentation of shao yang is fire, the presentation of tai yin is damp and the presentation of jue yin is wind. Only the presentation of shao yin does not move to heat rather than cold, because there is heat when fire prevails and there is cold when water prevails. However, water can overcome fire, whereas fire is unable to overcome water when there is a disease in shao

> yin. Therefore, the presentation of shao yin moves towards cold following water in the urinary bladder rather than moves towards heat following the king fire in the heart.
>
> As to yang ming, the transformation of qi moves towards dryness following the metal of the large intestine when yang is excessive but moves towards damp following the earth of the spleen when yin is excessive. It does not always transform to excessive dryness. This is why the first part of the chapter of yang ming disease is related to the disorders of excessive dryness, while the second part of the chapter of yang ming disease is related to the disorders of excessive damp. As to shao yang, fire prevails when yang is excessive and the progression moves towards fu organs, while the progression moves towards zang organs when yang is deficient. It does not always transform to excessive fire.[41]

Enlightened by the diagram drawn by Zhang Jie-Bin (see Figure 6.2), Chen Nian-Zu (also known as Chen Xiu-Yuan, 1753–1823) pointed out:

> The qi transformation in six qi is not always caused by excess but also deficiency. One should be aware that excess can make trouble for qi transformation but one should also know that qi transformation does not take place when there is deficiency. Qi in six conformations can sometimes be excessive or deficient. Qi transformation can be too much when qi is excessive. Qi transformation does not occur when qi is deficient.[42]

Chen tried to use the concepts of 本氣 *běn qì*, 標氣 *biāo qì* and 中氣 *zhōng qì* in the theory of qi transformation in The Yellow Emperor's Inner Classic to elaborate pathologies for six conformations and their various syndromes. For example, he explained:

> 本氣 *běn qì* in yang ming is dryness qi and its 標氣 *biāo qì* is yang. If it fails to get balance from damp qi of tai yin, its 中氣 *zhōng qì*, the dryness qi and yang heat will prevail, leading to the disease of excess in the stomach and large intestine.[43]

Also, following the idea from Zhang Zhi-Cong that qi circulates between the exterior and interior, Chen clearly classified three yang diseases into

---

41 Huang Yuan-Yu. *Explanation for Difficult Questions in Discussion of Cold Damage* (*shāng hán xuán jiě*). In Li Yu-Bin (ed.) *Study of Discussion of Cold Damage by Huang Yuan-Yu* (*huáng yuán-yù dú shāng hán*). Beijing: People's Military Medical Press, 2010: 14–15

42 Chen Nian-Zu. *Section Two of New Annotation and Collation for Books by Chen Xiu-Yuan* (*xīn jiào zhù chén xiū-yuán yī shū dì èr jí*). Fuzhou: Fujian Scientific and Technological Publishing House, 2003: 15

43 Ibid., p.224

channel syndrome and fu syndrome in Discussion of Cold Damage, which combines the theory of qi transformation with zang-fu organs and channels and makes the theory of qi transformation more objective and practical. For example, he writes:

> What is channel syndrome in yang ming disease? The answer is feverish body, painful eyes, dry nose, inability to fall into asleep, aversion to heat...What is called fu syndrome in yang ming disease? The answer is tidal fever, delirious speech, persistent sweating of hands, feet and armpits, fullness in the abdomen and hard stool.[44]

Noticing that the theory of qi transformation in six conformations cannot be elucidated thoroughly without addressing substantial zang-fu organs and channels, Tang Zong-Hai (1847–1897), a well-known scholar who put forward integration of Chinese medicine and Western medicine, pointed out:

> Zhang Zhi-Cong and Zhang Ling-Shao [also known as Zhang Xi-Ju, c. 1644] made an effort to explore the theory of qi transformation comprehensively. Their discussion is quite detailed. However, they ignored that qi must attach to substantial things (zang-fu organs and channels). Therefore, the approach to studying the theory of qi transformation without addressing substantial things is absolutely incorrect.[45]

Tang attached great importance to substantial things, i.e. zang-fu organs and channels, for exploring the theory of qi transformation in six conformations of Discussion of Cold Damage. For example, he wrote:

> Tai yang is the greatest yang in the heavens. It is this kind of yang qi that can mingle with "the ten thousand things." It indeed originates from water under the earth, though it spreads in the universe. What we have most on the earth is water. It is this plenitude of water that generates a great quantity of qi and mingles with "the ten thousand things"... Corresponding to water in nature is the fu organ of the urinary bladder of tai yang in the human body. Since the urinary bladder governs all water in the body, it is called fu organ of cold and water. Although water is cold in nature, the urinary bladder is called the tai yang channel because qi

44 Ibid., p.225

45 Tang Zong-Hai. *Notes on the Use of The Book for Correction for Preliminary Commentary for Discussion of Cold Damage* (*shāng hán lùn qiān zhù bǔ zhèng fàn lì*). In *Five Types of Medical Works in Relation to Connection Between Chinese Medicine and Western Medicine* (*zhōng xī huì tōng yī xué wǔ zhòng, wǔ jí*). Shanghai: Publishing House of Selling Thousands of Books, 1908: 8

> that is generated from this water reaches to the exterior for defending the body and becomes the greatest yang, this is why it is called the tai yang channel. As a matter of fact, this kind of qi is not produced by the urinary bladder itself. It is generated by fire descended from the heart to warm and steam water.
>
> Like the sun in the heavens, there is the heart in the human body. Sunlight shines on water on the earth and steams qi upward. Therefore, the fire in the heart descends to the urinary bladder, steaming qi upward. The way for the heart to descend to the urinary bladder is through the small intestine, which is a fu organ of the heart...This is how the urinary bladder and small intestine can generate qi to defend the body, and they are called the tai yang channel.[46]

Obviously, Tang applied what happens in qi transformation in the universe to the human body, especially three yin, three yang and their related organs and channels. This approach made the theory of qi transformation in six conformations of Discussion of Cold Damage no longer purely imaginary but more tangible, relatively practical and easily understandable.

Wan You-Sheng (1917–2003), a well-known scholar who studied Discussion of Cold Damage, put forward exploration of the theory of qi transformation in six conformations based on the function of zang-fu organs and channels. He pointed out:

> The theory of three yin and three yang in Discussion of Cold Damage indeed demonstrates the activity of qi transformation according to the material base of zang-fu organs, channels and collaterals. The activity of qi transformation takes zang-fu organs as its root while using channels as its pathways. Therefore, the theory of three yin and three yang must include channels, collaterals, zang-fu organs and qi transformation. None of them can be absent in this theory. We should pay attention to pathological reaction on channels and collaterals, but great importance should be attached to the activity of qi transformation on channels and collaterals.[47]

Based on the discussion above, one might learn that the theory of qi transformation in six conformations in studying Discussion of Cold Damage is a product made by some ancient scholars. It is one of the important schools in studying Discussion of Cold Damage. Questions might be raised, such as the following:

---

46 Ibid., pp.1–2

47 Wan You-Sheng. *Key Points to Learn in Discussion of Cold Damage* (*shāng hán lùn zhī yào*). Nanchang: Jiangxi People's Publishing House, 1982: 13

- How is this theory applied to elaborate the pathology, clinical manifestations, differentiations and treatment approaches in six conformations in Discussion of Cold Damage?
- What do these applications mean for our daily practice, especially using differentiations and treatments discussed in Discussion of Cold Damage?

These questions are answered in the next section.

Applications of the theory of qi transformation in six conformations in Discussion of Cold Damage and their clinical significance

As mentioned above, scholars who belong to the school of qi transformation in six conformations in studying Discussion of Cold Damage have applied the theory of qi transformation in The Yellow Emperor's Inner Classic for studying the etiologies, pathologies, differentiations and treatment approaches given in this classic for more than 400 years. They have found that the theory of 本氣 *běn qì*, 標氣 *biāo qì* and 中氣 *zhōng qì* is very important for differentiations in six conformations in Discussion of Cold Damage as diseases in six conformations commonly show the dysfunction of qi transformation, though they are also related to pathological changes in zang-fu organs and channels. Below is a summary of those scholars' insightful thoughts and my own study.

Tai yang disease

The 本氣 *běn qì* for tai yang is cold qi. Its 標氣 *biāo qì* is yang that is warm in nature. Its 中氣 *zhōng qì* is heat qi from shao yin. Qi in tai yang is produced by its 中氣 *zhōng qì* acting on water in tai yang. Normally, heat qi from shao yin (heart and kidney) warms up and steams cold water in the urinary bladder, producing tai yang qi. Tai yang qi distributes and circulates in the most outer layer of the body to prevent the body from being attacked by pathological factors. The trend of the qi transformation of tai yang can move towards either 標氣 *biāo qì* (yang) or 本氣 *běn qì* (cold). It is this special physiology and qi transformation in tai yang that makes tai yang disease present with fighting between pathological factors and the defensive qi, stagnation of the defensive qi and failure of the defensive qi to warm the body surface at the very beginning. This is why Zhang Ji states "[the typical manifestations of the onset of] tai yang disease are a floating pulse, headache, ache and stiffness on the nape and aversion to cold" in the first line of tai yang disease. It is this special physiology and qi transformation in tai yang that makes tai yang disease present with cold, heat and water-accumulation syndromes when there are disorders of tai yang qi.

It is this special physiology and qi transformation in tai yang that determines the basic treatment principle for tai yang, which is to promote sweating with acrid and warm herbs, acrid, cool and/or cold herbs, and promote urination with acrid, warm and bland herbs. For example, Zhang Ji not only discussed wind-cold syndrome treated with Cinnamon Twig Decoction (*guì zhī tāng*) in line 12 and by Ephedra Decoction (*má huáng tāng*) in line 35 but also talked about many heat syndromes, like warm pathogen disease in line 6 and stagnant heat syndromes treated with Pueraria, Scutellaria, and Coptis Decoction (*gé gēn huáng qín huáng lián tāng*), Major Bluegreen Dragon Decoction (*dà qīng lóng tāng*), Ephedra, Apricot Kernel, Licorice and Gypsum Decoction (*má huáng xìng rén gān cǎo shí gāo tāng*) and Gardenia and Prepared Soybean Decoction (*zhī zǐ chǐ táng*) in lines 34, 38, 63 and 76, respectively. Moreover, several water-accumulation syndromes or phlegm due to water accumulation have been treated with Cinnamon Twig Decoction minus Cinnamon Twig plus Poria and White Atractylodes (*guì zhī qù guì jiā fú líng bái zhú tāng*) in line 28, Minor Bluegreen Dragon Decoction (*xiǎo qīng lóng tāng*) in line 40 and Five-Ingredient Powder with Poria (*wù líng sǎn*) in line 71.

Since the production of tai yang qi is very dependent on its 中氣 *zhōng qì*, heat qi from shao yin (heart and kidney), tai yang disease can easily progress to shao yin, leading to cold and deficiency syndromes in shao yin. These progressions can be seen in the treatment implemented by Cinnamon Twig and Licorice Decoction (*guì zhī gān cǎo tāng*) in line 64 for yang deficiency in the heart, Frigid Extremities Decoction (*sì nì tāng*) in lines 29 and 91, Cinnamon Twig plus Aconite Accessory Root Decoction (*guì zhī jiā fù zǐ tāng*) in line 20, Cinnamon Twig Decoction minus Peony plus Aconite Accessory Root (*guì zhī qù sháo yào jiā fù zǐ tāng*) in line 22, and Dry Ginger and Aconite Accessory Root Decoction (*gān jiāng fù zǐ tāng*) in line 61 for yang deficiency in the kidney. In line 86, there is a more severe scenario in which water accumulation can be caused by yang deficiency in the kidney, which is treated with True Warrior Decoction (*zhēn wǔ tāng*).

Of course, the treatment for tai yang, especially promotion of sweating, should be used with extreme caution in order not to damage the yang (heat qi) of shao yin, its 中氣 *zhōng qì*, leading to cold and yang deficiency in shao yin. For example, when applying Major Bluegreen Dragon Decoction (*dà qīng lóng tāng*), the strongest formula to promote sweating in tai yang disease, Zhang Ji repeatedly reminds us:

> If there are feeble and weak pulses, sweating and aversion to wind, this formula cannot be ingested. Otherwise, there will be spread of cold feeling from the hands and the feet to the limbs, jerking of tendons and twitching of muscles. These indicate the wrong treatment (line 38).
>
> If there is no shao yin syndrome. Major Bluegreen Dragon Decoction (*dà qīng lóng tāng*) should be used to promote (sweating) and disperse pathological factors (line 39).

Also, since tai yang qi is produced by heat qi from the kidney and heart to warm cold water in the urinary bladder, Zhang Ji has specially chosen Cinnamomi Ramulus (*guì zhī*), which is the chief herb to warm yang for the heart, to group with Poria (*fú líng*), Atractylodis macrocephalae Rhizoma (*bái zhú*), Polyporus (*zhū ling*) and Alismatis Rhizoma (*zé xiè*)—herbs to make Five-Ingredient Powder with Poria (*wù líng sǎn*) for treating accumulation of water in the urinary bladder.

Yang ming disease

Dryness qi, which belongs to yin, is 本氣 *běn qì* for yang ming, while its 中氣 *zhōng qì* is damp qi. If one only looks at the properties of yang ming, which are dryness qi and that it belongs to two yangs, one can easily understand why there are so many excess, heat and dryness syndromes in yang ming disease discussed by Zhang Ji in the chapter of yang ming disease. However, this is not a comprehensive view for yang ming disease in Discussion of Cold Damage, because Zhang Ji discusses cold syndromes, cold-damp syndromes and cold-damp syndromes with yang deficiency in the spleen in many lines in the chapter of yang ming disease. Moreover, unlike the first line, which only discusses the outline of a disease in other chapters, Zhang Ji mentions several presentations of yang ming disease including the syndrome of constrained spleen, which clearly proves that the spleen is an important player in yang ming disease. Why is the spleen so critical for yang ming disease? Because both dryness qi and damp qi belong to yin, and the qi transformation in yang ming tends to move towards its 中氣 *zhōng qì*, i.e. damp qi that relates to the spleen. Clearly, damp qi, its 中氣 *zhōng qì*, plays an important role in this qi transformation. If damp qi is weak and fails to balance dryness qi and two yangs in yang ming, excess heat and dryness syndromes will prevail. Chen Nian-Zu pointed out:

> 本氣 *běn qì* for yang ming is dryness qi and its 標氣 *biāo qì* is yang. If they are not balanced by damp qi in tai yin, both dryness qi and yang will be excessive, leading to excess in the stomach (and large intestine).[48]

However, if damp qi is too strong due to improper treatments or the body's constitution, the disease would progress to cold, damp and yang deficiency, which belong to tai yin disease. For example, inability to eat in lines 190, 191 and 194 indicates that damp is getting strong and there is a possibility for yang ming disease to progress to cold, damp and yang deficiency in tai yin disease. Of course, "if purging is used to eliminate heat, there will be hiccup. The reason for this consequence is there is deficiency and cold in the stomach (line 194)." In clinical condition, the syndrome of cold and damp in tai yin disease can be seen in the following case:

> After the promotion of sweating for Cold Damage, there is yellow color in the eyes and over the body. The reason is because interior cold and damp have not been resolved. Therefore, purging cannot be employed and the treatment should be focused on cold and damp (line 259).

Zhang Zhi-Cong (also known as Zhang Yin-An, 1616–1674) offered a good summary for the progression of yang ming disease based on the theory of qi transformation:

> In yang ming disease, when there is fever, thirst, dry and hard stool, these indicate that a disorder locates in the yang aspect of yang ming disease. When there is cold and deficiency in the stomach, leading to inability of separating the clear from the turbid, vomiting after eating, a slow pulse and intolerance of cold, these indicate that the disease has progressed to yin and damp, which is 中氣 *zhōng qì* of yang ming.[49]

Since there is such progression based on the theory of qi transformation in six conformations in Discussion of Cold Damage, Zhang Ji was

48 Chen Nian-Zu, op. cit., p.226

49 Liu Du-Zhou first cited this statement in his article which said that the statement comes from Zhang Zhi-Cong; however, I have not found this statement in the book Zhang Zhi-Cong wrote. See Liu Du-Zhou, "The theory of qi transformation in Discussion of Cold Damage." *New Chinese Medicine*, 1983 (2): 4

extremely careful to apply purging method for excess, dryness and heat for fu organ syndrome in yang ming disease. For example, he frequently reminds practitioners that "in yang ming disease, if there is fullness and hard feeling in the epigastric region, purging cannot be applied. If there is incessant diarrhea after purging, the patient will die (line 205)." "If there is absence of passing gas, it indicates that only the first part of the stool is hard but the rest of it is loose. If purging is applied for this condition, there will be distention and fullness in the abdomen and inability to eat (line 209)." And in the footnote for Major Order the Qi Decoction (*dà chéng qì tāng*) and Minor Order the Qi Decoction (*xiǎo chéng qì tāng*), the main purging formulas for fu organ syndrome in yang ming disease, there is a caution provided by Zhang Ji: "If there is defecation, the rest of the decoction should not be taken."

Shao yang disease

It is well know that alternating chills and fever are keys to identify shao yang disease. Interestingly, Zhang Ji did not put them in line 263, which is called the outline for shao yang disease, but wrote that "[the typical manifestations of the onset of) shao yang disease are bitter taste in the mouth, dry throat and dizziness," which has been largely ignored by contemporary practitioners in the West in their daily practice. Why did Zhang Ji attach more importance to bitter taste in the mouth, dry throat and dizziness than alternating chills and fever to identify shao yang disease in this line? To answer this question, the theory of qi transformation must be consulted. Shao yang's 本氣 *běn qì* is fire qi and its 標氣 *biāo qì* is yang. Wind qi, its 中氣 *zhōng qì*, belongs to yang. All of these three bear yang and the interaction among these three would make shao yang move towards its 本氣 *běn qì*, fire qi. In this interaction, wind qi can facilitate fire qi. It is special qi transformation in shao yang that makes yang in shao yang easily agitated, leading to the flare up of fire. As Zhang Zhi-Cong (also known as Zhang Yin-An, 1616–1674) states, "Fire qi is in charge in shao yang. Bitter taste in the mouth and dry throat are signs of the transformation of fire qi. Dizziness is caused by upper attack of heat."[50] Zhang Ji probably noticed this trend of qi transformation and chose bitter

50 Zhang Zhi-Cong. *Ancestor Stamp for Discussion of Cold Damage* (*shāng hán lùn zōng yìn*). In Zheng Lin et al. (eds) *Complete Medical Works by Zhang Zhi-Cong* (*zhāng zhì-cōng yī xué quán shū*). Beijing: China Publishing House of Traditional Chinese Medicine, 2005: 750

taste in the mouth, dry throat and dizziness, all symptoms in the upper part of the body, to demonstrate that the fire qi from shao yang has flared up quickly after severe stagnation instead of increasing gradually.

Liu Du-Zhou (1917–2003), a well-known scholar who specialized in Discussion of Cold Damage, summarized it as the following:

> Bitter taste in the mouth, dry throat and dizziness, and other heat symptoms and signs demonstrate that the qi transformation has followed fire qi, its 本氣 *běn qì*. Discomfort and fullness in the chest and hypochondriac region, and taciturnity with no desire to eat, are signs of qi stagnation of the gall bladder, and "dizziness" shows that wind qi is involved.[51]

According to Ke Qin's study, shao yang disease based on the theory of qi transformation in six conformations can move towards its 中氣 *zhōng qì*, wind qi and jue yin, rather than only towards its 本氣 *běn qì*, fire qi, because there are some similarities between shao yang and jue yin in regard to qi transformation, pathology and clinical presentations. He explains:

> Jue yin relates to the liver, while the gall bladder is attached to the inside of the liver. Therefore, heat syndromes in jue yin disease are caused by internal invasion from the disorder of ministerial fire of the gall bladder. One should be aware that both shao yang and liver are related to the ministerial fire. When the disorder of this fire invades the inside of body, it can induce jue yin disease. When it moves to the outside of the body, it can induce shao yang disease. The dry throat in shao yang disease is the prelude to excessive thirst in jue yin disease; discomfort and fullness in the chest and hypochondriac region in shao yang disease is the prelude to feeling of qi surging to the chest, pain and burning in the chest; absence of desire to eat is the root for hunger with no desire to eat; sick and discomfort in the stomach and frequent nausea is the prelude to vomiting with round worms.[52]

Concerning the treatment approaches for shao yang disease, since the 本氣 *běn qì* for shao yang is fire and its 標氣 *biāo qì* is yang, the treatment for shao yang should clear and disperse heat with acrid, bitter and cold herbs.

51 Chen Ming et al. *Liu Du-Zhou's Clinical Guidance to Apply Theories and Formulas in Discussion of Cold Damage* (*liú dù-zhōu shāng hán lín zhèng zhǐ yào*). Beijing: Learning Garden Publishing House, 1998: 223

52 Ke Qin. *Discussion of Special Topic in Surviving with Cold Damage* (*shāng hán lái sū jí, shāng hán lùn yì*). Shanghai: Shanghai Science and Technology Publishing House, 1978: 45

Tai yin disease

The 本氣 *běn qì* for tai yin is damp qi and its 標氣 *biāo qì* is yin. Tai yin and its 本氣 *běn qì*, damp qi, share the same energy, yin, which are compatible with each other. Also, damp qi produces tai yin, therefore tai yin tends to move towards yin, especially its 本氣 *běn qì*, damp qi. It is this special qi transformation that makes tai yin disease present with cold-damp when it is attacked by pathological factors, which is described by the outline of tai yin disease as follows: "[The typical manifestation of the onset of] tai yin disease is fullness in the abdomen and vomiting, poor appetite, progressive severe diarrhea and abdominal pain at times" (line 273). This is probably why the pathologies discussed in all eight lines in tai yin disease are most related to cold-damp or cold-damp with yang deficiency. However, Zhang Ji recorded that there is a chance for the disease to progress from tai yin to yang ming, the organ that bears dryness qi (中氣 *zhōng qì* for tai yin). For example, in line 278, Zhang Ji wrote:

> On day seven or eight after suffering from the [tai yin] disease, the diarrhea must automatically stop despite there having been sudden vexation and diarrhea more than ten times a day, because the yang of the spleen recovers and putrid and turbid things have been eliminated by bowel movement.

Since there is cold-damp, which is a group of two yin pathological factors, Zhang Ji set up the following treatment principle, which implies that acrid, sweet and hot herbs must be used, in line 277: "If there is automatically diarrhea without thirst, it belongs to tai yin disease since there is cold in this organ. One should warm the organ and the family of Frigid Extremities Decoction (*sì nì tāng*) is appropriate."

Shao yin disease

Similar to the qi transformation of tai yang, the qi transformation in shao yin tends to move towards either 標氣 *biāo qì* (yin) or 本氣 *běn qì* (heat qi), because the tendency of the movement between them depends much on the results from the interaction between yin and heat qi in shao yin with the mediation of 中氣 *zhōng qì*, tai yang (cold qi). With cold qi from tai yang, yin in shao yin overcomes heat qi, and the transformation will move towards cold qi; otherwise, the transformation will move towards heat qi. It is this special qi transformation that makes shao yin disease present with either cold syndromes or heat syndromes, which follow either its

標氣 *biāo qì* or its 本氣 *běn qì* to cause disease when there are disorders in shao yin. For example, the cold and yang deficiency syndromes can be seen in the following lines: "in shao yin disease, when there is general pain, cold hands and feet, pain in joints and a deep pulse, Aconite Accessory Root Decoction (*fù zǐ tāng*) should be prescribed (line 305)" and "in shao yin disease, when there is a deep pulse, warm method should be applied immediately, Frigid Extremities Decoction (*sì nì tāng*) might be used (line 323)." Moreover, heat syndromes can be seen in lines 303, 310–312. In line 303, Zhang Ji writes that "after suffering from shao yin disease for more than two or three days, there is vexation in the heart and inability to fall asleep. Coptis and Ass-Hide Gelatin Decoction (*huáng lián ē jiāo tāng*) should be prescribed."

Like tai yin disease, the role the 中氣 *zhōng qì*, tai yang, play in the progression of shao yin disease is also recorded by Zhang Ji in the chapter on shao yin disease, as there are a few lines which discuss when shao yin disease has regressed from shao yin to tai yang, especially the urinary bladder. For example, the cold and yang deficiency in the kidney can affect the function of the urinary bladder, leading to dysuria and/or pain in the lower abdomen, which is described in lines 282 and 316, respectively. Moreover, the heat syndrome can also transmitted to the urinary bladder, as stated in line 293: "In shao yin disease, when there is feverish feeling in the whole body, hands and feet on the eighth or ninth days, this indicates that there is heat in the urinary bladder. There must be blood in the urine." Of course, one can see from the discussion above that the treatment for shao yin disease should warm and tonify yang, or nourish yin and clear deficient heat accordingly.

Jue yin disease

Like the qi transformation in yang ming, the qi transformation in jue yin moves towards its 中氣 *zhōng qì*, fire qi, because among wind qi (本氣 *běn qì*), jue yin (標氣 *biāo qì*) and fire (中氣 *zhōng qì*), there are two yangs and one yin, which make their movement towards yang. Wind qi and its 中氣 *zhōng qì*, shao yang, has mother-son relationship (wood can produce fire according to mutual production relationship in the theory of five elements) and share the same energy, i.e. yang. It is this special qi transformation in jue yin that causes so many heat syndromes in jue yin disease. However, one might notice that there are cold syndromes, heat syndromes and a combination of heat and cold syndromes recorded in the chapter on jue yin disease in Discussion of Cold Damage. But why did Zhang Ji only choose heat syndrome as the outline for jue yin syndrome such as excessive thirst, feeling of qi surging to the chest, pain and burning in the chest and hunger with no desire to eat in line 326, though there are cold syndromes, heat syndromes and a combination of heat and cold syndromes in jue yin disease? Based on his study for qi transformation in six conformations, Zhang Zhi-Cong (also known as Zhang Yin-An, 1616–1674) offered a good answer:

> [The typical manifestation of the onset of] jue yin disease is excessive thirst, feeling of qi surging to the chest, pain and burning in the chest. This indicates that the disease has turned into fire due to the theory that jue yin moves towards its 中氣 *zhōng qì*, fire qi.[53]

Based on the discussion above, one might deduce that there is a principle for qi transformation in six qi and that Discussion of Cold Damage does prove that there are presentation and progression for three yin and three yang diseases in six conformations according to this principle. Knowing this would have great benefit for our differentiation and treatment. The Yellow Emperor's Inner Classic sums up this clinical significance as follows:

> Among hundreds of diseases, the presentation can start at the disorder of 本氣 *běn qì*, the disorder of 標氣 *biāo qì* and the disorder of 中氣 *zhōng qì*. Therefore, one can get good results from treating 本氣 *běn qì*, 標氣 *biāo qì* and 中氣 *zhōng qì*, respectively, or 本氣 *běn qì* and 標氣 *biāo qì* simultaneously… Therefore, it is said that "knowing the theory of 本氣 *běn qì* and 標氣 *biāo qì*, one would not fail in one's clinical practice."[54]

Zheng Shou-Quan (also known as Zheng Qin-An, 1824–1911), an ancestor for the school of supporting yang who lived in Sichuan, further pointed out:

> In six conformations, each conformation has its own 標氣 *biāo qì*, 本氣 *běn qì* and 中氣 *zhōng qì*. When pathological factors invade the body, there are possibilities to present syndromes following 中氣 *zhōng qì*; syndromes following 標氣 *biāo qì* rather than 中氣 *zhōng qì*; syndromes following 本氣 *běn qì*. Therefore, 標氣 *biāo qì* would be involved at the beginning when pathological factors invade a conformation, but it can

53 Zhang Zhi-Cong, op. cit., p.749

54 Wang Bing, op. cit., p.533

> affect 中氣 *zhōng qì* shortly. If practitioners do not study the theory of qi transformation, they will not know how a syndrome starts and where it goes.[55]

However, since there is deficiency or excess in terms of yin and yang among zang-fu organs and variety in regard to pathological factors, the presentation and/or progression of disease in six conformations might fail to follow this principle discussed in the theory of qi transformation. Zhang Ji noticed these exceptions and recorded that each disease might present or progress differently rather than only according to its 本氣 *běn qì*, 標氣 *biāo qì* and 中氣 *zhōng qì*. The exceptional presentation or progression does not mean that there is no necessity to learn the principle for qi transformation for differentiations and treatment approaches for diseases in six conformations. According to Zhang Deng-Ben and Sun Li-Jun, applying the principle of qi transformation in six conformations bears the following three clinical significances:[56]

1. It highlights common syndromes, such as more damp syndromes, than other syndromes in tai yin disease due to its 本氣 *běn qì* being dampness qi and 標氣 *biāo qì* being yin in tai yin; more heat syndromes than other syndromes in shao yang disease due to its 本氣 *běn qì* being fire qi and 標氣 *biāo qì* being yang in shao yang.

2. It stresses the complications of disease. For example, there are heat syndromes and cold syndromes in shao yin disease. There are exterior cold syndromes and occurrence of exterior and interior cold syndromes in tai yang disease because tai yang can move towards its 本氣 *běn qì*, cold qi, leading to the syndrome treated by Ephedra, Asarum, and Aconite Accessory Root Decoction (*má huáng xì xīn fù zǐ tāng*). There is the combination of heat and cold syndrome as tai yang moves towards both 標氣 *biāo qì* and 本氣 *běn qì*, leading to the syndrome treated by Major Bluegreen Dragon Decoction (*dà qīng lóng tāng*).

3. It highlights the syndrome that has been ignored by practitioners. For example, heat syndromes are commonly seen in yang ming

55 Zheng Shou-Quan and Tang Bu-Qi. *Explanation for Works of Zheng Qin-An* (*zhèng qīn-ān yī shū chán shì*). Chengdu: Sichuan Publishing House, 1996: 66

56 Zhang Deng-Ben and Sun Li-Jun. "Applications of the theory of biao, ben and zhong qi in differentiation and treatment for diseases in six conformations in Discussion of Cold Damage." *Journal of Shanxi College of Traditional Chinese Medicine*, 2002 (9): 1

disease, but if the qi transformation moves towards its 中氣 *zhōng qì*, there will be cold and damp syndromes.

Besides the content of qi transformation discussed in the previous paragraphs, some scholars who specialized in Discussion of Cold Damage strongly believed that the theory of opening, closing and pivot could also be applied to study and practice for diseases in six conformations of Discussion of Cold Damage. They put forward that the theory of opening, closing and pivot is part of the theory of qi transformation in six conformations, though it might not be related to the theory of qi transformation in The Yellow Emperor's Inner Classic. Deng Shao-Xian (also known as Deng Xu-Cheng, 1898–1971), a well-known specialist in studying Discussion of Cold Damage from Chengdu University of Traditional Chinese Medicine and a chief writer for the second edition of the national textbook for Discussion of Cold Damage, offered very valuable thoughts for studying Discussion of Cold Damage in this regard. Unfortunately, his thoughts have not been published but have been recorded by Prof. Chen Zhi-He, another well-known scholar in studying Discussion of Cold Damage, in his class notes from his apprentice study. I was very fortunate to have read and made a copy of these class notes in 1981 called "Mr. Deng Shao-Xian Discusses Some Issues to Learn Discussion of Cold Damage." The following paragraph is related to the theory of opening, closing and pivot recorded in these class notes:

> Master Deng points out that "what is called the opening, closing and pivot is to summarize the different function and relationship among three yin and three yang." Chapter 6 of Basic Questions in The Yellow Emperor's Inner Classic states that "tai yang is supposed to open, yang ming to close, while shao yang serves as a pivot. Tai yin is supposed to open, jue yin to close, while shao yin serves as a pivot." Wang Bing (also known as Qi Xuan-Zi, 710–804) explains as follows: "The opening, closing and pivot is related to the different quantity and functions among three yang (the three yin have the same thing). The opening refers to the beginning of qi movement, closing refers to the power to control, and the pivot is in charge of turning of qi elegantly."[57]
>
> In the normal condition of the human body, three yang tend to move out while three yin tend to move in. However, because qi in three yin and three yang are different in terms of quantity and function, the author of The Yellow Emperor's Inner Classic used the opening, closing and

57 Wang Bing, op. cit., p.50

pivot to summarize these different functions. In fact, opening refers to outward qi movement, closing refers to the inward qi movement and the pivot controls the key for opening and closing. They cooperate with each other and form a whole system. For example, qi of tai yang circulates on the body surface and defends it, while qi of tai yin is supposed to be transported and distributed by the spleen and lung, respectively. Both tai yang and tai yin are in charge of outward qi movement on the body surface and inside of the body, respectively; therefore, their functions falls into the category of opening.

Yang ming is supposed to ripen food and transform it into qi and blood, which enter the channels. While jue yin is supposed to store blood, it looks like fire in wind, which is contained and not bright and hot. Both yang ming and jue yin are in charge of inward qi movement and their function falls into the category of closing.

Shao yang governs ministerial fire, which circulates in the three burners, and locates in the half exterior and half interior. Shao yin governs water and fire, and they are the places where true yin and true yang are stored. The fire from shao yin can warm tai yin and its water can nourish wood. It locates between tai yin and jue yin and makes qi circulate constantly between tai yin and jue yin. Therefore, the functions of shao yang and shao yin fall into the category of the pivot.

When there is invasion of pathological factors, tai yang will be the first one to be attacked which commonly leads to the dysfunction of opening for tai yang. If tai yang opens too much, excessive sweating will be produced; if tai yang fails to open, there will be absence of sweating. Therefore, Cinnamon Twig Decoction (*guì zhī tāng*) and Ephedra Decoction (*má huáng tāng*) are two basic formulas to treat cold syndromes in tai yang disease. Other formulas like Half Cinnamon Twig and Half Ephedra Decoction (*guì zhī má huáng gè bàn tāng*), Two-Parts Cinnamon Twig Decoction with One-Part Ephedra Decoction (*guì zhī èr má huáng yī tāng*), Cinnamon Twig Decoction plus Pueraria (*guì zhī jiā gé gēn tāng*) and Pueraria Decoction (*gé gēn tāng*) are just modifications for these two formulas according to the severity of the syndromes and associated conditions. If tai yang fails to open and the disease progresses to the inside of the body, transmuted syndromes like chest-binding syndrome, pi syndromes, water-accumulation syndrome and blood-amassment syndrome will present depending on the body's constitution and where the disease progresses. Therefore, at the early stage in Cold Damage, proper management of Cinnamon Twig Decoction (*guì zhī tāng*) and Ephedra Decoction (*má huáng tāng*) bears important clinical significance, which can cure disease when it locates in tai yang or reduce the possibility for the disease to progress to the inside of the body.

If yang ming fails to close, there will be abdominal fullness, constipation, vomiting or diarrhea. The treatment principle is no more than recovering its closing function by use of Order the Qi Decoction (*chéng qì tāng*),[58] Gardenia and Prepared Soybean Decoction (*zhī zǐ chǐ táng*), White Tiger Decoction (*bái hǔ tāng*) and Pueraria Decoction (*gé gēn tāng*).

Dysfunction of the pivot of shao yang can present with alternating chills and fever, discomfort and fullness in the chest and hypochondriac region, taciturnity with no desire to eat, sick and discomforting feeling in the stomach and frequent nausea with the following possible symptoms and signs: vexation in the chest and other possible symptoms and signs. The application of Minor Bupleurum Decoction (*xiǎo chái hú tāng*) is just to recover its pivot function.

If tai yin fails to process food by the spleen and distribute it to the lung, there will be sinking of clear qi and rebellion of turbid qi, leading to abdominal fullness, vomiting, diarrhea and so on. A formula like Frigid Extremities Decoction (*sì nì tāng*) should be prescribed for recovery of the opening function of tai yin. When there is dysfunction of shao yin, there will be deficiency of fire and water, leading to thin and feeble pulses and the desire to sleep. The progression of the disease can move to either cold or heat conditions based on cold qi and fire qi transformation. Frigid Extremities Decoction (*sì nì tāng*) is recommended for recovering yang for the former condition, while Coptis and Ass-Hide Gelatin Decoction (*huáng lián ē jiāo tāng*) is used to nourish yin and clear heat for the latter condition. Both approaches are no more than recovering the function of fire and water.

Jue yin is on the edge of the end of yin but the restarting of yang and contains fire in wood. If it fails to close, ministerial fire will not be contained, leading to the combination of heat and cold syndromes. Its progression is very dependent on the body's constitution. If the patient has a relatively yang body constitution, the disease will transform into heat syndromes; if the patient has a relatively yin body constitution, the disease will transform into cold syndromes. Since it has complicated presentations in the regard of pathology, its treatment varies accordingly. This is why it said that eight treatment approaches can be applied for jue yin disease. However, the approach that combines both cold and warm herbs is commonly used for jue yin disease.

The paragraphs above simply list examples for the application of the theory of opening, closing and pivot. Besides these examples, one must

58 This refers to the family of Order the Qi Decoction (*chéng qì tāng*) such as Major Order the Qi Decoction (*dà chéng qì tāng*) and Minor Order the Qi Decoction (*xiǎo chéng qì tāng*).

> pay attention to the relationship between opening, closing and pivot. They can affect each other when there is a disease. For example, failure of tai yang to open can affect the closing function of yang ming, and vice versa. Therefore, there is the approach of treating dysfunction of opening in tai yang for the closing function in yang ming. Moreover, the function of opening in tai yang and closing in yang ming is relevant to the function of pivot in shao yang. For example, the reason to discuss Minor Bupleurum Decoction (*xiǎo chái hú tāng*) in the chapter on tai yang disease is that it tends to recover the normal function of tai yang and eliminate pathological factors by working on the pivot function of shao yang. Also, the approach to treat shao yang for the combination of three yang diseases has the same meaning. The relationship among three yin share the same relationship in terms of opening, closing and pivot, and the approaches used in three yang can be applied for the disorders in three yin. Furthermore, one should notice that opening, closing and pivot function between three yin and three yang affect each other. For example, the opening function of tai yang relies on the opening function of tai yin, and the closing function of yang ming depends on the closing function of jue yin. The pivot function of shao yang relates to the pivot function of shao yin. All of these facts are no more than demonstrations that the human body should be viewed as a whole. The relationship between three yin and three yang are that they support each other physiologically and affect each other pathologically. Therefore, understanding these relationships comprehensively will benefit our clinical practice.[59]

Overall, the theory of opening, closing and pivot can be used to elaborate the pathologies and presentations in diseases in six conformations, elucidate the progressions for diseases in six conformations and guide the treatment for diseases in six conformations. The school of qi transformation in studying Discussion of Cold Damage consists of two parts: the theory of 本氣 *běn qì*, 標氣 *biāo qì* and 中氣 *zhōng qì* in six conformations and theory of opening, closing and pivot in six conformations. It is one of the important schools to study Discussion of Cold Damage. Unfortunately, it has been largely ignored by contemporary scholars and practitioners, especially scholars in the West, for quite a long period of time. This school began in the twelfth century and flourished from the seventeen to the nineteen century. Scholars and practitioners in those centuries applied the theory of 本氣 *běn qì*, 標氣 *biāo qì* and 中氣 *zhōng qì* and the theory of opening, closing and pivot for exploring the principle of differentiation

59 Chen Zhi-Heng and Deng Shao-Xian, personal communication, 1981

and treatments for diseases in six conformations in Discussion of Cold Damage based on the principle that the human body corresponds to nature. They strongly believed that diseases in six conformations are the disorders in six qi. The greatest achievement made by the school of qi transformation is that it has highlighted the importance of the qi transformation in six conformations in the studying of Discussion of Cold Damage based on the theories of zang-fu organs and channels. It has offered a quite insightful approach to study Discussion of Cold Damage, especially for resolving some difficult issues in studying this classic and applying its treatment approaches clinically, approaches which have gradually been understood and valued by more contemporary scholars and practitioners. Naturally, studying six conformations in Discussion of Cold Damage is indispensable, though, of course, none of the theories are perfect. We have to admit that some pathologies, progressions and clinical manifestations cannot be completely explained by the theories of this school. However, it is this imperfect explanation that drives us to continually improve the theories of this school based on our study and clinical practice of these theories.

7

HALF EXTERIOR AND HALF INTERIOR, HARMONY AND SHAO YANG

Everyone who studies Chinese medicine must be familiar with the term "half exterior and half interior (半表半裡 *bàn biǎo bàn lǐ*)," as it must be discussed in Eight Diagnostic Parameters in basic theory, though he or she may not have studied Discussion of Cold Damage. This term was never popular until Discussion of Cold Damage was published and research related to this classic was carried out. As a matter of fact, the term "half exterior and half interior" was not originally recorded in Discussion of Cold Damage. However, a similar term, "half in the interior and half in the exterior (半在裡半在外 *bàn zài lǐ bàn zài wài*)," can be found in line 148 of the book. What does "half in the interior and half in the exterior" mean in this line? Zhang Ji points out that "there must be interior symptoms and signs as well as exterior symptoms and signs." What kind of treatment approach would be appropriate for the condition of "half in the interior and half in the exterior? He states that "Minor Bupleurum Decoction (*xiǎo chái hú tāng*) can be prescribed to treat this condition."

Cheng Wu-Ji (1063–1156), the first scholar to offer commentary on Discussion of Cold Damage, first introduced the term "half exterior and half interior (半表半裡 *bàn biǎo bàn lǐ*)" for study of this classic. In his book, Annotating and Explaining Discussion of Cold Damage (註解傷寒論 *zhù jiě shāng hán lùn*) published in 1144, he makes the following comment about the treatment for the condition in line 148: "Minor Bupleurum Decoction (*xiǎo chái hú tāng*) might be prescribed to eliminate pathological factors located in half exterior and half interior."[1] Based on information given by Zhang Ji and commentary made by Cheng Wu-Ji, Minor Bupleurum Decoction (*xiǎo chái hú tāng*) can fulfill the goal

1 Cheng Wu-Ji. *Annotating and Explaining Discussion of Cold Damage* (*zhù jiě shāng hán lùn*). Beijing: People's Health Publishing House, 1978: 151

of dealing with this half exterior and half interior condition. But how this formula deals with both "interior symptoms and signs as well as exterior symptoms and signs" simultaneously, and why Zhang Ji does not choose herbs to release the exterior to treat tai yang and clear the interior to treat this condition rather than recommend Minor Bupleurum Decoction (*xiǎo chái hú tāng*), must be two big questions in the reader's mind. In order to answer these questions, several important concepts related to this formula must be carefully studied.

The first one is the concept of harmony, and harmonization (和法 *hé fǎ*), the treatment approach that stems from the concept of harmony. "Harmony" is one of the common translations for the Chinese character "和 *hé*," which is a very popular and indispensable philosophical and cultural concept in Chinese history. It is also a very important concept practiced in Chinese medicine and in regular life in China for several thousand years. One might remember that at the opening ceremony of the 2008 Olympic Games held in the Beijing more than 3000 dancers used small wooden boxes to form the Chinese character "和 *hé*." If you pay a visit to the Forbidden City in Beijing, one of the largest halls you cannot miss is called "Great Harmony Hall (太和殿 *tài hé diàn*). This hall was used to hold a grand ceremony for an emperor to ascend the throne and was also used for an emperor to accept greetings from his ministers. Interestingly, two large halls behind Great Harmony Hall which are used to practice rites and hold important state banquets also use the character "和 *hé*" in their names, i.e. "Neutral Harmony Hall (中和殿 *zhōng hé diàn*) and "Protect Harmony Hall (保和殿 *bǎo hé diàn*)." In fact, not only emperors and royal family but also ordinary people in China attach great importance to harmony in their daily life. It is said that "if you have harmony in a family, everything will prosper (家和萬事興 *jiā hé wàn shì xīng*)." Being one of the important treatment approaches that stems from the concept of harmony (和 *hé*) and brings the body back into a harmonious condition, harmonization has been a hot topic in studying Discussion of Cold Damage, especially in studying shao yang disease. In order to fully comprehend the concept of harmony and harmonization, and the method based on the concept of harmony, one has to answer the following questions first:

- What does the character "和 *hé*" mean in Chinese culture and philosophy?

- Why is the concept of this character so popular that it is indispensable in Chinese daily life?

As early as 1100 BC, this character was one of more than 4500 characters carved on the scapular of a cow or the bone of a turtle, and these characters were called "inscription on bone" or "oracle bone" (甲骨文 *jià gŭ wén*). The meaning of the character "和 *hé*" has been encoded in the original inscription on the bone.

In his book, 500 Cases for Changes to Chinese Characters (漢字演變五百例 *hàn zì yán biàn wŭ băi lì*) published in 2002, Li Le-Yi points out that the character "和 *hé*" on the oracle bone is depicted by a pictograph of an ancient musical instrument (Figure 7.1), which is called "龠 *yuè*." It comprises several bamboo pipes that are played by the mouth. The mouth blows in this instrument and makes a harmonious chord.[2]

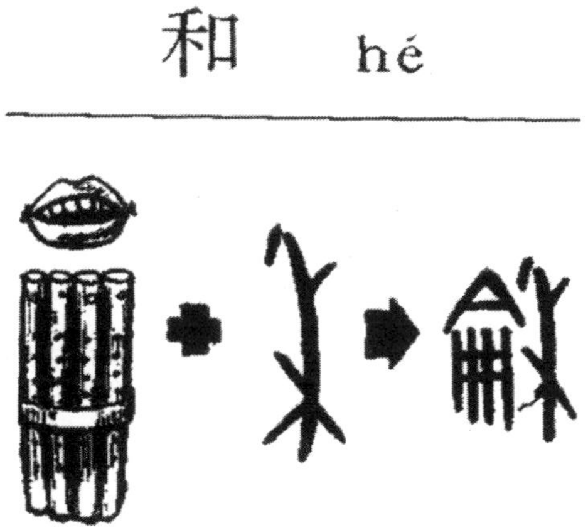

FIGURE 7.1 THE CHARACTER "和 *HÉ*" ON THE ORACLE BONE

According to Xu Shen (also known as Xu Shu-Zhong, c. 100 AD) in his book, Explanation for Chinese Characters (說文解字 *shuō wén jiĕ zì*) published in 122 AD, which was the first book that discussed the four methods for ancient Chinese characters to be created, the method to create this character was called phonetic complex (形聲字 *xíng shēng zì*) in ancient China,[3] i.e. the left part of the character gives the picture that

2 Li Le-Yi. *Five Hundred Cases for Changes to Chinese Characters* (revised edition) (*hàn zì yán biàn wŭ băi lì*). Beijing: Publishing House of Beijing Language University, 2002: 129

3 Xu Shen. *Explanation for Chinese Characters* (*shuō wén jiĕ zì*). Beijing: Chinese Publishing House, 1963: 314

shows what a thing looks like and encodes some meaning, while the right part of the character gives the sound of the character and how to pronounce it. Apparently, the picture of the character "和 *hé*" demonstrates how to blow different notes and make harmonious chords. Therefore, it is reasonable to assume that this character originally carried the meaning of combining different things and making them balanced. Interestingly, one of the meanings of "harmony" is "notes of music combined in writing in a pleasant-sounding way."[4]

Historically, many well-known ancient philosophers and writers have paid great attention to this meaning and offered many famous statements that have exerted great influence on our thinking. Zuo Qiu-Ming (c. 422 BC), a well-known writer, offered an exceptional statement to explain why harmony (和 *hé*) is so important for our life by citing some natural phenomena in his book, Brief Historical Stories for States (國語 *guó yŭ*). He wrote:

> Harmony, which combines different things and makes them balanced, indeed creates things, while identification, which simply adds or heaps things, gets what is the same as the original one in terms of quality. Therefore, kings of the past combined earth with metal, wood, water and fire to generate hundreds of things, and mixed sour, bitter, sweet, pungent and salty flavors to make delicious food, and combined different notes to make a masterpiece of music…If sound has the same tone, it is not attractive to the ears. If colors are the same, one cannot create a beautiful painting.[5]

In Chapter 42 of his book, Morals Classic (道德經 *dào dé jīng*), published at the end of the Spring and Autumn period, Lao Zi (also known as Li Er or Li Dan, c. 471 BC) first applied the principle of harmony (和 *hé*) to explain the relationship between yin and yang. He writes: "The Dao begot the one, the one begot two, two begot three and three begot the myriad things. The myriad things bear yin and embrace yang. Yin and yang mingle and endorse each other for achieving harmony."[6]

---

4 Paul Procter et al. *Longman Dictionary of Contemporary English*. London: Pitman Press, 1978: 517

5 Wang Ji-Min et al. *Translation and Comments for Brief Historical Stories of States* (*guó yŭ yì zhù*). Guangzhou: Hundreds Flower Island Literature and Arts Publishing House, 1992: 329

6 Sha Shao-Hai and Xu Hong. *Complete Explanation for Lao Zi* (*lăo zĭ quán yì*). Guiyang: Guizhou People's Publishing House, 1989: 87

In his book, Analects of Confucius (論語 *lùn yǔ*), published in the early Warring States period,[7] and in the Book of Rites (禮記 *lǐ jì*), written and published by a later follower of his, Confucius (also known as Kong Zi or Kong Qiu, 551–479 BC) concluded that "harmony (和 *hé*) is a basic principle for everything in nature,"[8] and "in the application of rites, harmony is most important."[9] Because the doctrines of Daoism and Confucianism have had a tremendous influence on Chinese philosophy and culture, the concept of harmony, which blends different things and makes them balanced, has become an indispensable concept that is practiced in Chinese daily life.

Of course, harmonization (和法 *hé fǎ*) stems from the concept of harmony (和 *hé*) and is one of the most common treatment approaches one comes across when reading ancient medical literature and practicing medicine every day. It includes harmonizing or adjusting the relationship between the nutritive qi and the defensive qi, between the liver and spleen, harmonizing shao yang and so on. Historically, the character "和 *hé*" was first recorded in Fifty-two Diseases and Their Formulas (五十二病方 *wǔ shí èr bìng fāng*), which was published later in the Warring States period[10] and before The Yellow Emperor's Inner Classic (黃帝內經 *huáng dì nèi jīng*).[11] In this book, the character "和 *hé*" appears 22 times, among which 20 times it means "mix with" in preparing medicine, one time it means "suitable" and one time it means "divide" in administering medicine.

Around 190 BC, scholars and practitioners first used the character "和 *hé*" to describe pathologies and treatment approaches, the contexts of which call for the character to be translated as "appropriate" and "balance." These applications were found on the bamboo slips dug out

---

7 The Warring States period started in 476 BC and ended in 221 BC.

8 Yang Tian-Yu. *Comments and Explanation for Book of Rites* (*lǐ jí yì zhù*). Shanghai: Shanghai Ancient Literature Publishing House, 2004: 691

9 Xu Zhi-Gang. *Complete Explanation for the Analects of Confucius* (*lùn yǔ tōng shì*). Beijing: People Literatures Publishing House, 1997: 6

10 Zhang Zheng-Yao and Xin Bo. "Textual research for the publishing time of 'Fifty-two Diseases and Their Formulas Written on Silk'." *Journal of History for Cultural Relics*, 2007 (6): 9

11 Ma Ji-Xing and Li Xue-Qin. *Fifty-two Diseases and Their Formulas in Books Written on Silk from Tombs in Han Dynasty at Ma Wang Dui* (*má wáng duī hàn mù bó shū, wǔ shí èr bìng fāng*). In *The Panel to Recover Books Written on Silk from Tombs in Han Dynasty at Ma Wang Dui*. Beijing: Publishing House of Cultural Relics, 1979: 179 (These are the earliest formulas discovered in China thus far.)

from tombs from the early Western Han Dynasty (206 BC to 24 AD). The slips state:

> The reason for wealthy people to suffer from disease is lack of appropriate joy and anger. Joy indicates excess of yang qi; anger indicates excess of yin qi. Therefore, in order to balance these emotions, the person who knows how to preserve health quickly exhales hot qi when there is joy and quickly exhales cold qi when there is anger.[12]

Later, there were wider applications of the character "和 *hé*" in The Yellow Emperor's Inner Classic (黃帝內經 *huáng dì nèi jīng*) and Difficult Questions (難經 *nàn jīng*), two classics that Zhang Ji mentioned in his preface as the reference books for his writing Discussion of Cold Damage. In Difficult Questions, the character "和 *hé*" appears nine times, which is used to describe the physiology and pathology of organs, orifices and pulses. However, the usage of this character flourishes in The Yellow Emperor's Inner Classic, since this character appears as many as 121 times in the book and is widely used to describe the following seven aspects: balance in nature, preserving health, physiology, pathology, treatment (in which twice it is related to reaction after treatment, five times it is related to normalization after treatment) and the rest of the time it is related to the detailed approaches for the preparation and administration of medicine (see Table 7.1 for further details). The meaning of the character "和 *hé*" has been largely expanded—it is not only limited to "mix with," "suitable" and "divided" in Fifty-two Formulas (五十二病方 *wǔ shí èr bìng fāng*) but also applies its original meaning, "harmony," in Chinese medicine and introduces other meanings like "exchange (intercourse)," "adjust," "balance," "moderate," "modest," "adapt," and "response."

Since Zhang Ji mentions in the preface of his book that he consulted The Yellow Emperor's Inner Classic when writing Discussion of Cold Damage, two questions might be raised:

- Does Zhang Ji use the character "和 *hé*"?
- How did The Yellow Emperor's Inner Classic influence his usage if Zhang Ji indeed used this character?

12 Gao Da-Lun. *Study on Qi Cultivation: Book on Bamboo Slips Dug from Tombs in Han Dynasty at Zhang Jia Mountain* (*zhāng jiā shān hàn jiǎn yǐn shū yán jiū*). Chengdu: Bashu Publishing House, 1995: 170

Table 7.1 Summary of usage for the character "和 *hé*" in The Yellow Emperor's Inner Classic

Usage	Balance in nature	Preserving health	Physiology	Pathology	Treatment			Preparation of medicine	Administration of medicine
Presentation frequency	13	7	41	10	48			1	1
					Reaction to treatment	Condition back to normal after treatment	Treatment approaches		
					2	5	41		

According my calculations, there are a total of 40 times in 31 lines that Zhang Ji uses this character in Discussion of Cold Damage. The usage of this character can be classified into the following seven categories:

1. It refers to physiology and can be translated into "harmony" or "harmonious" as in "the nutritive qi is in harmony" and "the nutritive qi is harmonious" in line 53, and "if there is harmony in the stomach" in line 265.
2. It is used to describe pathology such as "the defensive qi is not in harmony with the nutritive qi" in line 53 or "the defensive qi is not harmonious" in line 54. Other lines that demonstrate such application of this character are lines 29, 152, 157, 265 and 304.
3. It is used to describe clinical manifestations and means abnormality, and the translation can vary depending on the clinical manifestations to which it relates. For example, "the pulses are harmonious" appears twice in line 105. Other lines that demonstrate such application of this character are lines 252 and 304.
4. It is used to describe that the physical condition has returned to normal after treatment, and this character can be translated into "harmony" or "normal" such as "The recovery will be achieved with harmony between the defensive qi and the nutritive qi from

further promotion of sweating" in line 53 and "If yin and yang can harmonize spontaneously, there will be automatic recovery" in line 58. Other lines that demonstrate such application of this character are lines 49, 93, 131, 211 and 230.

5. It is used to describe treatment approaches and can be translated into "harmonize" but can imply "purging" or "moistening" as in "One should harmonize the stomach, Regulate the Stomach and Order the Qi Decoction (*tiáo wèi chéng qì tāng*) might be prescribed" in line 70, and "A small amount of water might be given to harmonize qi in the stomach and to ensure the recovery of the disease" in line 71 and "Cinnamon Twig Decoction (*guì zhī tāng*) is appropriate to slightly adjust or harmonize the defensive qi and nutritive qi" in line 387. Other lines that demonstrate such application of this character are lines 208, 209, 250 and 251.

6. It refers to the method of preparing formulas and can be translated into "mix with" as in "Grind Natrii Sulfas (*máng xiāo*) and Armeniacae Semen Amarum (*xìng rén*), make it look like fat and then mix them with the powder of Rhei Radix et Rhizoma (*dà huáng*) and Lepidii/Descurainiae Semen (*tíng lì zǐ*)" in line 131. Other lines that demonstrate such application of this character are lines 166, 247, 315, 338, 352 and 386.

7. It refers to the method of administering a formula and can be translated into "mix into" or "mix with" as in "Grind the five ingredients above into powder and mix 6–9 grams of powder with rice soup" in line 71 and "Grind the ingredients into powder and mix 6–9 grams of powder with boiling water and take it" in line 141A. Other lines that demonstrate such application of this character are lines 141B, 313, 318 and 395.

Based on the study above, Zhang Ji adapted five applications of the character "和 *hé*" from The Yellow Emperor's Inner Classic when writing Discussion of Cold Damage, applications which use this character for physiology, pathology, treatment, preparation of medicine and administration of medicine. According to his preface, Discussion of Cold Damage was written originally to deal with diseases, and Zhang Ji did not use the character "和 *hé*" to describe balance in nature and preservation of health. It is for this reason that Zhang Ji first used this character to describe clinical manifestations. From this analysis, one can see that Zhang Ji did take The Yellow Emperor's Inner Classic as a reference when writing his book. However, his mind was not constricted by this classic. He not only adapted the thinking and ideas from The Yellow Emperor's Inner Classic but also developed them.

Concerning treatment, there are a total of six times that Zhang Ji used the character "和 *hé*" to discuss treatment methods. Interestingly, none of them are recorded to be relevant to shao yang diseases or harmonizing shao yang among these six applications of this character. Rather, they can be classified into two categories:

1. It implies purging in lines 70, 208, 209, 250 and 251 since purging formulas such as Regulate the Stomach and Order the Qi Decoction (*tiáo wèi chéng qì tāng*) and Minor Order the Qi Decoction (*xiǎo chéng qì tāng*) are employed to implement this treatment approach, respectively, and the character "和 *hé*" alludes to "purging."

2. It refers to moistening in line 71 since the method to implement this approach is that "a small amount of water might be given to harmonize qi in the stomach and to ensure the recovery of the disease."

Besides these two applications of the character "和 *hé*," lines 53 and 387 might imply the meaning of harmonizing the nutritive qi and defensive qi, because the formula to carry out this treatment method is Cinnamon Twig Decoction (*guì zhī tāng*). Naturally, questions arise such as the following:

1. When was harmonization as a treatment approach first introduced for shao yang disease in the history of studying and applying theory from Discussion of Cold Damage?

2. Who was the first person to apply harmonization?

3. Why should harmonization be applied in shao yang?

Cheng Wu-Ji (1063–1156), the first scholar to offer commentary on Discussion of Cold Damage, first adapted the concept of harmonization and then connected this concept to shao yang disease and Minor Bupleurum Decoction (*xiǎo chái hú tāng*) when he commented on line 266, which is in the chapter on shao yang disease. In his book, Annotating and Explaining Cold Damage (註解傷寒論 *zhù jiě shāng hán lùn*) published in 1144, he wrote:

> The disease has progressed from tai yang to shao yang, which indicates that pathological factors have entered inside the body. When there are hard feeling and fullness in the hypochondriac region, dry heave and inability to eat, alternating chills and fever, they indicate that pathological factors exist in half exterior and half interior. The deep and tight pulses would indicate interior excess in fu organs due to progression of pathological factors if vomiting and purging methods have been applied. If not, the pathological factors have not entered fu organs and the exterior condition has not been resolved yet, though the deep and tight pulses indicate they are progressing to the interior. Minor Bupleurum Decoction (*xiǎo chái hú tāng*) might be employed to harmonize shao yang.[13]

In another of his books, Understanding the Truth for Discussion of Cold Damage (傷寒明理論 *sháng hán míng lǐ lùn*) published in 1156, he further elaborates on why harmonization is suitable for shao yang disease:

> When pathological factors locate on the exterior, one should cook a formula to promote sweating; when pathological factors locate in the interior of the body, one should purge them by provoking diarrhea; when pathological factors do not locate solely either on the exterior or in the interior, but rather in the half exterior and the half interior, in this case, promotion of sweating is not appropriate, and promotion of vomiting and purging are not good either. It is suitable to apply harmonization. Minor Bupleurum Decoction (*xiǎo chái hú tāng*) is an agent to harmonize both the exterior and the interior.[14]

Six hundred years later, Ke Qin (also known as Ke Yun-Bo, c. 1669) echoed Cheng's idea and further pointed out that "this formula [Minor Bupleurum Decoction (*xiǎo chái hú tāng*)] is a remedy to harmonize the pivot of shao yang, and it is a principal formula to harmonize the exterior and interior."[15] Because Both Cheng Wu-Ji and Ke Qin were famous scholars who commented on Discussion of Cold Damage, their interpretations for the relationship among shao yang, harmonization and Minor Bupleurum Decoction (*xiǎo chái hú tāng*) had a tremendous influence on studying and practicing the theories from Discussion of Cold Damage and have been well received by subsequent scholars and practitioners.

13 Cheng Wu-Ji, op. cit., p.151

14 Ibid., p.51

15 Ke Qin. *Supplementary on Surviving with Discussion of Cold Damage* (*shāng hán lái sū jí, shāng hán fù yì*). Shanghai: Shanghai Science and Technology Publishing House, 1978: 44

Around 1636, Zhang Jie-Bin (also known as Zhang Jing-Yue, 1563–1640), a famous scholar in the Ming Dynasty, expanded the concept of harmonization and offered a broader sense for it. In the book, Annotation and Commentary for Complete Medical Works by Jing-Yue (校注景岳全書 *jiào zhù jǐng-yuè quán shū*), he elaborates:

> Harmonization is designed for abnormalities in diseases. When the condition associates with deficiency, one should tonify for harmonization; when the condition associates with stagnation in qi and blood, one should promote circulation for harmonization; when the condition associates with cold, one should warm the body for harmonization; when the condition associates with heat, one should clear heat for harmonization, and the meaning of harmonization is variable.[16]

In his book, Medical Comprehension (醫學心悟 *yī xué xīn wù*) published in 1732, Cheng Guo-Pen (also known as Cheng Zhong-Ling, 1662–1735), who first put harmonization among Eight Treatment Principles in Chinese medicine, i.e. promotion of sweating, promotion of vomiting, purging, harmonization, warming, clearing, dissipating and tonifying, echoed Zhang's idea that one should only address one approach when discussing harmonization. He wrote:

> There is harmonization that is implemented by clearing; there is harmonization that is realized by warming; there is harmonization that is achieved by dissipating; there is harmonization that is implemented by tonifying; there is harmonization that is realized by drying; there is harmonization that is achieved by moistening; there is harmonization that is gained by relieving the exterior; there is harmonization that is gained by purging.[17]

In fact, Dai Tian-Zhang (also known as Dai Lin-Jiao, c. 1660), a famous scholar and physician who specialized in warm-pathogen disease, noticed that it is not proper to just address one approach when discussing harmonization and first put two approaches that opposed each other for understanding harmonization. In his book, Clear Differentiation for Warm-Pathogen and Pestilential Diseases (溫疫明辨 *wēn yǐ míng biàn*) published in 1675, he pointed out that "combining cold and warm agents is called harmonization; blending agents of tonifying and reducing is

16 Zhao Li-Xun et al. *Annotation and Commentary for Complete Medical Works by Jing-Yue (jiào zhù jǐng yuè quán shū)*. Beijing: People's Health Publishing House, 1991: 1242

17 Cheng Guo-Pen. *Medical Comprehension (yī xué xīn wù)*. Changchun: Liaoning Science and Technology Publishing House, 1997: 7

called harmonization; relieving the exterior and interior simultaneously is called harmonization; reducing hyperactivity is called harmonization."[18] He Bing-Yuan (also known as He Lian-Chen, 1861–1919), Dai's follower and a famous scholar who specialized in warm-pathogen disease, summarized this idea in his book, Revised and Expanded Discussion of Warm-Pathogen Disease (重訂廣瘟熱論 *chóng dìng guáng wēn rè lùn*) first published in 1960, as the following:

> All methods that deal with the exterior and interior simultaneously, combining cold and warm herbs, mixing bitter and cold agents, the combination of tonifying and reducing, elimination of residual or recurrent pathogens, and adjustment of qi and blood, are called harmonization. What is called harmonization is to treat both sides.[19]

In her article, "On 'Harmonization' in Discussion of Cold Damage" published in 2002, Nie Hui-Min, a famous professor who specializes in Discussion of Cold Damage at Beijing University of Traditional Chinese Medicine, clearly classifies harmonization into two categories; a narrow sense and a broad sense:

> Harmonization in a broad sense refers to the treatment principle that has functions to adjust the hyperactivity, eliminate cold and heat pathogens, and tonify the deficiency for expelling pathological factors and curing diseases… Harmonization in a narrow sense specially refers to treatment approaches, and it is one of the eight basic treatment approaches. It attends the treatment goal through harmonization such as harmonization of pivot, harmonization of the nutritive qi and defensive qi, harmonization of the spleen and stomach, harmonization of ascending and descending, and harmonization of the interior and the exterior.[20]

Since 2003, some scholars have even expanded the concept of harmonization to include adjustment of qi and blood, balance of yin and yang, harmonization of the liver and spleen, and harmonization of the liver and stomach. Obviously, these interpretations for harmonization have expanded to the point that it seems the concept of harmonization encompasses every treatment approach without limitation and causes

18 Dai Tian-Zhang. *Clear Differentiation for Warm-Pathogen and Pestilential Diseases* (*wēn yì míng biàn*). Shanghai: Shanghai Science and Technology Publishing House, 1959: 67

19 He Bing-Yuan. *Revised and Expanded Discussion of Warm-Pathogen Disease* (*chóng dìng guáng wēn rè lùn*). Beijing: People's Health Publishing House, 1961: 145

20 Nie Hui-Min. "On 'Harmonization' in Discussion of Cold Damage." *Journal of Chinese Medicine*, 2002 (17): 199

some confusion between harmonization in Discussion of Cold Damage and other treatment approaches in Chinese medicine since 2003.

Noticing the shortage of these interpretations for discussing harmonization in Chinese medicine, Ma Yi-Chao and colleagues have pointed out:

> Promotion of sweating, purging and harmonization represent basic treatment approaches in tai yang, yang ming and shao yang diseases, respectively, in Discussion of Cold Damage. Based on this fact, the concept of "harmonization" should be limited… However, scholars and practitioner after Zhang Ji have expanded the meaning of "harmonization," especially calling the treatment for the syndrome due to the disharmony between cold and heat, and the syndrome due to disharmony between the nutritive qi and the defensive qi, "harmonization."
>
> This must be discussed clearly. For example, the disharmony between cold and heat actually refers to the syndrome of the mixture of cold and heat. Since it is the syndrome of the mixture of cold and heat, what is called "adjust and harmonize" cold and heat actually refers to the method to employ "warm (herbs)" and "cold (herbs)" at the same time, i.e. it "adjusts and harmonizes" cold and heat by employing warming and clearing methods, which still fall into the category of using warm herbs to deal with a cold condition and using cold herbs to treat a heat condition… Harmonization is paralleled with the promotion of sweating and purging. Only the methods that employ Bupleurum Decoctions for shao yang disease can be called "harmonization."
>
> Since jue yin is on the hinge of yin and yang and bears the function of the pivot in the body, it also makes sense to call the approach that soothes qi of the liver in the formulas such as Frigid Extremities Powder (*sì nì săn*)[21] and Rambling Powder (*xiāo yáo săn*)[22] as 'harmonization'."[23]

As mentioned at beginning of this chapter, the character "和 *hé*" originally depicts bamboo pipes by one mouth blowing. The mouth blows these pipes while the holes on these pipes are opened and closed by putting the

---

21 Frigid Extremities Powder contains Bupleuri Radix (*chái hú*), Paeoniae Radix Alba (*bái sháo*), Aurantii Fructus Immaturus (*zhǐ shí*) and Glycyrrhizae Radix Preparata (*zhì gān căo*). See line 318 for further details.

22 Rambling Powder contains Bupleuri Radix (*chái hú*), Paeoniae Radix Alba (*bái sháo*), Angelicae Sinensis Radix (*dāng guī*), Atractylodis Macrocephalae Rhizoma (*bái zhú*), Poria (*fú líng*), Zingiberis Rhizoma Recens (*shēng jiāng*), Menthae Haplocalycis Herba (*bò hé*) and Glycyrrhizae Radix Preparata (*zhì gān căo*).

23 Ma Yi-Chao, Jiang Jian-Guo and Lu Xiao-Ming. "Discussion of several issues related to formulas of Bupleurum decoctions, their syndromes and harmonization." *Journal of Shandong University of Traditional Chinese Medicine*, 2003 (1): 21

finger tips on and off of them. Without letting qi in and out by closing and opening these holes, harmonious music cannot be produced. Similarly, without letting qi move in and out or up and down through some structures in the body, the harmonization, and the treatment that brings harmony back to the body, cannot be realized.

It might be argued that adjusting the nutritive qi and defensive qi should be called the approach of harmonization and Cinnamon Twig Decoction (*guì zhī tāng*) should be considered as the agent to do this job, because Zhang Ji does state in line 53:

> This is because the defensive qi is not in harmony with nutritive qi, since the defensive qi circulates outside of the vessels while the nutritive qi moves in the vessels. The recovery will be achieved with harmony between the defensive qi and the nutritive qi from further promotion of sweating (regardless of there having already been sweating). Cinnamon Twig Decoction (*guì zhī tāng*) is appropriate.

This implies the function of this formula in this line is supposed to harmonize the nutritive qi and defensive qi. What is more, Zhang Ji clear states in line 387 that "Cinnamon Twig Decoction (*guì zhī tāng*) is appropriate to slightly adjust or harmonize defensive qi and nutritive qi." Yes, this is a good argument and the method and formulas that deal with the disharmony between the nutritive qi and the defensive qi should fall into the category of harmonization. But why do some scholars, like Ma Yi-Chao, not recognize the method and its formula mentioned in lines 53 and 387 as harmonization though Zhang Ji has clearly stated that? I believe that there are two reasons for them to come to such a conclusion. First, the qi movement invigorated by this method, especially implemented by Cinnamon Twig Decoction (*guì zhī tāng*), goes in one direction, because the whole formula tends to be warm in nature and acrid in flavor, which makes qi, particularly the nutritive qi, move from inside of vessels to the body surface (see Chapter 8 for further details). Second, as mentioned at beginning of this chapter, the character "和 *hé*" originally depicts the bamboo pipes by one mouth blowing, which implies "to combine different things and make them balanced." In order to balance two things, two directions of movement, i.e. in and out and/or up and down, are needed to allow two things to meet and interact with each other. Without these two directions of movements, which are opposed to each other yet move towards each other, how can two things meet and interact with each other for their balance? Without their meeting and interacting with each other, how can the harmony between them take place? Obviously, the method and formula mentioned in lines 53 and 387 fail to bring qi in and out and/or up and down for harmony simultaneously, which is a basic requirement for understanding the concept of the character "和 *hé*" and harmonization (和法 *hé fǎ*). It mainly moves qi out to the body surface with one direction for adjusting the relationship between the nutritive qi and the defensive qi. Therefore, the treatment implemented by Cinnamon Twig Decoction (*guì zhī tāng*) cannot be called harmonization.

However, readers might still have the following question in their mind, which has not been answered by the discussion above: How does harmonization work on two different things, especially for half interior and half exterior, or interior symptoms and signs as well as exterior symptoms and signs simultaneously?

To answer this question, the second important concept in this chapter must be introduced, which is "樞 *shū* (pivot)." According to Chapter 5 of Morals Classic (道德經 *dào dé jīng*), "the space between heaven and earth is like a bellows."[24] Of course, to become a functional bellows, qi must move in and out and/or up and down. Based on the basic natural principle in Chinese philosophy and culture, which states "as above, as below," the human body would also function as a bellows in which qi should move in and out and/or up and down. In order to make qi move in and out and/or up and down, there must be something opening and closing that lets qi perform these movements. Therefore, the theory of the "樞 *shū* (pivot)" for shao yang has been introduced in Chinese medicine.

The statement related to the theory of the pivot for shao yang can be found in Chapter 6 of Basic Questions and Chapter 5 of Spiritual Pivot in The Yellow Emperor's Inner Classic. It states that "shao yang serves a '樞 *shū* (pivot)' for the body."[25, 26] What does this character "樞 *shū* (pivot)" mean? According to Explanation for Chinese Characters (說文解字 *shuō wēn jiě zì*) published in 122 AD, it means "door hinge."[27] This explanation can be proved by a couple of books published before

24 Sha Shao-Hai and Xu Zi-Hong. *Complete Translation for Lao Zi* (*lǎo zǐ quán yì*). Guiyang: Guizhou People's Publishing House, 1989: 9

25 Wang Bing. *Basic Questions of The Yellow Emperor's Inner Classic* (*huáng dì nèi jīng sù wèn*). Beijing: People's Health Publishing House, 1963: 50

26 Anonymous. *Spiritual Pivot* (*líng shū jīng*). Beijing: People's Health Publishing House, 1963: 16

27 Xu Shen. *Explanation for Chinese Characters* (*shuō wén jiě zì*). Beijing: Chinese Publishing House, 1963: 120

that book. For example, A Pulse Book (脈書 *mài shū*) that was buried in tombs c. 106 BC first introduced this meaning in medicine. It states:

> If one of five signs for death presents, practitioners should first save the patient. The water that flows never gets rotted and the door hinge that moves is never damaged by worms, because they continually exercise. Exercise can make limbs strong and blood in organs flow smoothly. And smooth blood flow would be beneficial for the body.[28]

Historically, many scholars have talked about the door hinge function for shao yang that makes qi go in and out and have ignored its function to make qi move up and down. For example, Zhang Jie-Bin (known as Zhang Jing-Yue, 1563–1640), a famous scholar who made commentary for The Yellow Emperor's Inner Classic, wrote that "the reason to call shao yang a pivot is that it means qi can move in and out between the exterior and interior like a door hinge."[29] This explanation can be proved by the feature of the gall bladder. The gall bladder is classified as an "extraordinary fu organ" by The Yellow Emperor's Inner Classic. There is general agreement that the reason to classify it as an extraordinary fu organ is because it can store and discharge essence and qi, though the original text in this classic did not prove it.[30] Given this interpretation, the gall bladder can let qi in and out like a door hinge. However, it fails to demonstrate dynamic movement of qi. In fact, some scholars have ignored the explanation made by Wang Bing (also known as Qi Xuan-Zi, 710–804 AD), another well-known scholar who made commentary for The Yellow Emperor's Inner Classic. In his book, Basic Questions of The Yellow Emperor's Inner Classic (黄帝内經素問 *huáng dì nèi jīng sù wèn*) first published in 762 AD, he presented a good definition for the character "樞 *shū*," in terms of qi moving in a dynamic way, when he explained this statement related to shao yang in Chapter 6 of Basic Questions of The Yellow Emperor's Inner Classic. He wrote that "what is called '樞 *shū* (pivot)' means that

---

28 Gao Da-Lun. *Annotation and Explanation on Pulse Book on Bamboo Slips Dug from Tombs in Han Dynasty at Zhang Jia Mountain* (*zhāng jiā shān hàn jiǎn mài shū jiào shì*). Chengdu: Bashu Publishing House, 1992: 94

29 Zhang Jie-Bin. *Classified Classic* (*lèi jīng*). Beijing: People's Health Publishing House, 1982: 287

30 According to original text from Chapter 11 of *Basic Questions of The Yellow Emperor's Inner Classic*, "the brain, marrow, bone, vessels, uterus and gall bladder are generated by qi on the earth. They function like earth and store without discharge." See Wang Bing, op. cit., p.77

[shao yang] governs turning of qi elegantly."[31] In fact, the character "樞 *shū*" bears meaning of center or important part, which was used by Zhuang Zi (also known as Zhuang Zhou and Zhuang Zi-Xiu, 369–286 BC),[32] a famous writer and philosopher of the early Warring States period. Therefore, it is better to understand the concept of the character "樞 *shū*" dynamically and translate it, especially when it refers to shao yang as a pivot rather than a door hinge, which means the action of turning in various directions on a point.

Some scholars or readers might argue that since the character "樞 *shū*" is not recorded in Discussion of Cold Damage at all, how do you know that Zhang Ji did pay attention to qi moving in and out and/or up and down and applied the theory of pivot for shao yang disease in Discussion of Cold Damage? In order to answer this question, several lines related to shao yang disease in Discussion of Cold Damage have to be carefully studied. The first line one must examine is line 96, which is the first line to systematically discuss clinical manifestations of shao yang disease and its treatment, Minor Bupleurum Decoctions (*xiǎo chái hú tāng*), in detail, though it is recorded in the chapter on tai yang disease. In this line, Zhang Ji writes:

> After suffering from zhong feng syndrome in Cold Damage for five or six days, there is alternating chills and fever, discomfort and fullness in the chest and hypochondriac region, taciturnity with no desire to eat, sick and discomforting feeling in the stomach and easy vomiting, and with the following possible symptoms and signs: vexation in the chest and absence of nausea, or thirst, or abdominal pain, or distention and hardening below the hypochondriac region, or palpitation in the epigastrium and abnormal urination, or absence of thirst and slight fever in the body, or cough. Minor Bupleurum Decoction (*xiǎo chái hú tāng*) should be prescribed.

There are two groups of symptoms and signs that are relevant to the pivot function of shao yang which let qi move in and out and/or up and down. The first one is alternating chills and fever, which is considered as a main manifestation for shao yang disease in Chinese medicine. It has been very popular to hold the fighting between pathological factors and anti-pathogenic qi accountable for the presentation of alternating chills and fever. According to this opinion, fever presents when anti-pathogenic

31 Wang Bing, op. cit., p.50

32 Editorial Department of Business Publishing House. *Origin of Chinese Characters* (*cí yuán*). Beijing: Business Publishing House, 1980: 1622

qi overcomes pathological factors, and aversion to cold manifests when pathological factors prevail. But this explanation would be challenged by the following question: Such fighting and such waxing and waning between pathological factors and anti-pathogenic qi can also occur in any diseases like tai yang, yang ming, tai yin, shao yin and jue yin diseases, so why does shao yang disease, rather than those diseases, have alternating chills and fever? To answer this question, one must examine the physiological function of shao yang, because how can one understand the pathology and clinical manifestation related to shao yang disease without understanding deeply the physiological function of shao yang? The reason for the patient with shao yang disease to have such presentation is dysfunction of the pivot function of shao yang. As mentioned above, the pivot function of shao yang is supposed to let qi move dynamically, i.e. in and out and/or up and down. When pathological factors prevail, yang qi from shao yang will not be able to reach the body surface from the interior of the body transversely and push pathological factors back to the body surface through the pivot of shao yang. Of course, there is not so much yang qi, which is warm in nature, to warm on the body surface, on the one hand, and there is not so much yang qi to be stagnated to produce fever on the body surface, on the other hand. Therefore, aversion to cold presents but fever is absent; when anti-pathogenic qi gets stronger, building-up yang qi bursts out and is able to reach the body surface from the interior of the body transversely yet still does not move smoothly since pathological factors have not gone. These pathological factors can depress yang qi to a certain degree, making yang qi stagnate and produce fever, leading to the absence of aversion to cold.

The second group of symptoms and signs have many possible presentations such as cough, thirst, abnormal urination, and slight fever. In the "Difficult or Doubtable Questions" for line 96, I elaborate that these manifestations mean that three burners, another organ of shao yang, is involved. To answer this question, it is better to classify these possible symptoms and signs into several groups to see what the location would be for them. According to my analysis, these symptoms and signs can be classified into four groups: (a) symptoms and signs belonging to the upper burner such as vexation in the chest and cough; (b) symptoms and signs belonging to the middle burner such as palpitation in the epigastrium, absence of retching, thirst and abdominal pain; (c) symptoms and signs belonging to the lower burner such as abnormal urination; and (d) symptoms and signs belonging to the body surface such as fullness and hardening below the hypochondriac region, and slight fever in the body.

Not only alternating chills and fever but also slight fever is an indication of disease in shao yang, and applying Minor Bupleurum Decoction (*xiǎo chái hú tāng*) is the treatment according to Zhang Ji's clinical experience. As a matter of fact, there are quite a few lines in Discussion of Cold Damage that demonstrate that fever and aversion to wind (line 99), slight chill without fever (line 148), tidal fever (line 229) and absence of fever and chills (lines 37 and 230) can be treated by Minor Bupleurum Decoction (*xiǎo chái hú tāng*), a principal formula to deal with shao yang disease. Based on the present author's study, alternating chills and fever is related to qi moving in and out transversely in the three burners, while other symptoms and signs, except fullness and hardening below the hypochondriac region, which relate to the gall bladder channel, and slight fever, which indicates the involvement of the exterior, are relevant to the three burners, especially the dysfunction of the pivot of three burners, to move qi up and down vertically.

Line 230 gives concrete evidence to prove that Zhang Ji did address this pivot function of the three burners. In this line, he writes:

> In yang ming disease, when there is a hard feeling and fullness in the chest and hypochondriac region, constipation and vomiting, and white tongue coating, one might prescribe Minor Bupleurum Decoction (*xiǎo chái hú tāng*), which can make qi in the upper burner move smoothly, body fluid descend and qi in the stomach harmonize, and bring recovery after persistent sweating.

Clearly, sweating, disappearance of the vomiting and smooth bowel movement indicates that qi has been directed to the four directions, i.e. in and out, up and down, after taking Minor Bupleurum Decoction (*xiǎo chái hú tāng*). In other words, the pivot (樞 *shū*) function of shao yang is indeed discussed in the context of this line in Discussion of Cold Damage. Also, the reaction (defecation) after taking this formula described in line 148 has demonstrated qi moving downward.

To understand this analysis deeply, I would like to introduce the third important concept in this chapter, "腠 *còu*," which appears in Zhang Ji's work and reviews of the relationship between internal organs, such as the three burners, kidney, uterus, and "腠 *còu*," based on the study of The Yellow Emperor's Inner Classic and Difficult Questions. Generally, "腠 *còu*" can be understood as the interstices that locate among the skin, muscles, tendons and bones, while in Chapter 8 of Basic Questions of The Yellow Emperor's Inner Classic the three burners is defined as a fu organ that "takes charge of adjusting water passage."[33] According to Chapter 66 of Difficult Questions, which is considered to have been published after The Yellow Emperor's Inner Classic but before Discussion of Cold Damage:

> The moving qi between the kidneys is original vital qi for life and it is the root for the twelve channels. Therefore, this qi is called source qi. The three burners is another missionary who can distribute source qi over the body.[34]

However, where and how the source qi is distributed has been largely ignored by many scholars. In fact, in Spiritual Pivot (靈樞經 *líng shū jīng*) and Basic Questions (素問 *sù wèn*) of The Yellow Emperor's Inner Classic, the scholars who wrote this classic first disclosed the secret relationships among the kidney, urinary bladder, three burners, interstices among the skin, muscles, tendons and bones, and hair on the skin, and they laid out the road map for the distribution of the source qi carried by the three burners, one component of shao yang. They pointed out that "the kidney corresponds with the three burners and urinary bladder. And the three burners and urinary bladder correspond with the interstices and the hairs on the skin,"[35] and "clear yang qi can reach the interstices among the skin, muscles, tendons, and bones…and nourish limbs."[36]

Based on his study and clinical experience, Zhang Ji found that not only qi but also blood is distributed by the three burners, and the interstices among the skin, muscles, tendons and bones are a gate where pathological factors invade. In Chapter 1 of Essentials and Formula Discussions from the Golden Cabinet (金匱要略方論 *jīn gùi yào lüè fāng lùn*), a companion book for Discussion of Cold Damage, Zhang Ji states:

> If one can take good care of one's body…does not make the body weak, pathological factors will not invade the body through the 腠理 *còu lǐ*. The 腠 *còu* is a structure in the body where the three burners convey and

33 Wang Bing, op. cit., p.58

34 Nanjing College of Traditional Chinese Medicine et al. *Annotation and Explanation for Difficult Questions* (*nàn jīng jiào shì*). Beijing: People's Health Publishing House, 1979: 144

35 Anonymous, op. cit., p.92

36 Wang Bing, op. cit., p.32

> converge source qi, and a place where qi and blood are distributed, while the 理 *lǐ* is the texture on the skin, zang and fu organs.[37]

Zhang Jia-Li and colleagues have offered an insightful explanation for the relationship between the 腠 *còu* (interstice), skin, three burners and other zang-fu organs:

> "腠理 *còu lǐ*" is a kind of structure in the body that is predominated by the three burners and has relation to the skin and zang-fu organs. It is the place where source qi and true qi meet, and qi and blood are distributed.[38]

In line 97, Zhang Ji further describes:

> When there is deficiency of both qi and blood, the 腠理 *còu lǐ* are open and then pathological factors invade, leading to the fighting between anti-pathogenic qi and pathological factors, resulting in accumulation of pathological factors under the hypochondriac region.

Also, he noticed that pathological factors can even progress to the chong and uterus, affecting menstruation (see lines 143–145 for further details) through this structure, and recommended Minor Bupleurum Decoction (*xiǎo chái hú tāng*) to get rid of these pathological factors via recovering the pivot function of shao yang. Based on the discussion above, we can draw a figure (Figure 7.2) to illustrate the skin, interstices (腠 *còu*), three burners, kidney, and the chong and uterus.

Figure 7.2 is based on the description from The Yellow Emperor's Inner Classic and Zhang Ji's works, including Discussion of Cold Damage and Essentials and Formula Discussions from the Golden Cabinet, as well as the elaboration from later commentators, such as Zhang Jia-Li and colleagues. It has been illuminated that the three burners indeed serve as a pivot for qi, blood and body fluid moving between the body surface and inside of the body. Understanding Figure 7.2, one could be able to explain why women could be easily attacked by cold during menstruation and how pathological factors can affect menstruation and/or urination when catching a cold. Besides viewing the three burners as serving as a pivot for qi, blood and body fluid moving between the body surface and inside of the body, there are two other ways to understand the meaning of the pivot

37 Zhang Ji. *Essentials and Formula Discussions from the Golden Cabinet* (*jīn guì yào lüè fāng lùn*). Textually researched and annotated by Wen Di. Beijing: Chinese Publishing House, 1993: 2

38 Zhang Jia-Li. *Selected Reading for Essentials and Formula Discussions from the Golden Cabinet* (*jīn guì yào lüè xuǎn dú*). Beijing: Chinese Medicine Publishing House, 1999: 18

function for shao yang, i.e. understanding the pivot function for shao yang based on the yang qi condition and its circulation, and understanding it as a symbolic image for the movement of orifices in the upper part of the body.

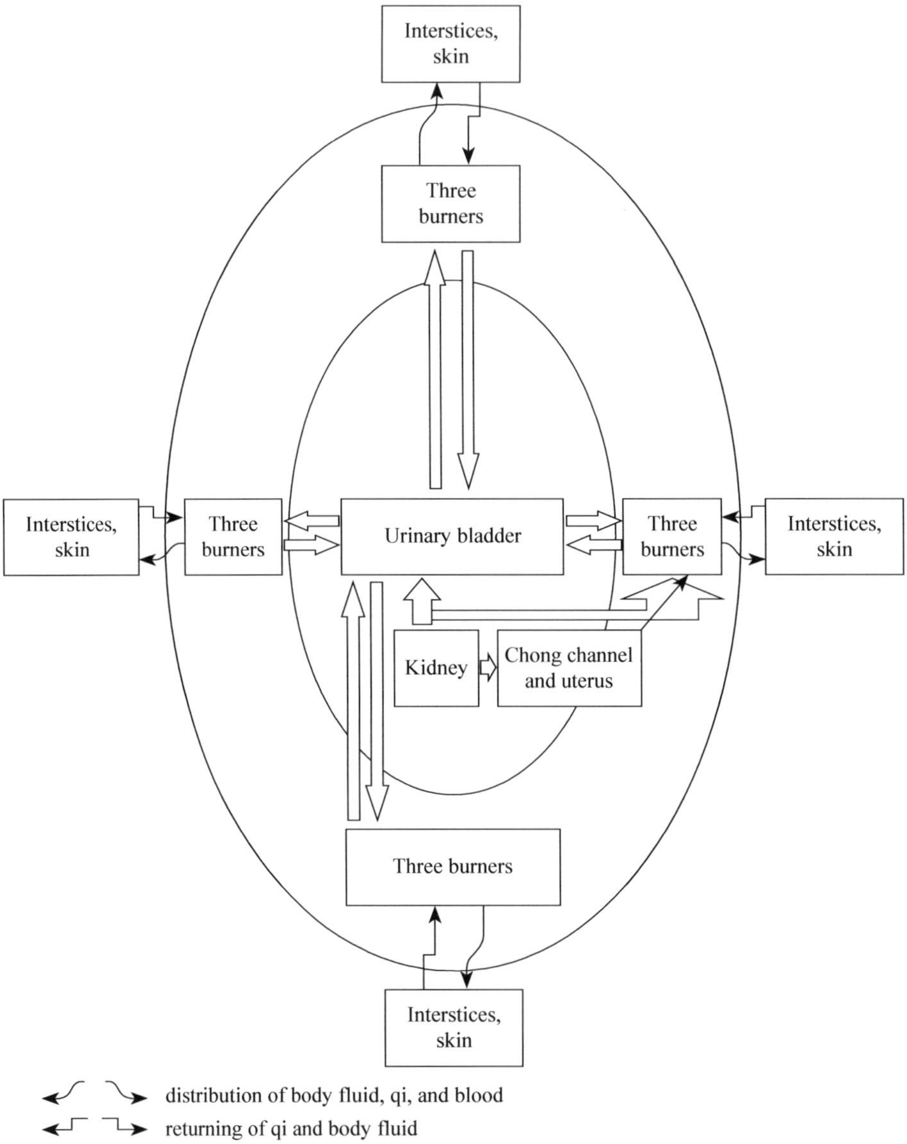

Figure 7.2 Relationship among the interstices (腠 *còu*), three burners, kidney, urinary bladder, chong channel and uterus with regard to dynamic movement for qi, blood and body fluid

According to Chapters 7, 66 and 74 of Basic Questions of The Yellow Emperor's Inner Classic and comments from Wang Bing,[39] yang can be further classified into tai yang that is called "three yangs" as it bears the strongest yang qi, yang ming that is called "two yangs" as it bears relatively strong yang qi, and shao yang that is called "one yang" as it bears the least yang qi among three yang. Yin can also be further classified into tai yin, shao yin and jue yin. Tai yin is called "three yins" as it contains the strongest yin qi, shao yin is called "two yins" as it contains relatively strong yin qi, and jue yin is called "one yin" as it contains the least yin qi. Because these yangs and yins are believed to wax and wane and connect to each other in the body, the flow of qi in these three yang and three yin can be represented as shown in Figure 7.3.

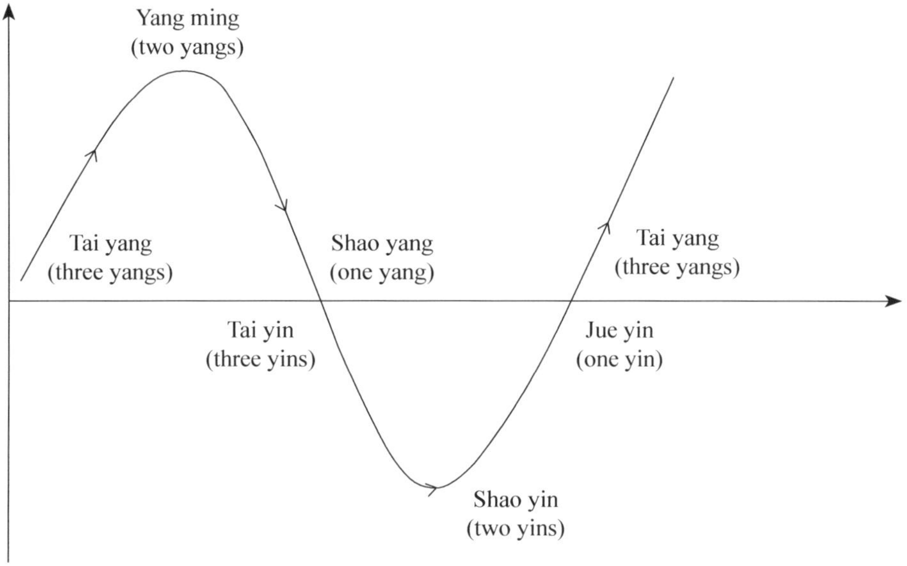

FIGURE 7.3 YIN AND YANG FUNCTION AND CIRCULATION AMONG THREE YINS AND THREE YANGS

From Figure 7.2 and 7.3 one should learn that shao yang, especially the three burners, is not only the pivot for body fluid, qi and blood circulation in and out and/or up and down between the body surface and inside of the body, but that it also serves as the pivot between three yin and three yang. Since its yang qi is the weakest among the three yang and its defensive ability is least strong, if pathological factors have progressed to shao yang,

39 Wang Bing, op. cit., pp.53–56, 365, 528–529

they will easily progress to the three yin and present three yin diseases. This is why Zhang Ji especially reminds us that "after suffering from Cold Damage for three days, the involvement of three yang should end and three yin should be attacked by pathological factors" in line 270, the line of the chapter on shao yang disease in Discussion of Cold Damage, and he would employ Ginseng Radix (*rén shēn*), Jujubae Fructus (*dà zǎo*) and Glycyrrhizae Radix Preparata (*zhì gān cǎo*), which are used to tonify qi of the spleen, for preventing such progression. In other words, shao yang is also a pivot that connects yang and yin in three yin and three yang. It can make yang qi enter yin to warm yin and yin qi come out to yang and support yang qi. Understanding the pivot function for shao yang, one can work on shao yang for mingling yin and yang when there is disconnection between them.

Now one might be able to understand why the harmonization belongs to shao yang, because the character "和 *hé*" implies "to combine different things and makes them balanced." In order to balance two things, two directions of movement, i.e. in and out and/or up and down, are needed for them to meet and interact with each other. Without these two directions of movements, which are opposed to each other, how can two things meet? Without such meeting and interaction, how can the harmony between them take place? Only shao yang can fulfill this goal, i.e. harmonization can only be brought about by shao yang.

I have been frequently asked by students that according to distribution of channels, because the channels of foot shao yang and hand shao yang locate between the channels of tai yang and yang ming (both foot and hand), can we call shao yang the pivot or door hinge for tai yang and yang ming in this way? It is correct that the shao yang channel goes between the tai yang and yang ming channel when we look at anatomical location of three yang channels. Also, it is correct that yang qi has decreased gradually from tai yang (three yangs) to shao yang (one yang) through yang ming (two yangs). But such explanation, especially for the decreasing of yang qi, would not be supported by the fact that it only addresses one direction of qi (declining yang qi), which does not meet the requirement for the pivot or even the door hinge. However, this anatomical distribution is quite useful to localize where a disease is clinically.

Historically, there is another interpretation for shao yang as the pivot based on symbolic thinking. According to Ke Qin (also known as Ke Yun-Bo, c. 1669), orifices on the head demonstrate the symbol of the pivot for shao yang as they can open and close and let something in and out. In his book, Discussion of Special Topic in Surviving with Cold Damage (傷寒來蘇集 • 傷寒論翼 *shāng hán lái sū jí* • *shāng hán lùn yì*) first published in 1674, Ke wrote:

> Shao yang locates half exterior and half interior, takes charge of circulation of ministerial fire in the three burners. The reason to use bitter taste in the mouth, dry mouth and dizziness as the outline for its disease is to attach great importance to the pathology. Mouth, throat and eyes are orifices where essence and qi in zang-fu organs distribute, through which the human connects with qi in nature. Shao yang cannot be called either the exterior or the interior. It is a place where [qi and essence] enter the interior and reach the exterior, which is called half exterior and interior. All of these three orifices can open and close. They can be seen when they open and cannot be seen when they close. They just look like and function like the symbol of the pivot.[40]

Ke's insightful interpretation for the disorders of the mouth, throat and eyes is supported by the text of line 263, which is called the outline for shao yang disease. If one reads the lines in the chapter on shao yang disease carefully, the ear can be considered as the symbol of the pivot for shao yang as deafness in the ears is called zhong feng syndrome in shao yang disease by Zhang Ji in line 264. If one opens his or her mind based on Ke's thoughts, any orifice including the eyes, ears, mouth, throat and nose can be viewed as the symbol of the pivot for shao yang. I have applied these thoughts in my clinic to treat sinusitis and allergy and gained good results. Based on the discussion above, Zhang Ji attached great importance to following three groups of symptoms and signs for identifying dysfunction of the pivot in shao yang: alternating chills and fever; symptoms and signs related to the three burners; and manifestation in upper orifices, especially eyes, throat, mouth and ears.

We have discussed what harmonization is and what "腠 *còu*" and the pivot related to harmonization means. How does Minor Bupleurum Decoction (*xiǎo chái hú tāng*) in Discussion of Cold Damage implement the treatment principle and recover the pivot function of shao yang by harmonization? In order to understand how this formula works for the pivot function of shao yang, much attention should paid to Bupleuri Radix (*chái hú*) since the formula is named after this herb and the dosage of

40 Ke Qin. *Discussion of Special Topic in Surviving with Cold Damage* (*shāng hán lái sū jí, shāng hán lùn yì*). Shanghai: Shanghai Science and Technology Publishing House, 1978: 33–34

Bupleuri Radix (*chái hú*) is at least twice as much as the dosages of the other herbs in this formula. According to Materia Medica by Shen Nong (神農本草經 *shén nóng běn cǎo jīng*), one of the classics to which Zhang Ji referred when he wrote Discussion of Cold Damage (especially the base for him to employ the herb):

> Bupleuri Radix (*chái hú*) is bitter in flavor and neutral in nature and can treat disorders in the heart and abdomen, deal with stagnant qi in the intestines and stomach, food stagnation, externally contracted cold and heat pathological factors, and can eliminate old things and generate new things.[41]

Bupleuri Radix (*chái hú*) has a neutral nature. According to the theory of nature (氣 *qì*) and flavor (味 *wèi*), nature occurs first and then flavors are produced by qi in universe. Qi, the nature of herbs, is first established when the seeds of herbs start to grow. They can be cold, cool, hot and warm or neutral in nature at the beginning. As they grow, they develop different flavors but their nature remains unchanged. For example, both Nelumbinis Folium (*hé yè*) and Nelumbinis Semen (*lián zǐ*) are neutral in nature. Nelumbinis Folium (*hé yè*) is bitter in flavor, which makes it the herb to deal with dampness. Nelumbinis Semen (*lián zǐ*), the fruit of Nelumbinis Folium (*hé yè*), is sweet in flavor, which changes its function from treating dampness to tonifying qi of the spleen. According to yin yang theory, warm nature and hot nature belong to yang, which is likely to reach to the exterior of the body as the exterior is yang, while cool nature and cold nature belong to yin, which is likely to stay inside the body. Of course, the neutral nature would stay in the middle or center part of the body. Therefore, qi, the nature of herbs, determines where herbs reach primarily in the body and the flavor and other properties it develops determine where it might go later. The neutral flavor of a herb means it is not cold and cool and is not hot and warm. It is this nature that might makes herbs reach neither the exterior nor the interior but the middle point or center in the body, which is the pivot in the body.

Based on the discussion above, with neutral nature, Bupleuri Radix (*chái hú*) can reach shao yang, the pivot in the body, first. The bitter flavor and light property that develop later can make this herb work on the pivot function of shao yang by going different directions, i.e. light quality makes qi move out and upward, while bitter quality makes qi

---

41 Anonymous. *Materia Medica by Shen Nong* (*shén nóng běn cǎo jīng*). Beijing: Scientific and Technological Literature Publishing House, 1996: 15

move down and inward. Because of its unique nature and flavor that work on the pivot of shao yang, Bupleuri Radix (*chái hú*) can be used to deal with both the exterior and interior illnesses such as "disorder in the heart and abdomen, stagnant qi in the intestines and stomach, food stagnation, and externally contracted cold and heat pathological factors" described in Materia Medica by Shen Nong (神農本草經 *shén nóng běn cǎo jīng*) and is an absolutely chief herb in Minor Bupleurum Decoction (*xiǎo chái hú tāng*).

Interestingly, Scutellariae Radix (*huáng qín*) and Pinelliae Rhizoma (*bàn xià*), two deputy herbs that assist Bupleuri Radix (*chái hú*) in the formula, are neutral in nature according to Materia Medica by Shen Nong (神農本草經 *shén nóng běn cǎo jīng*).[42] It is probably their nature that make these two agents specially selected to assist Bupleuri Radix (*chái hú*) to deal with the dysfunction of the pivot for shao yang. Scutellariae Radix (*huáng qín*) is considered bitter in this classic, and this raises a question: Why does Scutellariae Radix (*huáng qín*) not have the same ability as Bupleuri Radix (*chái hú*) for the pivot function of shao yang? The answer is that Scutellariae Radix (*huáng qín*) is heavier and more bitter than Bupleuri Radix (*chái hú*) and it does not have any ability to reach the body surface by itself. This is why almost all symptoms and signs mentioned in Materia Medica by Shen Nong that Scutellariae Radix (*huáng qín*) treats, such as jaundice due to heat, dysentery, diarrhea, water retention, amenorrhea due to blood stasis and carbuncle, belong to interior disorders. As for Pinelliae Rhizoma (*bàn xià*), it is acrid and can be used to treat Cold Damage, fever, chills, hardening sensation in the epigastrium, qi rebellion, swelling in the throat, dizziness, distention in the chest, cough, borborygmus and sweating according to this classic.

In summary, Minor Bupleurum Decoction (*xiǎo chái hú tāng*) is designed for recovering the pivot function of shao yang in the following way: Bupleuri Radix (*chái hú*), a chief herb, is used to reach the pivot of shao yang, letting the pivot turn by making qi move in and out and/or up and down. Scutellariae Radix (*huáng qín*) is employed to assist Bupleuri Radix (*chái hú*) to bring qi inward and downward while Pinelliae Rhizoma (*bàn xià*) is selected to help Bupleuri Radix (*chái hú*) to bring qi outward and upward. The way of these three herbs working for the pivot function of shao yang, i.e. Bupleuri Radix (*chái hú*) takes the main responsibility while Scutellariae Radix (*huáng qín*) and Pinelliae Rhizoma (*bàn xià*)

42 Ibid., pp.64, 92

assist it, appears in the exact pictorial image of the character "和 *hé* (harmony)": one mouth blows bamboo pipes and the fingers of two hands control the opening and closing of the holes on the bamboo pipes, for harmonious music.

Besides these three ingredients working for the goal of harmonization, Zhang Ji recommended a unique preparation method to enhance the effect of the harmonization for this formula. In the footnote for the formula, he wrote that the decoctions made from the formula should be decocted again. Both ancient and contemporary scholars have pointed out that the purpose for the second cooking is to make the properties from each of the ingredients get along with each other and make the flavor and nature for each ingredient not too strong and not too partial or biased (see "analysis of formula," line 96, for further details). Obviously, this unique preparation method is to balance the function of the formula, which can also be considered as one part of the harmonizing approach implemented by the formula.

Since the pivot function of shao yang would be recovered by Bupleuri Radix (*chái hú*), Scutellariae Radix (*huáng qín*) and Pinelliae Rhizoma (*bàn xià*), why did Zhang Ji employ Ginseng Radix (*rén shēn*), Zingiberis Rhizoma Recens (*shēng jiāng*), Jujubae Fructus (*dà zǎo*) and Glycyrrhizae Radix Preparata (*zhì gān cǎo*)? Yes, in most cases, Bupleuri Radix (*chái hú*) alone or these three herbs would be strong enough to recover the pivot function of shao yang. According to Chapter 3 of Basic Questions of The Yellow Emperor's Inner Classic, "yang qi is supposed to rise against to defend the body."[43] Shao yang bears one yang in terms of quantity and its yang qi is relative weak. It is a pivot for the body for letting qi move in and out and/or up and down including letting qi communicate between yin and yang as demonstrated in Figure 7.2. According to line 270, the disease might disappear in three yang and progress to three yin.

There are two reasons for Zhang Ji to add these four herbs on top of Bupleuri Radix (*chái hú*), Pinelliae Rhizoma (*bàn xià*) and Scutellariae Radix (*huáng qín*): the first is to tonify qi in the spleen, tai yin that bears three yins, and let qi from tai yin support shao yang by using Ginseng Radix (*rén shēn*), Jujubae Fructus (*dà zǎo*) and Glycyrrhizae Radix Preparata (*zhì gān cǎo*). The second reason is to adjust the disharmony between the stomach and shao yang by adding Zingiberis Rhizoma Recens (*shēng jiāng*) for treating poor appetite and vomiting caused by rebellion of qi in the stomach.

43 Wang Bing, op. cit., p.17

In summary, what is called "half interior and half exterior" was not recorded in the original text of Discussion of Cold Damage, but the similar description, "half in the interior and half in the exterior," can be found in line 148 of the book, which refers to "there must be interior symptoms and signs as well as exterior symptoms and signs." It is correct that the pathological factor can invade the shao yang, the pivot of the body, and the location of this disease is half interior and half exterior, which is proved by the context of line 96. However, understanding the meaning of the "樞 *shū*" function of shao yang bears very practical clinical significance. The character "樞 *shū*" cannot be only interpreted as "door hinge." It refers to the turning point dynamically and the word "pivot" is the correct one to convey this special meaning which makes qi move in and out and/or up and down. Bearing this idea in mind, one can understand why Minor Bupleurum Decoction (*xiǎo chái hú tāng*), a major formula to harmonize shao yang and recover the pivot function of shao yang, can be applied not only for half exterior and half interior (lines 96 and 266), which means the pivot function of shao yang is affected, but also the exterior condition alone (lines 231 and 394), interior condition alone (lines 100, 229 and 230) or the mixture of the exterior and interior syndromes (lines 98, 99 and 148). The latter three applications attach great importance to exercising the pivot function of shao yang, i.e. letting qi move in and out and/or up and down through the normal turning function of the pivot in shao yang for dealing with the exterior condition alone, or the interior condition alone, or a combination of both, though the pivot function of shao yang might not be affected by invasion of pathological factors. This might be one of the important clinical factors for understanding the meaning of half exterior, half interior and harmonization. Also, according to research from scholars who have studied Discussion of Cold Damage, the pivot in shao yang also refers to the upper orifices of the body like mouth, eyes, throat and ears, as they are held accountable for communication between the body and nature by closing and opening, which symbolize the pivot. In lines 263 and 264, Zhang Ji diagnoses the problems of these orifices as one of the shao yang syndromes and clinical applications have proved that these interpretations are quite insightful and helpful.

As mentioned at the beginning of this chapter, the character "和 *hé*" originally depicts the bamboo pipes by one mouth blowing, which implies "to combine different things and make them balanced." The way to make a piece of music by playing these pipes is accomplished by letting qi in and out through one mouth and the fingers of two hands. In order to balance two things, two directions of movement, i.e. in and out and/or up and down, are warranted for the two things to meet and interact with each other. Without these two directions of movements, which are opposed to each other, how can two things meet and interact? Without their meetings and interaction, how can the harmony between them occur? Among three yin and three yang, only shao yang can bring qi in and out and/or up and down from a very superficial level to a very deep level, as well as combine yin and yang; therefore, harmonization can only be brought about by working on shao yang. Because such qi movement through the pivot of the body cannot be achieved by one direction of movement performed by Cinnamon Twig Decoction (*guì zhī tāng*), and it cannot be brought about by the combination of tonifying and reducing, the adjustment of yin and yang, nor by adjusting qi and blood, which do not work on the pivot function of shao yang, it is not appropriate to call those methods harmonization (和法 *hé fǎ*).

8

NUTRITIVE QI, DEFENSIVE QI, TAI YANG QI AND THEIR TREATMENTS

Everyone who studies Chinese herbal medicine must know Cinnamon Twig Decoction (*guì zhī tāng*), a chief formula to adjust the nutritive qi and defensive qi for the disharmony between these two qi in tai yang disease. However, from where do these two qi, especially the defensive qi, come? How are the defensive qi and nutritive qi harmonized? These questions might be answered somewhat in textbooks for Discussion of Cold Damage in both Chinese and English. But these answers have not been comprehensive enough for understanding the function of Cinnamon Twig Decoction (*guì zhī tāng*). Furthermore, what exactly happens in the context of the disharmony between the nutritive qi and the defensive qi when wind-cold attacks the body? How do internal disorders (except kidney yin deficiency) cause the disharmony between the nutritive qi and the defensive qi? What difference is there between Cinnamon Twig Decoction (*guì zhī tāng*) and Ephedra Decoction (*má huáng tāng*) in working with the nutritive qi and defensive qi? These questions remain without clear answers. Based on reviewing Basic Questions of The Yellow Emperor's Inner Classic (*huáng dì nèi jīng sù wèn*), Discussion of Cold Damage, and related articles published since 1982, in this chapter I give relatively thorough answers to these questions.

From where does the defensive qi come? Does it originate in the upper burner or lower burner?

In Basic Questions of The Yellow Emperor's Inner Classic (*huáng dì nèi jīng sù wèn*), there are many instances in which the theory of the nutritive qi and defensive qi are quite intensively discussed. According to my calculations, there are a total of five chapters (Chapter 16, 18, 52, 59 and 72) devoted to discussion of the theory of the defensive qi and/or nutritive qi in Spiritual Pivot (靈樞經 *líng shū jīng*). Among these chapters, Chapter 18 is the most important, since it provides basic information for the production and circulation of the nutritive qi and defensive qi. In regard to the production of these two qi and their circulation, it states:

> The human body receives qi from [transformation of] food. Food enters the stomach and what is processed and absorbed from the food is transported to the lung. In this way, all five zang organs and six fu organs are nourished by this qi from food. The clear one in this qi is called the nutritive qi and the turbid one in this qi is called the defensive qi. The nutritive qi circulates in the vessels while the defensive qi circulates outside of the vessels… The Yellow Emperor says, "I would like to know the circulation of the nutritive qi and defensive qi, especially where they start." Qi Bo answers, "The circulation of the nutritive qi starts in the middle burner, while the circulation of the defensive qi starts in the lower burner (榮出中焦，衛出下焦 *róng chū zhōng jiāo, wèi chū xià jiāo*)."[1]

The word "starts" is the translation I use for the character "出 *chū*." Historically, there have been debates about where the defensive qi comes from based on how to interpret this character. According to Origin of Chinese Characters (辭源 *cí yuán*), "出 *chū*" bears two meanings in ancient literature: "something which comes out from inside" or "generates."[2] Scholars who believe that this character bears the former meaning would state that the defensive qi comes from the upper burner, while scholars who believe that this character bears the latter meaning would state that the defensive qi comes from the lower burner.

The first scholar who clearly put forward the idea that the defensive qi comes from the upper burner was Yang Shang-Shan (c. 666 AD). He writes that "the defensive qi starts at the upper burner and circulates towards the eyes…"[3] Yang's idea was echoed in ancient times by many famous scholars such as Sun Si-Miao, Wang Tao and Zhang Zhi-Cong. For example, in his work, Commentaries for Spiritual Pivot of The Yellow Emperor's Inner Classic (靈樞經集注 *líng shū jīng jí zhù*) published in 1672, Zhang Zhi-Cong points out:

> The character "下 *xià* (lower)" should be printed as "上 *shàng* (upper)" since the defensive qi is a kind of brave qi processed from food

1 Anonymous. *Spiritual Pivot* (*líng shū jīng*). Beijing: People's Health Publishing House, 1963: 51

2 Editorial Department of Business Publishing House. *Origin of Chinese Characters* (*cí yuán*). Beijing: Business Publishing House, 1980: 334

3 Yang Shang-Shan. *Simplicity of The Yellow Emperor's Inner Classic* (*huáng dì nèi jīng tài sú*). Beijing: People's Health Publishing House, 1955: 78

by yang ming and distributed to the exterior to defend the body from the upper burner.[4]

Many contemporary scholars who follow Yang's idea have found many sentences or paragraphs from The Yellow Emperor's Inner Classic to prove the truth of this statement. For example, Shi Zheng-Chu has cited the following paragraphs to demonstrate that this statement is indeed an idea recorded in this classic. He writes:

> In the chapter "Adjustment of Channels" of Basic Questions (Chapter 62), it states that "yang qi comes from the upper burner and the function of yang qi is to warm the skin and muscles." One can learn that yang qi in this paragraph includes the defensive qi from the sentence, "the function of yang qi is to warm the skin and muscles…" In the chapter "On Different Kinds of Qi" of Spiritual Pivot (Chapter 30), it states again that "the dispersing function of the upper burner is supposed to distribute what is processed from food for warming the skin, supporting the extremities, moistening hairs like moving fogs. This is called qi." The qi that warms the skin, supports the extremities and moistens hairs refers to the defensive qi.[5]

All of these original records in The Yellow Emperor's Inner Classic have made the statement that the defensive qi comes from the upper burner stand very well. However, it does not mean that the statement that the defensive qi comes from the lower burner is not true. Based on his research, especially checking Acupuncture Jia and Yi Classic (針灸甲乙經 *zhēn jiǔ jiǎ yǐ jīng*) written by Huang Fu-Mi (215–282 AD) and published c. 256 AD, Jiang You-Li points out:

> Acupuncture Jia and Yi Classic was written by Huang Fu-Mi based on compiling contents from Basic Questions, Spiritual Pivot and Keys to Choose Points for Acupuncture and Moxibustion from Bright Hall (明堂孔穴針灸治要 *míng táng kǒng xué zhēn jiǔ zhì yaò*). In this book, the sentence "the defensive qi comes from the lower burner" was clearly recorded. Since the time when Hung was alive was not so far from the time when The Yellow Emperor's Inner Classic was completed, what it recorded should be convincing. Therefore, the sentence that the defensive

4 Zhang Zhi-Cong. *Collection of Commentaries on Spiritual Pivot of The Yellow Emperor's Inner Classic* (*líng shū jīng jí zhù*). In Zheng Lin et al. (eds) *Complete Medical Works by Zhang Zhi-Cong* (*zhāng zhì-cōng yī xué quán shū*). Beijing: China Publishing House of Traditional Chinese Medicine, 2005: 449

5 Shi Zheng-Chu. "Discussion of the relationship between 'The Defensive Qi Comes from the Lower Burner' and 'The Defensive Qi Comes from the Upper Burner'." *The Journal of Wen Zhou Medical College*, 1982 (2): 79

> qi comes from the lower burner is indeed the original text in The Yellow Emperor's Inner Classic.[6]

Similarly, scholars who hold it to be true that the defensive qi comes from the lower burner have also cited much concrete evidence to prove this statement. Yang Dian-Xing, a scholar from Chengdu University of Traditional Chinese Medicine, has pointed out:

> Circulation of the defensive qi, especially moving in and out, is related to the kidney. The chapter "Invasion of Pathological Factors" [Chapter 71] of Spiritual Pivot states that "[the defensive qi] circulates in the yang part of the body during the day and in the yin part of the body during the night. It often moves from the foot shao yin channel to the other zang-fu organs."
>
> The chapter "Circulation of the Defensive Qi" [Chapter 76] of Spiritual Pivot states that "the defensive qi circulates in the yang part of the body during the day and in the yin part of the body during the night." When it enters the yin part of the body, it often moves from the foot shao yin channel to the kidney, from the kidney to the heart, from the heart to the lung, from the lung to the liver, from the liver to the spleen and from the spleen back to the kidney to complete a cycle of the circulation.[7]

Furthermore, the following citation from The Yellow Emperor's Inner Classic might be strong enough to show how the defensive qi moves from the kidney to reach the body surface:

> The kidney corresponds to the three burners and urinary bladder. And the three burners and urinary bladder correspond with the interstices and hairs on the skin...[8] Clear yang qi can reach the interstices between the skin, muscles, tendons and bones...and nourish limbs.[9]

Based on this special relationship between the body surface, three burners, urinary bladder and kidney in regard to the production and distribution of the defensive qi, the disease progression from tai yang to shao yin is discussed in Chapter 33 of Basic Questions:

---

6 Jiang You-Li. On "The defensive qi comes from the lower burner." *Journal of Traditional Chinese Medicine*, 1981 (12): 13

7 Yang Dian-Xing. "Exploring how the defensive qi originates from the lower burner." *Sichuan Journal of Traditional Chinese Medicine*, 1989 (3): 2

8 Anonymous, op. cit., p.92

9 Wang Bing. *Basic Questions of The Yellow Emperor's Inner Classic* (*huáng dì nèi jīng sù wèn*). Beijing: People's Health Publishing House, 1963: 32

> Tai yang is in charge of the defensive qi and is first attacked by exogenous pathological factors. Because tai yang and shao yin are related to each other externally and internally, when shao yin is affected by the heat in tai yang, its qi can follow this heat to rebel, leading to wind-jue syndrome.[10]

Since the stomach is mentioned in the production of the defensive qi, historically, some scholars like Zhang Deng-Ben asserted that "the defensive qi comes from the middle burner."[11] Because the lung, stomach, spleen and kidney are involved in different periods of the distribution of the defensive qi, it is not a mistake to state that the defensive qi comes from the upper, middle and lower burners. However, because the different burners play different roles in the initial, middle and final distribution of defensive qi, it would be more precise to state that the defensive qi originates from the kidney in the lower burner, is supported and nourished by the spleen and stomach in the middle burner and is dispersed by the lung in the upper burner.

As is generally known, Zhang Ji did study The Yellow Emperor's Inner Classic for writing Discussion of Cold Damage and formulating the six conformations differentiation. Of course, his work reflects this study, especially the theory of the nutritive qi and defensive qi set up by The Yellow Emperor's Inner Classic. Although Zhang Ji did not talk of the physiological functions of these two qi directly, one can assume that he indeed used this theory in his analysis and treatment for externally contracted diseases. In Discussion of Cold Damage, he uses the terms "defensive qi" and "nutritive qi" quite a few times in lines 53, 54 and 95. In line 3 of Chapter 5 of Essentials and Formula Discussions from the Golden Cabinet (金匱要略方論 *jīn gùi yào lüè fāng lùn*), a companion book to Discussion of Cold Damage written by him, he writes:

> The pulses are slow and relatively weak on the distal position. The slow pulse indicates the invasion of cold, while the relatively weak pulse denotes deficiency. If there are deep and relatively weak pulses, it indicates the deficiency of the nutritive qi, which can develop into blood deficiency; if there are floating and relatively weak pulses, it indicates the deficiency of the defensive qi, which can be subject to the invasion of wind.[12]

10 Ibid., p.195

11 Zhang Deng-Ben. "Answers to questions regarding 'The Defensive Qi Comes from the Lower Burner'." *Shanxi Journal of Traditional Chinese Medicine*, 1981 (6): 41

12 Zhang Ji. *Essentials and Formula Discussions from the Golden Cabinet* (*jīn gùi yào lüè fāng lùn*). Textually researched and annotated by Wen Di. Beijing: Chinese Publishing House, 1993: 28

Obviously, Zhang Ji applied the theory of nutritive qi and defensive qi, especially that the defensive qi is in charge of defending the body and the nutritive qi is part of the composition of the blood, to disease differentiation in his clinical practice. Interestingly, Zhang Ji likes to mention both terms, especially putting them together in one sentence or even one phrase in tai yang disease. Why did Zhang Ji do so in Discussion of Cold Damage? This question was answered by research from ancient scholars, the idea that "tai yang is a fence for the body as it contains the nutritive qi and defensive qi, and defends the body surface." In his book, Treatise on Discussion of Cold Damage (傷寒論條辨 *shāng hán lùn tĭao biàn*) published in 1592, Fang You-Zhi (1523–1594), a famous scholar who commented on this classic, first put forward this idea. He writes:

> Tai yang refers to the channel of the urinary bladder...[the urinary bladder channel] is a big one among six channels. It governs the skin and is in charge of the nutritive qi and defensive qi. Therefore, tai yang is the first layer to be attacked by exogenous pathological factors.[13]

Fang's idea for interpretation of the function of tai yang has had tremendous influence on both ancient and contemporary scholars in their studies for Discussion of Cold Damage and has been well received by them. However, this idea has been challenged by the following question raised by Xue Zhen-Bin:

> Someone wants to prove this idea based on the fact that tai yang is the biggest and longest channel and connects to Du 16. But foot tai yang channel is only one of the channels over the body and it is just a partial way for the circulation of the nutritive qi and defensive qi. It can fall into the category of tai yang [Zhang] Zhong-Jing set up. But it would be difficult to convince one that the foot tai yang channel is in charge of the nutritive qi and defensive qi and governs the body surface![14]

Facing such challenge, scholars who wrote the reference book of Discussion of Cold Damage for students in medical colleges avoided use of the term "tai yang channel" and introduced the term "tai yang" to present this idea. They wrote that "tai yang governs the body surface and is in charge of

---

13 Fang You-Zhi. "Treatise on Discussion of Cold Damage (*shāng hán lùn tĭao biàn*)." In Business Publishing House (ed.) *Three Books on Discussion of Cold Damage* (*shāng hán lùn zhù sān zhŏng*). Beijing: Business Publishing House, 1957: 7

14 Xue Zhen-Bin. "Preliminary exploration of the idea that tai yang is in charge of the nutritive qi and defensive qi." *Shanxi Journal of Traditional Chinese Medicine*, 1985 (10): 434

the nutritive qi and defensive qi. It provides the protection for the body surface."[15] What does the term "tai yang" mean when studying Discussion of Cold Damage? Based on the theory of qi transformation, tai yang does not only mean the foot and hand tai yang channels. It does not only refer to the urinary bladder and small intestine either. It includes all of them and other organs such as the heart, lung, spleen and kidney, especially in terms of the production and movement of the defensive qi. In order to understand tai yang comprehensively, it is necessary to introduce the term "tai yang qi" or "qi of tai yang." Based on the discussion above, there is agreement that the nutritive qi and defensive qi are main components for tai yang qi regardless of it referring to the narrow sense of tai yang, i.e. only the channel, or the broad sense of tai yang, i.e. all things involved in the production and movement of these two qi. But where does this tai yang qi come from and how does it affect the differentiation and treatment for diseases in Discussion of Cold Damage? This question is answered in the next section.

Tai yang qi in six conformations in Discussion of Cold Damage

No one can find the term "tai yang qi" or come across any line to discuss the production and movement of tai yang qi in Discussion of Cold Damage. What we can do is to review the lines related to proving whether or not Zhang Ji followed the theory of the nutritive qi and defensive qi discussed in The Yellow Emperor's Inner Classic and develop some new ideas for this theory.

First, Zhang Ji did apply the theory of the nutritive qi and defensive qi recorded in The Yellow Emperor's Inner Classic. He consciously knew that nutritive qi is part of the composition of blood since he wrote in line 50:

> When the pulse is floating and tight, there should be general aches and pain. It is suitable to resolve the illness by the promotion of sweating. However, if the pulse is slow at the proximal position, one cannot promote sweating. On what basis does one know this? It is because the nutritive qi is not sufficient and blood is deficient.

Based on the treatment including herbs and administration of herbs, we can see that Zhang Ji clearly understood that tai yang qi comes from the

15 Li Pei-Sheng et al. *Teaching Reference Books for Traditional Chinese Medical Colleges: Discussion of Cold Damage (gāo děng zhōng yī yuàn xiào jiào xué cān káo shū: shāng hán lùn)*. Beijing: People's Health Publishing House, 1987: 10

lung, heart, spleen and kidney, which locate in the upper, middle and lower burners, respectively. In line 35, he proposed Ephedra Decoction (*má huáng tāng*) for the complete obstruction of the nutritive qi and defensive qi due to invasion of wind-cold, in which Ephedrae Herba (*má huáng*) is considered most important agent that can distribute the defensive qi from the lung to the skin to support tai yang qi. In lines 64, 112, 117 and 118, he recorded that tai yang disease would progress to yang deficiency of the heart if the fire needle is mistakenly used or sweating is mistakenly promoted. This progression is evidenced by applying formulas in which Cinnamomi Ramulus (*guì zhī*), a herb to enter the heart and warm the channel, serves as a chief agent. This indicates that tai yang qi, especially the nutritive qi, is related to the heart as the heart pumps the blood, and the nutritive qi is part of the blood. Ke Qin, a scholar who specialized in Discussion Cold Damage in the seventeenth century, paid much more attention to the relationship between tai yang qi and the heart and lung. He writes:

> The nutritive qi and defensive qi circulate on the body surface but they originate from the heart and the lung. Therefore, when tai yang is attacked, the nutritive qi and defensive qi will not function well. If there is dysfunction of the nutritive qi and defensive qi, the heart and lung will be in trouble.[16]

In line 12, not only Zingiberis Rhizoma Recens (*shēng jiāng*) and Jujubae Fructus (*dà zǎo*), which are considered to tonify and adjust qi for the spleen and stomach, are chosen to formulate Cinnamon Twig Decoction (*guì zhī tāng*), but also rice porridge, a diet formula to support the middle burner is used in seeking help from the spleen and stomach for supporting the nutritive qi and defensive qi. Many more examples can be found in the text of Discussion of Cold Damage for proving that Zhang Ji was very fond of the idea that the defensive qi comes from the lower burner and developed his unique way to deal with the syndromes related to the disorders of the defensive qi. Interestingly, Zhang Ji did not use Astragali Radix (*huáng qí*) and Codonopsis Radix (*dǎng shēn*), agents with sweet and warm properties, to tonify the lung and spleen for supporting the defensive qi; rather, he specially chose Aconiti Radix Lateralis (*fù zǐ*), an acrid and hot herb to warm and tonify the yang of the kidney for the deficiency of the defensive qi. Obviously, he strongly believed that the root of the defensive

---

16 Ke Qin. *Discussion of Special Topic in Cold Damage* (*shāng hán lái sū jí, shāng hán lùn yì*). Shanghai: Shanghai Science and Technology Publishing House, 1978: 27

qi stemmed from the kidney in the lower burner and tried to strengthen the defensive qi through warming and tonifying yang in the kidney. Such practices can be found in lines 20, 22, 68, 91, 92 and 155.

Second, Zhang Ji noticed that tai yang qi has something to do with shao yang, chong and uterus, based on his observation of the progression of tai yang disease. In lines 143–145, Zhang Ji recorded that Minor Bupleurum Decoction (*xiǎo chái hú tāng*) would work very well for what is called "the syndrome of invasion of the blood chamber (the uterus and chong channel) by heat," in which there is fever or alternating chills and fever due to the stagnation of the defensive qi. The elegant approach that makes this treatment effective is that it attaches great importance to shao yang, the pivot that helps qi move from the kidney to the body surface through the pivot function of shao yang, rather than the lung, heart, spleen and stomach in the upper and middle burners, respectively, for normalizing the defensive qi. Because chong channel originates from the kidney and uterus and attaches to the kidney, once qi in the kidney moves to the body surface through the pivot of shao yang, not only heat in the blood chamber will be pushed out through this pivot, but also the defensive qi will be reinforced and circulation of the defensive qi will be normalized for eliminating the stagnation of the defensive qi on the body surface.

Since invasion of the blood chamber by heat can give rise to fever or alternating fever and chills due to the stagnation of the defensive qi and effective treatment is to work on the pivot function of shao yang, it is reasonable to assume that the circulation of the defensive qi, one part of tai yang qi, is related to the pivot function of shao yang, chong and uterus, i.e. the defensive qi originates from the kidney, moves to the chong channel and uterus, and further circulates to the skin through shao yang and interstices (腠 *còu*), its corresponding part on the body surface. This is just one route for the defensive qi to move from the kidney to the body surface. Unfortunately, this route has been largely ignored by scholars and practitioners in their studies and practices, though it has been present in Discussion of Cold Damage for more than 1800 years. Knowing this circulation route for the defensive qi can help explain why women easily catch cold particularly during their menstruation. This is the first route for the production and distribution of the defensive qi. The second one is that it moves from the kidney to the spleen and the body surface and is dispersed to the body surface by the lung. The third one is from the kidney to the urinary bladder and its channel before finally reaching the body surface.

Another contribution made by Zhang Ji for the distribution of the defensive qi is that he noticed that the chest can serve as a pathway for this qi distributed from the heart and/or the lung to the body surface. These relationships can be proven by the fact that tai yang disease can progress to the chest, leading to either stagnant heat in the chest and diaphragm or the chest-binding syndrome (see lines 76–79, 131 and 134–138 for further details).

In summary, there are three routes for the qi to move from the kidney to the body surface and distribute the defensive qi. They all originate from the kidney. All information related to these three routes is illustrated in Figure 8.1.

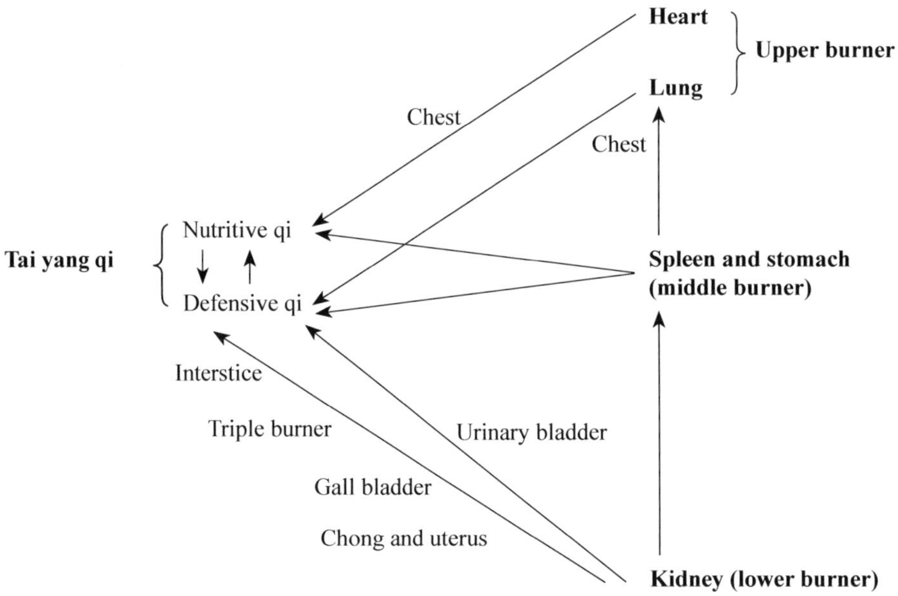

FIGURE 8.1 THE PRODUCTION AND DISTRIBUTION OF TAI YANG QI

Bearing Figure 8.1 in mind, one can predict the possible progressions from tai yang disease and know how to ask questions to check or rule out these progressing possibilities. Having studied the chapter that deals with tai yang disease in Discussion of Cold Damage, I found that Zhang Ji indeed observed progressions due to the disorder of the production and/or distribution of tai yang qi in his clinical practice. Table 8.1 on page 196 summarizes these progressions in tai yang disease.

According to Chapter 18 of Spiritual Pivot of The Yellow Emperor's Inner Classic, the defensive qi circulates outside the vessels while the nutritive qi circulates inside the vessels. Does the defensive qi only circulate outside the vessels and the nutritive qi only circulate inside the vessels? How does one treat the disorders of the nutritive qi and defensive qi simultaneously? These questions are answered in detail in the next section.

Relationship between the nutritive qi and the defensive qi and the treatments for their disorders

Readers who have carefully read Discussion of Cold Damage might notice that Zhang Ji paid much attention to the relationship between these two qi as evidenced by lines such as "this is because the defensive qi is not in harmony with the nutritive qi" (line 53), "this means that the defensive qi is not harmonious" (line 54) and "weakness of the nutritive qi and unreasonable strength of the defensive qi…" (line 95). As a matter of fact, the authors who wrote The Yellow Emperor's Inner Classic noticed that the nutritive qi and the defensive qi do not completely separate outside and inside the vessels. In Chapter 52 of Spiritual Pivot (靈樞經 *líng shū jīng*), a chapter titled "On the Defensive Qi," they write:

> In essence, qi processed from food, the qi that circulates outside the vessels, is called the defensive qi, while the very delicate one that circulates inside the vessels is called the nutritive qi. They flow with each other like yin and yang and connect to each other outside and inside the vessels like a loop.[17]

Zhao Yi-Kong, a scholar who lived c. 1934, further explained how these two qi connect to each other. He explained that "although the defensive qi circulates outside the vessels, it interacts with the nutritive qi inside the vessels; although the nutritive qi circulates inside the vessels, it interacts with the defensive qi outside the vessels."[18] However, detailed information in this context has not been provided by past scholars. Based on my study and clinical practice for more than three decades, the following explanation for the harmonious relationship between the nutritive qi and the defensive qi is offered:

17 Anonymous, op. cit., p.100

18 Cai Lu-Xian. Section 16 of *Collections of Chinese Medical Literature* (*zhōng guó yī yào huì hǎi shí liù juàn*). Shanghai: Chinese Publishing House, 1941: 228

Table 8.1 Progressions and treatments in tai yang disease caused by the disorder of production and distribution of tai yang qi

Cause for progression	Organ(s) in which progression occurred	Line(s) in Discussion of Cold Damage	Formulas recommended
After improper promotion of sweating, purging and vomiting	Lung	41, 42	Minor Bluegreen Dragon Decoction (*xiǎo qīng lóng tāng*)
	Heart	64	Cinnamon Twig and Licorice Decoction (*guì zhī gān cǎo tāng*)
	Interstices	39, 40	Major Bluegreen Dragon Decoction (*dà qīng lóng tāng*)
	Shao yang	37, 96	Minor Bupleurum Decoction (*xiǎo chái hú tāng*)
	Chest and diaphragm	76–79	Gardenia and Prepared Soybean Decoction (*zhī zǐ chǐ táng*)
	Chest	21, 22	Cinnamon Twig Decoction minus Peony (*guì zhī qù sháo yào tāng*), Cinnamon Twig Decoction minus Peony plus Aconite Accessory Root (*guì zhī qù sháo yào jiā fù zǐ tāng*)
	Chest	131, 134–137	Major Decoction [for pathogens] Stuck in the Chest (*dà xiàn xiōng tāng*)
	Chest	138	Minor Decoction [for pathogens] Stuck in the Chest (*xiǎo xiàn xiōng tāng*)
	Spleen	163	Cinnamon Twig and Ginseng Decoction (*guì zhī rén shēn tāng*)
	Spleen	29	Licorice and Dry Ginger Decoction (*gān cǎo gān jiāng tāng*)

	Spleen	67	Poria, Cinnamon Twig, Atractylodes, and Licorice Decoction (*fú líng guì zhī bái zhú gān cǎo tāng*)
	Stomach	26, 168, 169	White Tiger plus Ginseng Decoction (*bái hǔ jiā rén shēn tāng*)
	Spleen and stomach	149, 155, 157, 158	Pinellia Decoction to Drain the Epigastrium (*bàn xià xiè xīn tāng*), Fresh Ginger Decoction to Drain the Epigastrium (*shēng jiāng xiè xīn tāng*), and Licorice Decoction to Drain the Epigastrium (*gān cǎo xiè xīn tāng*)
	Small intestine and large intestine	34	Pueraria, Scutellaria, and Coptis Decoction (*gé gēn huáng qín huáng lián tāng*)
	Urinary bladder	71, 72	Five-Ingredient Powder with Poria (*wù líng sǎn*)
	Urinary bladder	106, 124–126	Peach Pit Decoction to Order the Qi (*táo hé chéng qì tāng*) Appropriate Decoction (*dǐ dàng tāng*), and Appropriate Pill (*dǐ dàng wán*)
	Uterus and chong channel	143–145	Minor Bupleurum Decoction (*xiǎo chái hú tāng*)
	Kidney	29	Frigid Extremities Decoction (*sì nì tāng*)
	Kidney	82	True Warrior Decoction (*zhēn wǔ tāng*)

In light of the theory of yin and yang, the nutritive qi, which belongs to yin, and the defensive qi, which belongs to yang, should communicate and promote each other. Therefore, some defensive qi enters the vessels to warm nutritive qi while most of it remains circulating outside the vessels. Nutritive qi and defensive qi meet inside the vessels where the defensive qi warms the nutritive qi, which is a precursor of the blood. After being warmed, there will be two things taking place for the nutritive qi: one is the nutritive qi that goes out of the vessels to support the defensive qi, which has already circulated there; another is that some of it will transform into body fluid, which also goes out of the vessels to moisten and nourish the tendons, muscles and skin. In turn, when the defensive qi is supported, it can protect the nutritive qi and make it mostly circulate inside the vessels. In this way, yin and yang, the nutritive qi and defensive qi, are in a state where they communicate with and support each other, making the skin and muscles warm, and nourishing the muscles and tendons.

Because the nutritive qi circulates mostly in the vessels and is a precursor of blood, it brings the spirit (神 *shēn*) back and forth between the body surface and the heart. When this harmonization condition is normal, one can have normal feeling on the skin, tendons and muscles. This is the harmonious condition between the nutritive qi and the defensive qi which takes place outside and inside the vessels. Figure 8.2 demonstrates the relationship between these two qi.

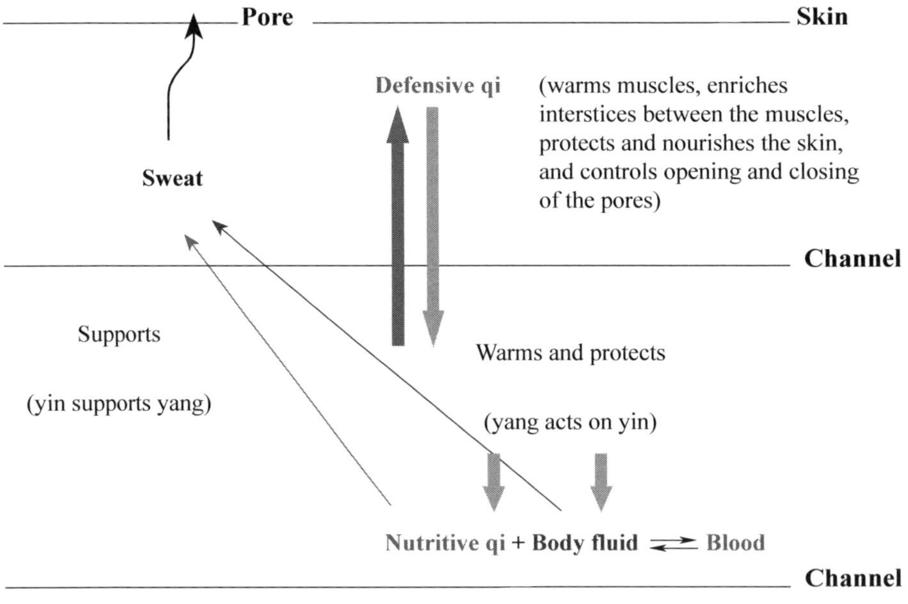

Figure 8.2 Normal relationship between the nutritive qi and the defensive qi

Since tai yang qi consists of the nutritive qi and defensive qi, which circulates on the body surface, the function of the nutritive qi, the defensive qi and their relationship are compromised when exogenous pathological factors attack the body surface. Therefore, some scholars who specialized in studying Discussion of Cold Damage would consider the disorders of these two qi as the main pathology of tai yang disease. In his book, True Classification and Analysis for Lines in Discussion of Cold Damage (傷寒論後條辨 *shāng hán lùn hòu tĭao biàn*) published in 1670, Cheng Ying-Mao pointed out that "when talking tai yang disease, one should know that the skin is attacked by pathological factors and the disease locates among the interstices, the nutritive qi and defensive qi."[19]

Han Xiang-Ling and colleagues have even used the theory of the nutritive qi and the defensive qi to explain the first line of the chapter on tai yang disease:

> The presentation of "a floating pulse, headache, ache and stiffness on the nape of the neck and aversion to cold" in the outline of tai yang disease are caused by the disharmony between the nutritive qi and the defensive qi. Tai yang governs the body surface where the nutritive qi and defensive qi circulate. Therefore, tai yang would be first attacked when wind-cold invades the body. Because anti-pathogenic qi is strong, it is capable of fighting with wind-cold on the body surface.
>
> The nutritive qi and defensive qi circulate inside and outside the vessels, respectively, and they rise up against wind-cold, leading to a floating pulse. Wind-cold attacks the channel of tai yang and interferes with the circulation of the nutritive qi and defensive qi since the nape of the neck is the place where the tai yang channel goes. Obstruction of qi produces pain. Therefore, there is ache and stiffness on the nape. When both qi fight with wind-cold, the circulation of the defensive qi is stagnated, leading to inability of the defensive qi to warm the muscles, resulting in aversion to cold. Therefore, it can be stated that tai yang disease is caused by the disharmony between the nutritive qi and the defensive qi.[20]

19 Cheng Ying-Mao. *True Classification and Analysis for Lines in Discussion of Cold Damage and Supplementary After-Reading Discussion of Cold Damage* (*shāng hán lùn hòu tiáo biàn, dú shāng hán lùn zhuì yú*). Beijing: China Publishing House of Traditional Chinese Medicine, 2009: 174

20 Han Xiang-Ling et al. "The disharmony between the nutritive qi and the defensive qi, and Cinnamon Twig Decoction (*guì zhī tāng*)." *Tianjin Journal of Traditional Chinese Medicine*, 2000 (6): 35

According to He Xin-Hui, there are four types of disharmony between the nutritive qi and the defensive qi discussed in Discussion of Cold Damage. They are unreasonable strength of the defensive qi and weakness of the nutritive qi (line 12), weakness of the defensive qi and harmony of the nutritive qi (lines 53 and 54), weakness of both the nutritive qi and the defensive qi (lines 42, 240 and 387) and the unreasonable strength of the defensive qi and stagnation of the nutritive qi (line 35).[21] I agree with these classifications but offer a different interpretation for "the nutritive qi is in harmony" in line 53, as it is merely a literal translation. One should understand that the nutritive qi does not function as well; otherwise, it would not make any sense to use the character "和 *hé* (harmony)," which means at least normal interaction between two things (see line 53, and Chapter 7 of the present book, for further details.) The subsequent discussion would focus on two typical syndromes of the disharmony between the nutritive qi and the defensive qi caused by invasion of wind-cold.

When there is more than one pathological factor of invasion, one should identify which is predominant. Therefore, when there is wind-cold attack, Zhang Ji demonstrated this detailed differentiation skill and classified the attacks into what is called "中風 *zhòng fēng*" and "傷寒 *shāng hán*," in which wind is predominant in "中風 *zhòng fēng*" and cold is predominant in "傷寒 *shāng hán*."

When wind is predominant, the pores on the skin will be forced to open, which makes an avenue for sweating since wind is characterized as outgoing in nature. Consequently, the defensive qi rises to fight against wind-cold and gets stagnation on the body surface. Finally, it fails to warm the skin, close and open pores on the skin properly and protect the nutritive qi, resulting in aversion to cold, chills, body ache, fever and spontaneous sweating. All of these symptoms compromise the communication between the nutritive qi and the defensive qi inside and outside the channels. This is one type of disharmony between the nutritive qi and the defensive qi. It is called "陽浮陰弱 *yáng fú yīn rùo*' in line 12, which can be translated into "floating yang and weakness of yin" or "營弱衛強 *róng rùo wèi qīang*," which means weakness of the nutritive qi and unreasonable strength of the defensive qi in line 95. (Weakness of nutritive qi merely means leakage of the nutritive qi and it by no means indicates deficiency of

21 He Xin-Hui. "Exploration of the syndrome of the disharmony between the nutritive qi and the defensive qi." *Forum for Chinese Medical Doctors*, 1998 (1): 4

the nutritive qi which requires tonification clinically, while unreasonable strength of the defensive qi means stagnation of the defensive qi.) It is this stagnation of the defensive qi that makes the defensive qi fail to do its job in warming the skin, closing pores on the skin and protecting nutritive qi, leading to spontaneous sweating. Figure 8.3 offers a picture for this kind of disharmony between the nutritive qi and the defensive qi in zhong feng syndrome, in which wind is predominant.

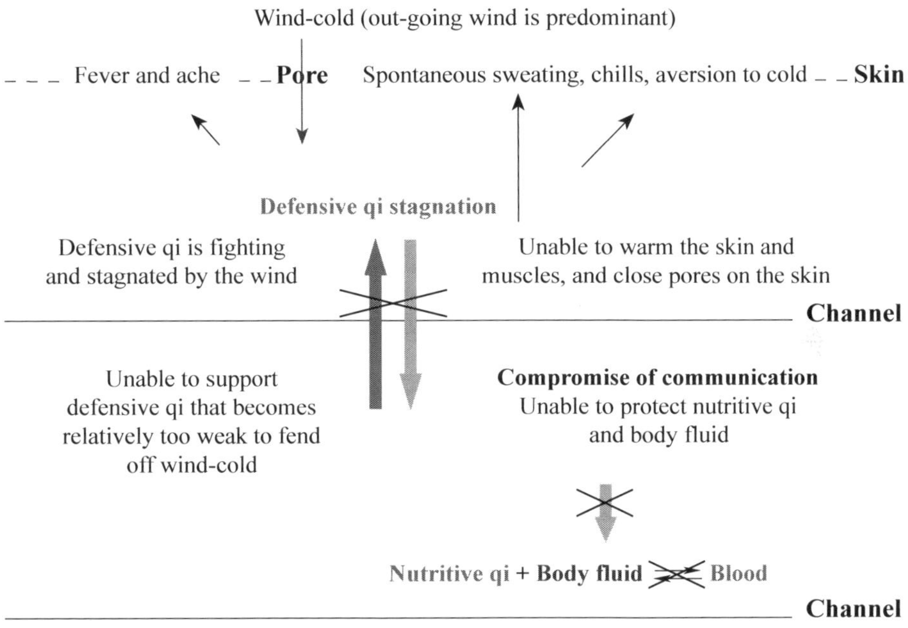

FIGURE 8.3 DISHARMONY BETWEEN THE NUTRITIVE QI AND THE DEFENSIVE QI IN ZHONG FENG SYNDROME DUE TO INVASION OF WIND-COLD IN WHICH WIND IS PREDOMINANT

When cold is predominant, the pores on the skin will be forced to close since cold is characterized by contraction. This makes broader and deeper obstructions on the body surface, i.e. not only congealment of the defensive qi but also the obstruction of the nutritive qi among the skin, muscle, tendons and bones, leading not only to fever and aversion to cold but also to absence of sweating, general ache and pain, muscle pain and joint pain, or even panting. All of these symptoms are caused by the obstruction of the nutritive qi and defensive qi. One can call this "complete obstruction of the nutritive qi and defensive qi," which is another type of disharmony between the nutritive qi and the defensive qi (see lines 3 and

35 for further details). Figure 8.4 demonstrates what happens for this kind of disharmony between these two qi in shang han syndrome, in which cold is predominant.

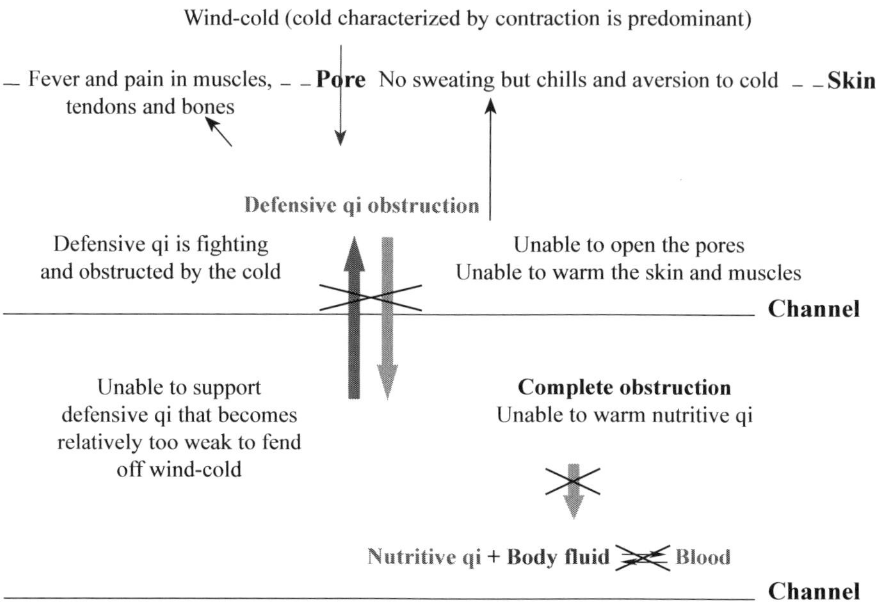

Figure 8.4 Disharmony between the nutritive qi and the defensive qi in shang han syndrome due to invasion of wind-cold in which cold is predominant

Comparing Figure 8.4 with Figure 8.3, one might notice that the location of the disease is slightly different, though both share the disharmony of the nutritive qi and defensive qi. The zhong feng syndrome caused by wind-cold, in which wind is predominant, only affects the muscles and skin, while the shang han syndrome caused by wind-cold, in which cold is predominated, affects the skin through to the bones. Why is there such difference in the regard of the location on the body surface? Because wind is a yang pathological factor and is likely to attack superficial parts of the body, while cold is a yin pathological factor and is likely to penetrate to deeper parts of the body. Figure 8.5 illustrates this rationale.

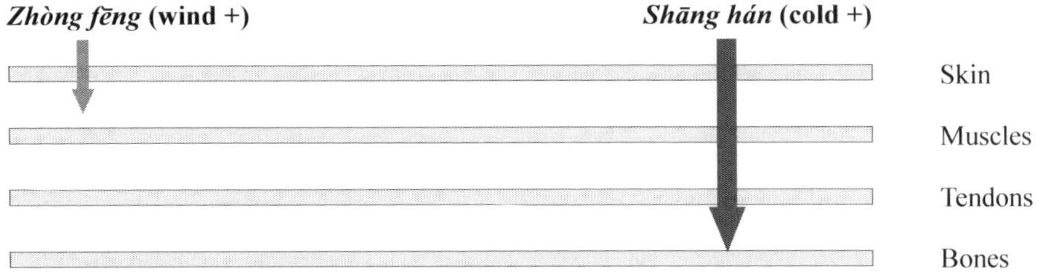

FIGURE 8.5 DIFFERENCE IN THE LOCATION OF TAI YANG DISEASE ON THE BODY SURFACE IN ZHONG FENG SYNDROME AND SHANG HAN SYNDROME DUE TO PREDOMINANCE OF WIND OR COLD

Because several internal organs, such as the kidney, urinary bladder, uterus, chong channel, shao yang, spleen, stomach, lung and heart, are involved in the production and distribution of tai yang qi, which includes the nutritive qi and the defensive qi, is there any chance that the disharmony between the nutritive qi and the defensive qi could be caused by the disorders of those organs? The answer is yes, theoretically. When there is no external pathological factor attack but internal disorder due to the dysfunction of any of those organs, disharmony between the nutritive qi and the defensive qi can occur. For example, I have used Cinnamon Twig Decoction (*guì zhī tāng*) to successfully cure women with feverish feeling and spontaneous sweating during menstruation, which bothered the patient for over 1.5 years.

In lines 12, 95 and 35, Zhang Ji offers two famous formulas to deal with two kinds of disharmony between the nutritive qi and the defensive qi discussed above. Based on my many years of study and practice, a relatively thorough analysis for comprehensively understanding how these two formulas recover the harmony function from these two kinds of disharmony is offered.

Cinnamon Twig Decoction (*guì zhī tāng*) is designed for weakness of the nutritive qi and unreasonable strength of the defensive qi, leading to compromise of communication between these two qi, the pathology of zhong feng syndrome in tai yang disease. With its red color, acrid flavor and warm nature, Cinnamomi Ramulus (*guì zhī*) enters the heart, which takes charge of blood circulation, warms the vessels, makes the nutritive qi warm and transforms it into the defensive qi and body fluid that becomes sweating, while slightly dispersing wind-cold. The sweating can serve as a substrate to carry wind-cold out of the body via the pores on the skin. With its sour and bitter flavor, Paeoniae Radix Alba (*bái sháo*) has three functions: to support the blood that can break into body fluid and the nutritive qi, to provide a source for the transformation mentioned above, especially a source of sweating initiated by Cinnamomi Ramulus (*guì zhī*), and to keep sweating in check to prevent damage to qi or body fluid. Zingiberis Rhizoma Recens (*shēng jiāng*) and Jujubae Fructus (*dà zǎo*) are used to reinforce the function of Cinnamomi Ramulus (*guì zhī*) and Paeoniae Radix Alba (*bái sháo*), respectively, in regard to dispersing wind-cold and nourishing the blood while seeking help for support of the nutritive qi and defensive qi from the spleen and stomach, which is one of the sources for the production of both types of qi. With its sweet flavor, Glycyrrhizae Radix Preparata (*zhì gān cǎo*) is not only a coordinator for this formula—it can also either support yin, which is the nutritive qi in this case, or support yang, which means the defensive qi in this case, because the combination of acrid and sweet can generate yang while the combination of sour and sweet can generate yin. After taking Cinnamon Twig Decoction (*guì zhī tāng*), wind-cold will be brought out by sweating and the harmonized relationship between the nutritive qi and the defensive qi will be recovered.

As discussed above, either invasion of wind-cold or internal disorders from organs related to the production or distribution of these two qi can be accountable for disharmony between them, leading to spontaneous sweating. In order to recover the harmonious relationship between these two qi, it is necessary to promote sweating again by Cinnamon Twig Decoction (*guì zhī tāng*), though the patient has already had spontaneous sweating. Clinically, some practitioners are afraid to use Cinnamon Twig Decoction (*guì zhī tāng*) for spontaneous sweating, because they do not understand the difference between sweating before and after treatment by Cinnamon Twig Decoction (*guì zhī tāng*) and worry that using it, which would promote sweating with warm nature and acrid flavor, can exacerbate the sweating the patient already has and damage qi or body fluid. Zhang Zhi-Cong first elaborated that "this line [line 53] discusses that Cinnamon Twig Decoction (*guì zhī tāng*) not only disperses the nutritive qi and defensive qi among qi and blood for sweating, but can also harmonize the nutritive qi and defensive qi among qi and blood to stop sweating."[22] Xu Da-Chun has further offered a very explicit explanation for the sweating before and after using Cinnamon Twig Decoction (*guì zhī tāng*):

> Spontaneous sweating and promoting sweating are quite different from each other. Spontaneous sweating is caused by the separation of the nutritive qi and defensive qi, while promotion of sweating is to make the nutritive qi and defensive qi harmonious. Spontaneous sweating will damage anti-pathological qi, while promotion of sweating will eliminate pathological factors. Making sweating again is for the sake of spontaneous sweating. In this way, the nutritive qi and defensive qi would be harmonized and the sweating would cease (rather than get worse after prompting sweating).[23]

Ephedra Decoction (*má huáng tāng*) is designed for the complete obstruction of the nutritive qi and defensive qi, the pathology of shang han syndrome in tai yang disease. With its acrid flavor and warm nature, Ephedrae Herba (*má huáng*) enters the lung, which governs the skin and hair, opens the pores on the skin, an indispensable avenue to dispel wind-cold, and makes the body surface ready for the sweating process promoted by Cinnamomi Ramulus (*guì zhī*). With its bitter flavor and warm nature, Armeniacae Semen Amarum (*xìng rén*) can descend the lung qi, which can indirectly enhance the dispersing function of Ephedrae Herba (*má huáng*) for the lung and elimination of wind-cold, as both the descending and dispersing functions of the lung rely on each other. Glycyrrhizae Radix Preparata (*zhì gān cǎo*) is not only a coordinator but it can also support yang when its sweet flavor mixes with the acrid flavor of Ephedrae Herba (*má huáng*). Compared with Cinnamon Twig Decoction (*guì zhī tāng*), Ephedra Decoction (*má huáng tāng*) is warmer and can vigorously activate yang since cold is predominant in this case. Without such warming nature and very active yang, the pores on the skin cannot be opened, complete obstruction of the nutritive qi and defensive qi inside and outside the vessels among the skin, muscles, tendons and bone cannot be resolved and there is no way for wind-cold, especially cold, to be eliminated from the body surface. Of course, Paeoniae Radix

22 Zhang Zhi-Cong, Collection of Commentaries for Discussion of Cold Damage (*shāng hán lùn jí zhù*), reproduced in Zheng Lin *et al.*, (ed.) Completed Medical Works by Zhang Zhi- Cong (*zhāng zhì-cōng yī xué quán shū*). Beijing: China Publishing House of Traditional Chinese Medicine, 2005: 638

23 Xu Da-Chun. *Classification of Formulas in Discussion of Cold Damage* (*shāng hán lùn lèi fāng*). Beijing: People's Health Publishing House, 1984: 5

Alba (*bái sháo*) is not appropriate since its sour flavor would exacerbate the obstruction of the nutritive qi and defensive qi and further trap wind-cold, therefore it is omitted in this formula. Because there is absence of sweating, the circulation of the nutritive qi and defensive qi is completely obstructed without any leakage of body fluid, there is no necessity to get a supply of the body fluid, the nutritive qi and defensive qi from the spleen and stomach. Therefore, Zingiberis Rhizoma Recens (*shēng jiāng*) and Jujubae Fructus (*dà zǎo*) are not employed for this case.

One might notice that the defensive qi is not always produced by the zang-fu organs internally, it can also be generated locally on the body surface, i.e. generated by the channels between the muscle, tendons and bones. Understanding this can benefit our treatment. For example, when the defensive qi is relatively weak but has not reached the point that is differentiated as deficiency, one can follow Zhang Ji's approach to add Cinnamomi Ramulus (*guì zhī*) and Paeoniae Radix Alba (*bái sháo*) to generate the defensive qi by acting on the nutritive qi in channels. Interestingly, the defensive qi does not always circulate with the nutritive qi along channels. In Chapter 43 of Basic Questions of Yellow Emperor's Inner Classic, another route of the circulation of the defensive qi is described as the following:

> The defensive qi is a brave qi generated from food. It moves smoothly and fast and is unable to enter the channels. Therefore, it circulates in the skin, among muscles, and steams to the membrane above the diaphragm and disperses in the chest and abdomen.[24]

A similar description for such circulation of the defensive qi can also be found in Chapter 71 of Spiritual Pivot of Yellow Emperor's Inner classic: "The defensive qi is a brave and fast-moving qi from food. It first circulates between the skins and muscles on extremities without stopping."[25] Apparently, the defensive qi has another route, which allows it to be distributed from the zang-fu organs directly to the body surface and do its job in warming muscles, enriching interstices between muscles, protecting and nourishing the skin, and controlling the opening and closing of the pores, rather than always circulating with the nutritive qi inside and outside the channels. As a matter of fact, if one reads Discussion of Cold Damage carefully, one might notice Zhang Ji demonstrates various ways

24 Wang Bing, op. cit., p.245

25 Anonymous, op. cit., p.244

to work with the defensive qi, i.e. dispersing it by Ephedrae Herba (*má huáng*) through the lung; supporting it by Aconiti Radix Lateralis (*fù zǐ*) through the kidney; distributing it by Bupleuri Radix (*chái hú*) through the pivot of shao yang; reinforcing it by Zingiberis Rhizoma Recens (*shēng jiāng*) and Jujubae Fructus (*dà zǎo*) through the spleen and the liver; harmonizing it by Cinnamomi Ramulus (*guì zhī*) and Paeoniae Radix Alba (*bái sháo*) through the heart and/or channels.

Since the defensive qi does not always circulate along the channels, there might be a chance that only the defensive qi is affected rather than both the defensive qi and nutritive qi, leading to a disharmony between them. For example, Chen Shi-Wen and colleagues recorded that wind can only attack the nose and throat, which are part of the lung system, leading to nose congestion and loss of voice, and this can be treated by Ephedrae Herba (*má huáng*), Armeniacae Semen Amarum (*xìng rén*) and Glycyrrhizae Radix Preparata (*zhì gān cǎo*), which is called Three-Unbinding Decoction (*sān ǎo tāng*).[26] Clinically, I have often used this formula to treat aversion to cold, cough or panting due to wind-cold attacks. Obviously, this is a modification of Ephedra Decoction (*má huáng tāng*), i.e. Ephedra Decoction minus Cinnamomi Ramulus (*guì zhī*). Why is Cinnamomi Ramulus (*guì zhī*) taken out from Three-Unbinding Decoction (*sān ǎo tāng*)? Because only the defensive qi and the lung are involved and the heart and the nutritive qi are normal, the treatment should focus on recovering the lung's function for the distribution of the defensive qi instead of normalizing the relationship between the nutritive qi and the defensive qi. Another example is the creation of Jade Windscreen Powder (*yù píng fēng sǎn*), which contains Astragali Radix (*huáng qí*), Atractylodis Macrocephalae Rhizoma (*bái zhú*) and Saposhnikoviae Radix (*fáng fēng*). This formula was originally recorded by Zhu Zhen-Heng (also known as Zhu Dan-Xi, 1281–1358) in his work, Teaching of (Zhu) Dan-Xi (丹溪心法 *dān xī xīn fǎ*) first published in 1465, and was designed to treat spontaneous sweating.[27] Wang Ang (also known as Wang Ren-An, 1615–1694) recorded that this formula can be used to treat a person who is vulnerable to catch cold due

26 Chen Shi-Wen, Chen Cheng and Pei Zong-Yuan (eds) *Imperial Grace Formulary of Tai Ping Era* (*tài píng huì míng hé jì jú fāng*). Beijing: People's Health Publishing House, 1959: 42

27 Zhu Zhen-Heng. *Teaching of (Zhu) Dan-Xi* (*dān xī xīn fǎ*). Beijing: China Publishing House of Traditional Chinese Medicine, 2008: 143

to the deficiency of the defensive qi.[28] Why did Zhu not use Cinnamon Twig Decoction (*guì zhī tāng*) to treat spontaneous sweating and why did Wang recommend it to prevent the body from being attacked by cold? Because they realized that the deficiency of the defensive qi in this case has nothing to do with the heart and/or the nutritive qi. The lung is the organ to be held accountable for the deficiency of the defensive qi. It is the qi deficiency of the lung which makes the lung unable to distribute its qi through the network of the lung to the body surface, leading to the deficiency of the defensive qi on the body surface and further giving rise to the susceptibility to cold. Since Astragali Radix (*huáng qí*) can tonify qi in the lung and strengthen the defensive qi, it is a perfect agent for this condition. Of course, Cinnamomi Ramulus (*guì zhī*), which works on the heart, the nutritive qi and blood in the channels, would not be a good choice for it.

In conclusion, there are two ways to produce the defensive qi, to generate it by the nutritive qi locally or by the organs internally, and several ways to distribute the defensive qi such as through lung, spleen, stomach, shao yang, urinary bladder and kidney. There are two ways to generate the nutritive qi—by warming the blood and the defensive qi locally, or working on the heart and spleen internally. Besides circulating with the nutritive qi inside and outside the channels, the defensive qi can circulate alone amongst the skin, muscles, chest and abdomen. When the defensive qi and nutritive qi circulate side by side outside and inside the channels, they mutually support each other for a harmonious relationship. In the clinic, good results come from precise differentiation and treatment accordingly. When the nutritive qi and/or the defensive qi are suspected of being involved in a disease, one should first figure out where the disease is located, then check whether or not the defensive qi alone, the nutritive qi alone or both are involved, and finally treatment can be focused on one or several aspects to recover the normal function of the nutritive qi and/or the defensive qi, the two components of tai yang qi

28 Wang Ang. *Collected Explanations for Medical Formulas* (*yī fāng jí jiě*). Shanghai: Shanghai Science and Technology Publishing House, 1959: 21

9

EXPLORATION OF THE RESOLVING TIME FOR DISEASES IN SIX CONFORMATIONS

Introduction

As everything in the universe goes through the process of starting, maturing, declining and dying or transforming into another thing, diseases in the human being must have the same process. Following this principle in the universe, scholars in ancient times recorded that not only internal disorders but also externally contracted diseases would take place and get better in a certain time frame. For example, according to Chapter 22 of Basic Questions of The Yellow Emperor's Inner Classic, the disease in each organ would start and then get worse, better or even be cured at a certain time of year[1] and febrile diseases due to attack of exogenous pathological factors would start and get better in a certain number of days.[2] Applying this thought in his daily practice, Zhang Ji found that this principle is also applied for diseases in six conformations and first put forward the resolving time for tai yang disease, yang ming disease, shao yang disease, tai yin disease, shao yin disease and jue yin disease in six conformations in lines 9, 193, 272, 275, 291, and 328, respectively. They are described as follows:

- Line 9: 太陽病欲解時，從巳至未上 *Tài yáng bìng yù jiě shí, cóng sì zhì wèi shàng* (The time when tai yang disease is about to resolve is from 9am to 3pm).
- Line 193: 陽明病欲解時，從申至戌上 *Yáng míng bìng yù jiě shí, cóng shēn zhì xū shàng* (The time when yang ming disease is about to resolve is from 3pm to 9pm).

1 Wang Bing. *Basic Questions of The Yellow Emperor's Inner Classic* (*huáng dì nèi jīng sù wèn*). Beijing: People's Health Publishing House, 1963: 143–146

2 Ibid., pp.183–186

- Line 272: 少陽病欲解時，從寅至辰上 *Shào yāng bìng yù jiě shí, cóng yín zhì chén shàng* (The time when shao yang disease is about to resolve is from 3am to 9am).
- Line 275: 太陰病欲解時，從亥至丑上 *Tài yín bìng yù jiě shí, cóng hài zhì chǒu shàng* (The time when tai yin disease is about to resolve is from 9pm to 3am).
- Line 291: 少陰病欲解時，從子至寅上 *Shào yín bìng yù jiě shí, cóng zǐ zhì yín shàng* (The time when shao yin disease is about to resolve is from 11pm to 5am).
- Line 328: 厥陰病欲解時，從丑至卯上 *Jué yīn bìng yù jiě shí, cóng chǒu zhì mǎo shàng* (The time when jue yin disease is about to resolve is from 1am to 7am).

In the original text, these 12 characters, 子 *zǐ*, 丑 *chǒu*, 寅 *yín*, 卯 *mǎo*, 辰 *chén*, 巳 *sì* , 午 *wǔ*, 未 *wèi*, 申 *shēn*, 酉 *yǒu*, 戌 *xū* and 亥 *hài*, are called "地支 *dì zhī* (Earthly Branches)" or "十二地支 *shí èr dì zhī* (Twelve Earthly Branches)." They have been used to designate years, months and hours since as early as 206 BC. According to Ren Ying-Qiu, a famous scholar at Beijing University of Traditional Chinese Medicine, "地支 *dì zhī* (Earthly Branches)" or "十二地支 *shí èr dì zhī* (Twelve Earthly Branches) was first and officially used to designate hours during day and night in 104 AD."[3]

Based on these Earthly Branches, the time during day and night is divided into 12 periods, and each period includes 2 hours as shown in Table 9.1.

Based on Zhang Ji's descriptions in the lines above, the allocation of the period of time for each disease to resolve in six conformations is summarized in Table 9.2.

3 Ren Ying-Qiu. *Collection of the Papers of Ren Ying-Qiu* (*rèn yìng-qiū wén jí*). Beijing: People's Army Physician Publishing House, 2009: 44

Table 9.1 Allocation of hours during day and night according to Twelve Earthly Branches (十二地支 *shí èr dì zhī*)

Twelve Earthly Branches (十二地支 *shí èr dì zhī*)	Hours
子 *zǐ*	11pm to 1am
丑 *chǒu*	1am to 3am
寅 *yín*	3am to 5am
卯 *mǎo*	5am to 7am
辰 *chén*	7am to 9am
巳 *sì*	9am to 11am
午 *wǔ*	11am to 1pm
未 *wèi*	1pm to 3pm
申 *shēn*	3pm to 5pm
酉 *yǒu*	5pm to 7pm
戌 *xū*	7pm to 9pm
亥 *hài*	9pm to 11pm

Table 9.2 Allocation of resolving time for diseases in six conformations

Disease	Resolving time
Shao yang	寅 *yín* – 辰 *chén* (3am to 9am)
Tai yang	巳 *sì* – 未 *wèi* (9am to 3pm)
Yang ming	申 *shēn* – 戌 *xū* (3pm to 9pm)
Tai yin	亥 *hài* – 丑 *chǒu* (9pm to 3am)
Shao yin	子 *zǐ* – 寅 *yín* (11pm to 5am)
Jue yin	丑 *chǒu* – 卯 *mǎo* (1am to 7am)

The facts of the resolving time for diseases in six conformations

From Table 9.2, one can learn the following facts related to the resolving time for diseases in six conformations:

1. Zhang Ji observed that the time for each disease to resolve is a total of 6 hours, which is broken down into three 2-hour periods:

   1) The times when shao yang disease is about to resolve are the 6 hours that cover 寅 *yín* (3am to 5am), 卯 *mǎo* (5am to 7am) and 辰 *chén* (7am to 9am).

   2) The times when tai yang disease is about to resolve are the 6 hours that cover 巳 *sì* (9am to 11am), 午 *wǔ* (11am to 1pm) and 未 *wèi* (1pm to 3pm).

   3) The times when yang ming disease is about to resolve are the 6 hours that cover 申 *shēn* (3pm to 5pm), 酉 *yǒu* (5pm to 7pm) and 戌 *xū* (7pm to 9pm).

   4) The times when tai yin disease is about to resolve are the 6 hours that cover 亥 *hài* (9pm to 11pm), 子 *zǐ* (11pm to 1am) and 丑 *chǒu* (1am to 3am).

   5) The times when shao yin disease is about to resolve are the 6 hours that cover 子 *zǐ* (11pm to 1am), 丑 *chǒu* (1am to 3am) and 寅 *yín* (3am to 5am).

   6) The times when jue yin disease is about to resolve are the 6 hours that cover 丑 *chǒu* (1am to 3am), 寅 *yín* (3am to 5am) and 卯 *mǎo* (5am to 7am).

2. The time for resolution in three yang diseases comprises nine 2-hour periods, i.e. 18 hours from 寅 *yín* (3am) to 戌 *xū* (9pm), while the time for resolution in three yin diseases comprises five 2-hour periods, i.e. 10 hours from 亥 *hài* (9pm) to 卯 *mǎo* (7am).

3. In three yang diseases, there is no overlapping time, while there *is* overlapping time in three yin diseases in regard to the time for resolution, i.e. tai yin disease shares 子 *zǐ* (11pm to 1am) and 丑 *chǒu* (1am to 3am) with shao yin disease, while shao yin disease shares 丑 *chǒu* (1am to 3am) and 寅 *yín* (3am to 5am) with jue yin disease. What is more, all three yin diseases can resolve in 丑 *chǒu* (1am to 3am), while 寅 *yín* (3am to 5am) and 卯 *mǎo* (5am to 7am) are the times shared by jue yin disease and shao yang disease.

4. The sequence of the time to resolve from yang disease to yin disease is from shao yang – tai yang – yang ming – tai yin – shao yin – jue yin, rather than the sequence of the chapters of each disease in Discussion of Cold Damage, i.e. tai yang – yang ming – shao yang – tai yin – shao yin – jue yin disease, which shows a possible order of progress in these diseases.
5. The connections between yang diseases and yin diseases when they are about to resolve are especially from yang ming to tai yin and from jue yin to shao yang.

The concept of the resolving time for diseases in six conformations

The debate about the length of time

Historically, some scholars argue that 4 hours should be considered for each disease to resolve in six conformations, though most scholars agree that 6 hours should be applied for these speculations. Qian Huang (also known as Qian Tian-Lai, c. 1707) is the first scholar who challenged 6 hours for each disease to resolve and wrote:

> Qi in shao yang flourishes between 寅 *yín* (3am to 5am) and 卯 *mǎo* (5am to 7am). At this time, its channel is full of qi, and anti-pathogenic qi can overcome pathological factors. Therefore, shao yang disease is about to resolve. When the time reaches to 辰 *chén* (7am to 9am), its qi starts to transform to the strongest yang qi and is going to become qi for tai yang. Its yang qi at this time is not less any more. Therefore, the time for shao yang disease to recover is from 寅 *yín* (3am to 5am) to 卯 *mǎo* (5am to 7am).[4]

Obviously, this interpretation views the character "上 *shàng*" as "前 *qián* (before, prior to)" in the sentence "從寅至辰上 *cóng yín zhì chén shàng*" and excluded 辰 *chén* (7am to 9am). According to textual research, there is a slight difference in these resolving times in Supplement to Thousand Ducat Formulas (千金翼方 *qiān jīn yì fāng*), a work written by Sun Si-Miao (581–682 AD). The book's contents, which are related to the material in Discussion of Cold Damage, are often used as important references to study this classic. In Supplement to Thousand Ducat Formulas, the character "上

4 Qian Huang. *Trace to Source for Discussion of Cold Damage* (*shāng hán sù yuán jí*). Shanghai: Shanghai Health Publishing House, 1957: 250

shàng" is replaced by the character "盡 *jìn*." For example, the sentence "太陽病欲解時，從巳至未上 *tài yáng bìng yù jiě shí, cóng sì zhì wèi shàng*" is recorded as "太陽病欲解時，從巳盡未 *tài yáng bìng yù jiě shí, cóng sì jìn wèi*."[5] Based on his study for the records related to the description of these resolving times in each disease of six conformations, Li Hang-Zhou stated that "what is called '盡 *jìn*' means '到 *dào* (to),' i.e. the time when tai yang disease is about to resolve from 巳 *sì* to未 *wèi*, in total, two 2-hour periods instead of three 2-hour periods."[6] Although the character "上 *shàng*" can mean "前 *qián*" (before, prior to), it does not mean that Zhang Ji applied this meaning of the character to the sentences related to the time to resolve in each disease of six conformations. According to my research, Zhang Ji used the character "上 *shàng*" 64 times in Discussion of Cold Damage. Among these 64 occurrences, there are four related to the description about time. They are:

- Line 7: 頭痛至七日以上自愈者 *tóu tòng zhì qī rì yǐ shàng zì yù zhě* (A headache lasts for more than seven days).
- Line 212: 不大便五六日，上至十餘日 *bù dà biàn wǔ liù rì, shàng zhì shí yù rì* (The bowel movement has been absent for five or six days to more than ten days).
- Line 303: 少陰病，得之二三日以上 *shào yīn bìng, dé zhī èr sān rì yǐ shàng* (Shao yin disease lasts for more than two or three days).
- Line 384: 却四五日，至陰經上 *què sì wǔ rì, zhì yīn jīng shàng* (Four or five days later, it is possible for the disease to progress to yin channel).

The phrase "至陰經上 *zhì yīn jīng shàng* (it is possible for the disease to progress to yin channel)" in line 384 shares the same structure with the phrase "巳至未上 *zhì wèi shàng*" in the sentence "從巳至未上 *cóng sì zhì wèi shàng*" in line 9. Therefore, the character "上 *shàng*" in the sentence "從巳至未上 *cóng sì zhì wèi shàng*" must mean that the time has reached 未 *wèi* (1pm to 3pm) rather than stopping before未 *wèi* (1pm

5 Sun Si-Miao. *Supplement to Thousand Ducat Formulas* (*qiān jín yì fāng*). Beijing: People's Health Publishing House, 1955: 98

6 Li Hang-Zhou. *Exploration for Balanced View of Qi Transformation Reflected by Resolving Time for Diseases in Six Conformation in Discussion of Cold Damage* (*shāng hán lùn liù jīng bìng yù jiě shí suǒ àn hán qì huà píng héng guān tān jiū*). Beijing: Beijing University of Chinese Medicine, 2011: 36

to 3pm). Like the sentences "不大便五六日，上至十餘日 *bù dà biàn wǔ liù rì, shàng zhì shí yù rì* (The bowel movement has been absent from five or six days to more than ten days)" in line 212, should Zhang Ji want to express that the time has not reached to 未 *wèi* (1pm to 3pm), he would not use the character "上 *shàng*" at the end of the sentence and write this sentence as "從巳上至未 *cóng sì shàng zhì wèi*" rather than "從巳至未上 *cóng sì zhì wèi shàng*" in line 9.

Given that the character "盡 *jìn*" indeed means "到 *dào* (to)," and that this character, instead of the character "上 *shàng*," was used originally in Discussion of Cold Damage (though this meaning has not been found in various dictionaries), this does not mean that this character must mean "到 *dào* (to)" in the sentence "從巳盡未 *cóng sì jìn wèi*." According to my calculations, there are 19 occurrences of this character, and besides that, it might be used to describe the resolving time for each disease in six conformations, which is recorded in Supplement to Thousand Ducat Formulas. Among these 19 occurrences, I found the phrase "盡劑 *jìn jì*" in the sentence "不必盡劑 *bù bì jìn jì*" in the footnote for Cinnamon Twig Decoction (*guì zhī tāng*) in line 12 shares the same structure and grammar with the phrase "盡未 *jìn wèi*" in the sentence "從巳盡未 *cóng sì jìn wèi*."

According to Chinese grammar in ancient times, the phrase "盡劑 *jìn jì*" means "finishing the decoction." Similarly, the phrase "盡未 *jìn wèi*" should be interpreted as "finishing the time related to 未 *wèi* (1pm to 3pm)," i.e. "going through the time related to 未 *wèi* (1pm to 3pm)," and the time related to 未 *wèi* (1pm to 3pm) must be involved, rather than excluded for the time when tai yang disease is about to resolve. Therefore, the sentence "太陽病欲解時，從巳盡未 *tài yáng bìng yù jiě shí, cóng sì jìn wèi*" must be understood as "the time when tai yang disease is about to resolve is from 9am to 3pm," i.e. three 2-hour periods, rather than "the time when tai yang disease is about to resolve is from 9am to 1pm," i.e. two 2-hour periods, though this sentence might be originally written in Discussion of Cold Damage. The speculations from Qian Huang and Li Hang-Zhou did not hold up well since they failed to reflect what Zhang Ji wanted to express.

But why is the period of time for each disease about to resolve limited to three 2-hour periods? Why is the time for the resolving in three yang diseases longer than the time for the resolving in three yin diseases? Why do all three yin diseases resolve in 丑 *chǒu* (1am to 3am)? All of these questions are answered in the next section.

Mechanism of the resolving time for diseases in six conformations

To answer the questions above, first one must answer why scholars in ancient China would divide day and night into 12 periods of time by the Twelve Earthly Branches shown in Table 9.1 and what these Twelve Earthly Branches mean for the human body, because Zhang Ji specially used them to predict the time for each disease in six conformations to resolve, and his secret must be encoded in these Twelve Earthly Branches. Ancient Chinese observers noted that life on earth, including human activity, is related to the movement of the sun. They noticed that time in each year and time in each day is affected by this movement. Yin and yang, in each season in a year and each hour during day and night, change according to this movement. For example, Chapter 4 of Basic Questions of The Yellow Emperor's Inner Classic states:

> There is yin within yang, and there is yang within yin. Take the elapse of day and night as an example. It belongs to yang in nature from the dawn to the midday and it is yang within yang. It belongs to yang in nature from midday to dusk, but it is yin within yang. It belongs to yin in nature from dusk to cockcrow and it is yin within yin. It belongs to yin in nature from cockcrow to sunrise and it is yin within yang. And the human being corresponds to them.[7]

Based on these observations for the change of yin and yang during day and night, ancient scholars designed these Twelve Earthly Branches to further divide the day and night into 12 periods. In order to demonstrate how yin and yang change during day and night, ancient scholars applied Twelve Declining and Growing Hexagrams (十二消息卦 *shí èr xiāo xī guà*) to explain these changes in detail, though Twelve Declining and Growing Hexagrams was first introduced during the Han Dynasty (206 BC to 220 AD) to elaborate for the change of yin and yang during a year.[8] Cheng Wu-Ji, one of the first scholars who commented on Discussion of Cold Damage, noticed that the condition of yin and yang at different times plays an important role in resolving disease in six conformations. He wrote:

---

7 Wang Bing, op. cit., p.24

8 Liu Yu-Jian. *Section One of Study on Symbols, Numbers and Doctrine of Book of Changes During West and East Han Dynasty* (*liáng hàn xiàng shù yì xué yán jiū*). Nanning: Guangxi Education Publishing House, 1995: 33

> Yang qi generates at 子 *zǐ* (11pm to 1am), and 子 *zǐ* (11pm to 1am) belongs to one yang, 丑 *chǒu* belongs to two yangs and 寅 *yín* (3am to 5am) belongs to three yangs. The reason for shao yin to resolve during these times is that the body with yin disease would get help from yang, and yin disease would resolve during these times.[9]

As far as I know, Qian Huang first combined Twelve Earthly Branches with Twelve Declining and Growing Hexagrams to explain the time when each disease is about to resolve. He stated:

> When there is attack of exogenous pathological factors, there must be qi deficiency. Since pathological factors have invaded tai yang channel, qi in the channel has been deficient and unable to eliminate the pathological factors, though they are about to leave. One must wait for the time when qi in the channel gets strong enough to eliminate the pathological factors. Tai yang belongs to the strongest yang and it reaches its peak during 巳 *sì* (9am to 11am) and 午 *wǔ* (11am to 1pm), and 巳 *sì* (9am to 11am), which is pure yang and is governed by hexagram one (乾 *qián guà*). Although one yin is generated at 午 *wǔ* (11am to 1pm), it is the time that yang qi is very strong…therefore, it is said that "the time when tai yang disease is about to resolve is from 巳 *sì* (9am to 11am) to 未 *wèi* (1pm to 3pm)."[10]

The twelve Declining and Growing Hexagrams was first introduced to describe the change of yin and yang in a year, but there is general agreement by ancient and contemporary scholars that the principle it demonstrates can still be applied to the change of yin and yang during day and night. In the following paragraph, I have combined Twelve Earthly Branches with Twelve Declining and Growing Hexagrams to explain them, because it is impossible to understand why Zhang Ji wrote the resolving time for each disease in six conformations without understanding the relationship between the sequence of time and the change of yin and yang in the heavens and on the earth and the human body during day and night.

According to the theory in Book of Changes (易經 *yì jīng*), the symbol, "▬▬▬" is called "陽爻 *yáng yáo*," which represents yang in the universe, while the symbol "▬ ▬" is called "陰爻 *yīn yáo*," which represents yin in the universe. There is general agreement that the creation of a trigram, which is the base for hexagrams, is based on observing the

9 Cheng Wu-Ji. *Annotating and Explaining Discussion of Cold Damage* (*zhù jiě shāng hán lùn*). Beijing: People's Health Publishing House, 1978: 156

10 Qian Huang, op. cit., p.6

movement of the sun during a year, and each hexagram consists of two trigrams, which locate on the upper part and lower part of the hexagram. The upper part or upper trigram is relevant to the heavens, while the lower part or lower trigram is related to the earth. The Twelve Declining and Growing Hexagrams are:

1. 复卦 *fù guà*

   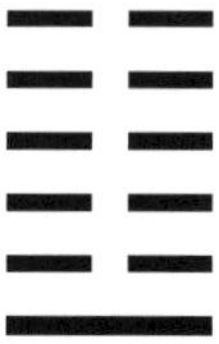

   The time to which it corresponds is 子 *zǐ* (11pm to 1am) and it demonstrates qi condition in the universe at this period of time. During this time one yang is generated and two yins remain on the earth while yang is hiding in the heavens. In other words, yang has returned and started to activate on the earth while the activity of yang is absent and yin prevails in the heavens, and more yin still descends on the earth.

2. 臨卦 *lín guà*

   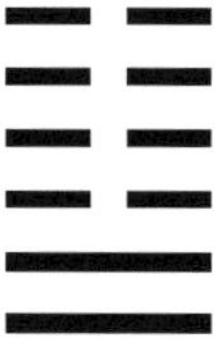

   The time to which it corresponds is 丑 *chǒu* (1am to 3am) and it demonstrates qi condition in the universe at this period of time. During this time two yangs are generated and one yin remains on the earth while yang is hiding in the heavens. In other words, yang is more active on the earth while the activity of yang is absent and yin prevails in the heavens, and yin still descends on the earth.

3. 泰卦 *tài guà*

   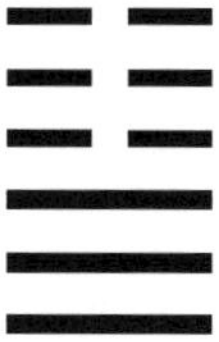

   The time to which it corresponds is 寅 *yín* (3am to 5am) and it demonstrates qi condition in the universe at this period of time. During this time three yangs are generated on the earth. Yang on the earth reaches its peak and yin is absent on the earth while yang in the heavens is still hiding in the heavens. In other words, yang on the earth becomes most active while the activity of yang is absent and yin prevails in the heavens. Yin in the heavens descends and yang on the earth ascends equally; yin and yang in the heavens and on the earth communicate well.

4. 大壯卦 *dà zhuàng guà*

The time to which it corresponds is 卯 *mǎo* (5am to 7am) and it demonstrates qi condition in the universe at this period of time. During this time one yang is generated in the heavens while yang on the earth reaches its peak. In other words, yang in the heavens has returned and become active. Overall yang qi between the heavens and the earth is getting stronger.

5. 夬卦 *guài guà*

The time to which it corresponds is 辰 *chén* (7am to 9am) and it demonstrates qi condition in the universe at this period of time. During this period, two yangs are generated in the heavens while yang on the earth reaches its peak. In other words, yang in the heavens becomes more active. Overall yang qi between the heavens and the earth is getting much stronger.

6. 乾卦 *qián guà*

The time to which it corresponds is 巳 *sì* (9am to 11am) and it demonstrates qi condition in the universe at this period of time. During this time three yangs are generated in the heavens. Yang between the heavens and the earth reaches its peak and becomes most active. From 复卦 *fù guà* to 乾卦 *qián guà*, yang has returned on the earth and gradually ascends from the earth to the heavens.

7. 姤卦 *gòu guà*

The time to which it corresponds is 午 *wǔ* (11am to 1pm) and it demonstrates qi condition in the universe at this period of time. During this time yang in the heavens reaches its peak while two yangs remain and one yin is generated on the earth. In other words, yin has started to return and descend on the earth and yang on the earth becomes less active while yang in the heavens prevails.

8. 遁卦 *dùn guà*

The time to which it corresponds is 未 *wèi* (1pm to 3pm) and it demonstrates qi condition in the universe at this period of time. During this time yang qi in the heavens reaches its peak while one yang remains and two yins are generated on the earth. In other words, more yin descends on the earth and yang on the earth becomes less active while yang in the heavens prevails.

9. 否卦 *pǐ guà*

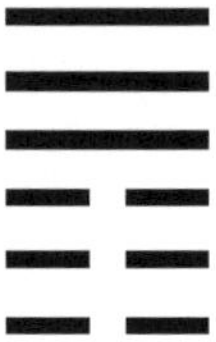

The time to which it corresponds is 申 *shēn* (3pm to 5pm) and it demonstrates qi condition in the universe at this period of time. During this time, yang qi in the heavens reaches its peak while three yangs are hiding and three yins are generated on the earth. In other words, most yin descends on the earth and yang on the earth becomes least active while yang in the heavens prevails.

10. 觀卦 *guān guà*

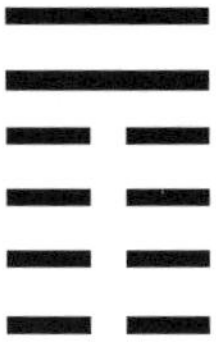

The time to which it corresponds is 酉 *yǒu* (5pm to 7pm) and it demonstrates qi condition in the universe at this period of time. During this time, two yangs remain and one yin is generated in the heavens and yang is hiding on the earth. In other words, most yin descends on the earth and the activity of yang on the earth is absent while yang in the heavens becomes less active too.

11. 剝卦 *bō guà*

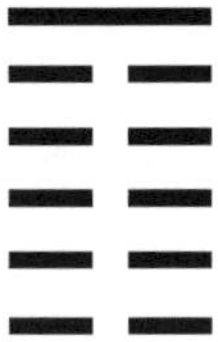

The time to which it corresponds is 戌 *xū* (7pm to 9pm) and it demonstrates qi condition in the universe at this period of time. During this time one yang remains and two yins are generated in the heavens and yang is hiding on the earth. In other words, most yin descends on the earth and the activity of yang on the earth is absent while yang in the heavens becomes much less active.

12. 坤卦 *kūn guà*

The time to which it corresponds is 亥 *hài* (9pm to 11pm) and it demonstrates qi condition in the universe at this period of time. During this time, there is only activity of yin qi in the heavens and on the earth. It is this activity of yin qi that makes qi accumulate and ready for the return of yang qi in the heavens and on the earth.

䷁

From the discussion above, one can learn that the Twelve Declining and Growing Hexagrams have demonstrated the change of yin and yang in the heavens and on the earth during day and night. A question might be raised: Did Zhang Ji notice the change of yin and yang during day and night and what is the evidence to support it? The answer is yes. In line 30, Zhang Ji observed that "when yang qi starts to recover at the middle of night, the feet should become warm." In line 60, Zhang Ji wrote that "the patient has vexation, agitation, sleeplessness during daytime and becomes peaceful at night," in line 104, he stated that "there is tidal fever around early evening" and in line 398, he recorded that "the patient's pulse has returned to normal but feels slight vexation in the evening." All of these lines prove that Zhang Ji indeed noticed there is a difference between day and night in regard to yang qi condition and he applied the knowledge of the change in yin and yang during day and night for the differentiation of diseases in six conformations.

But why is the period of time for each disease to resolve three 2-hour periods?

Number three is an important number in Chinese philosophy and culture. Lao Zi (also known as Li Er or Li Dan, c. 471 BC) stated: "The Dao begot the one, the one begot two, two begot three and three begot the myriad things. The myriad things bear yin and embrace yang. Yin and yang mingle and endorse each other for achieving harmony."[11] What does "three" mean? It means yin and yang mingle and endorse each other. Without this mingling and endorsing, yin and yang would be separate and nothing would be generated. Therefore, each cycle of time must contain three 2-hour periods for the production and maturation of qi during these

11 Sha Shao-Hai and Xu Hong. *Complete Translation for Lao Zi* (*lǎo zǐ quán yì*). Guiyang: Guizhou People's Publishing House, 1989: 87

times. However, this explanation is too vague to give a convincing answer for the question raised above.

Historically, there is another insightful interpretation first offered by Cheng Ying-Mao (also known as Cheng Jiao-Qian, c. 1669) in regard to the relationship between the five elements and the Twelve Earthly Branches. For example, he wrote that "although tai yang disease can resolve with help from strong yang qi during 巳 *sì* (9am to 11am) and 午 *wǔ* (11am to 1pm), it must get help from earth qi in 未 *wèi* (1pm to 3pm), because earth qi is harmonious qi."[12] According to the relationship between the five elements and Twelve Earthly Branches, 寅 *yín* (3am to 5am) and 卯 *mǎo* (5am to 7am) belong wood, 巳 *sì* (9am to 11am) and 午 *wǔ* (11am to 1pm) belong to fire, 申 *shēn* (3pm to 5pm) and 酉 *yǒu* (5pm to 7pm) belong to metal, 亥 *hài* (9pm to 11pm) and 子 *zǐ* (11pm to 1am) belong to water, and 辰 *chén* (7am to 9am), 未 *wèi* (1pm to 3pm), 戌 *xū* (7pm to 9pm) and 丑 *chǒu* (1am to 3am) belong to earth. Wang Hu (also known as Wang Ling-You, c. 1680) elaborated as follows:

> The time for each disease in six conformations takes three 2-hour periods. The time for tai yang disease to resolve is from 巳 *sì* (9am to 11am) to 未 *wèi* (1pm to 3pm). 未 *wèi* (1pm to 3pm) belongs to earth. The time for yang ming disease to resolve is from 申 *shēn* (3pm to 5pm) to 戌 *xū* (7pm to 9m). 戌 *xū* (7pm to 9pm) belongs to earth. The time for shao yang disease to resolve is from 寅 *yín* (3am to 5am) to 辰 *chén* (7am to 9am). 辰 *chén* (7am to 9am) belongs to earth. The time for tai yin disease to resolve ranges from 亥 *hài* (9pm to 11pm) to 丑 *chǒu* (1am to 3am), and the time for shao yin disease to resolve is from 子 *zǐ* (11pm to 1am) to 寅 *yín* (3am to 5am). The time for jue yin disease to resolve is from 丑 *chǒu* (1am to 3am) to 卯 *mǎo* (5am to 7am). The resolving time for all three yin disease also depends on earth [because they share 丑 *chǒu* (1am to 3am), which belongs to earth]. This is the absolute principle that cannot be challenged.[13]

But why is the earth element the indispensable one for every element? According to the numbers demonstrated in the river map in Figure 9.1, number five, the basic number for the earth element, is the crucial one for

12 Cheng Ying-Mao. *True Classification and Analysis for Lines in Discussion of Cold Damage and Supplementary After-Reading Discussion of Cold Damage* (*shāng hán lùn hòu tiǎo biàn, dú shāng hán lùn zhuì yú*). Beijing: China Publishing House of Traditional Chinese Medicine, 2009: 191–192

13 Wang Hu. *Commentary on Differentiation in Discussion of Cold Damage* (*shāng hán lùn biàn zhèng guáng zhù*). Shanghai: Shanghai Health Publishing House, 1958: 57

the mature number of every element, i.e. one plus five equals six, which is the mature number for water; two plus five equals seven, which is the mature number for fire; three plus five equals eight, which is the mature number for wood; four plus five equals nine, which is the mature number for metal; and five plus five equals ten, which is the mature number of the earth. Obviously, 未 *wèi* (1pm to 3pm), 戌 *xū* (7pm to 9pm), 丑 *chǒu* (1am to 3am) and 辰 *chén* (7am to 9am), the time for earth element, is allocated in each three 2-hour period of time and makes qi during this period mature for resolving the disease related, i.e. 寅 *yín* (3am to 5am), 卯 *mǎo* (5am to 7am) and 辰 *chén* (7am to 9am) consist of the period of time that relates to earth qi for the qi in shao yang to mature and shao yang disease to resolve; 巳 *sì* (9am to 11am), 午 *wǔ* (11am to 1pm) plus 未 *wèi* (1pm to 3pm) consist of the period of time that relates to earth qi for the qi in tai yang to mature and tai yang disease to resolve; 申 *shēn* (3pm to 5pm), 酉 *yǒu* (5pm to 7pm) and 戌 *xū* (7pm to 9pm) consist of the period of time that relates to earth qi for the qi in yang ming to mature and yang ming disease to resolve; 亥 *hài* (9pm to 11pm), 子 *zǐ* (11pm to 1am) and 丑 *chǒu* (1am to 3am) consist of the period of time that relates to earth qi for the qi in tai yin to mature and tai yin disease to resolve; 子 *zǐ* (11pm to 1am), 丑 *chǒu* (1am to 3am) and 寅 *yín* (3am to 5am) consist of the period of time that relates to earth qi for the qi in shao yin to mature and shao yin disease to resolve; and 丑 *chǒu* (1am to 3am), 寅 *yín* (3am to 5am) and 卯 *mǎo* (5am to 7am) consist of the period of time that relates to earth qi for the qi in jue yin to mature and jue yin disease to resolve.

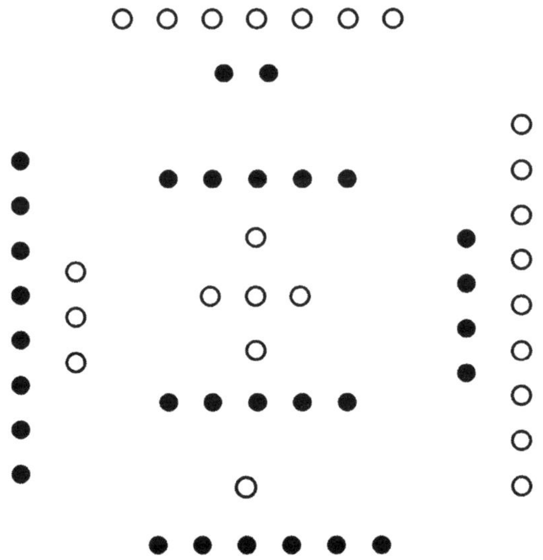

FIGURE 9.1 RIVER MAP

Twelve Declining and Growing Hexagrams also have allocated time and space during day and night, and this time and space during day and night is closely related to the movement of the sun, i.e. 子 *zǐ* (11pm to 1am) is related to midnight while 午 *wǔ* (11am to 1pm) is related to midday, and the sun rises around 卯 *mǎo* (5am to 7am) in the east and sets around 酉 *yǒu*(5pm to 7pm) in the west. However, this kind of sunrise and sunset can only be applied to the spring equinox and autumn equinox, and it does not work for the summer solstice and the winter solstice. Because the earth has its own angle of dip and circulates around the sun with an elliptical orbit, there is summer solstice, which has longer time during day than night, and winter solstice, which has longer time during night than day. In other words, the sun would rise in the northeast, which is 寅 *yín* (3am to 5am), and set in the northwest, which is 戌 *xū* (7pm to 9pm), at summer solstice, while the sun would rise in the southeast, which is 辰 *chén* (7am to 9am), and set in the southwest, which is 申 *shēn* (3pm to 5pm), at winter solstice.

In summary, the time for the sun rising is not limited to 卯 *mǎo* (5am to 7am) but can also be 寅 *yín* (3am to 5am) and 辰 *chén* (7am to 9am) depending on different seasons of the year. Likewise, the time for the sun setting is not limited to 酉 *yǒu* (5pm to 7pm) but can also be 申 *shēn* (3pm to 5pm) and 戌 *xū* (7pm to 9pm) depending on different seasons of the year. In other words, the change of qi in the universe and the human body might come either in one 2-hour period early or one 2-hour period later during summer solstice or winter solstice. Zhang Ji probably knew this change of qi in regard to different seasons in a year based on his observation and clinical practice, as he did not adhere to one 2-hour period, rather three 2-hour periods, which shows more flexibility and makes these predications more practical in clinical circumstances. But why does each three 2-hour period relate to the specific diseases in six conformations and how do they work?

One might notice that the discussion above mainly focuses on one 2-hour period instead of using three 2-hour periods to investigate what happens with respect to the change of yin and yang, particularly as this relates to the human being. At the beginning of this chapter, it was mentioned that the scholars who wrote The Yellow Emperor's Inner Classic recorded that not only internal disorders but also externally contracted diseases would take place or get better in certain time frames. The basis for this reasoning was that they realized each disease would have a chance to resolve by itself when its qi is supported by qi in the universe at the corresponding time. For example, in Chapter 22 of Basic Questions of The Yellow Emperor's Inner Classic, they wrote that "a disease will turn to the better or resolve when reaching the time of the element that associated itself."[14] Many ancient and contemporary scholars have followed this statement to explain why each disease in six conformations would resolve in a certain period of time. For example, Yu Chang (also known as Yu Jia-Yan, 1585–1644), wrote:

> When a disease is about to resolve, it must take place when qi in the conformation related is strong. Tai yang belongs to the strongest yang; therefore, it might resolve during 巳 *sì* (9am to 11am), 午 *wǔ* (11am to 1pm) and 未 *wèi* (1pm to 3pm) when qi in tai yang is very strong.[15]

However, this explanation is too obscure and one cannot know how exactly this theory works. This question remained until Han Xin-Bing and He Xin-Hui published their article, "Exploration of the Mechanism and Significance for the Time When Diseases Are About to Resolve in Discussion of Cold Damage," in 2009. In this article, they offer a relatively thorough explanation:

> The time during 巳 *sì* (9am to 11am), 午 *wǔ* (11am to 1pm) and 未 *wèi* (1pm to 3pm) is the period when yang in the heavens has reached its peak; the time during 申 *shēn* (3pm to 5pm), 酉 *yǒu* (5pm to 7pm) and 戌 *xū* (7pm to 9pm) is the period when yang in the heavens declines and the strength of yang is next to the time during 巳 *sì* (9am to 11am), 午 *wǔ* (11am to 1pm) and 未 *wèi* (1pm to 3pm); the time during 寅 *yín* (3am to 5am), 卯 *mǎo* (5am to 7am) and 辰 *chén* (7am to 9am) is the period when yang in the heavens increases yet its yang is most weak.
>
> In The Yellow Emperor's Inner Classic, it is stated that tai yang bears three yangs, yang ming bears two yangs, and shao yang bears one yang. Tai yang has the strongest yang, the strength of yang in yang ming is secondary to the one in tai yang, and the yang in shao yang is most weak. Therefore, the time during 巳 *sì* (9am to 11am), 午 *wǔ* (11am to 1pm) and 未 *wèi* (1pm to 3pm) corresponds to tai yang, the time during 申 *shēn* (3pm to 5pm), 酉 *yǒu* (5pm to 7pm) and 戌 *xū* (7pm to 9pm) corresponds to yang ming and the time during 寅 *yín* (3am to 5am), 卯 *mǎo* (5am to 7am) and 辰 *chén* (7am to 9am) corresponds to shao yang. According to the principle that the human being corresponds to nature, the change of

14 Wang Bing, op. cit., p.145

15 Yu Chang. *Writing on the Esteemed Discussion* (*shàng lùn piān*). In Yu Bo-Hai et al. (eds) *Collection of Famous Books on Discussion of Cold Damage, Essentials and Formula Discussions from the Golden Cabinet and Warm Disease* (*shāng hán jīn guì wēn bìng míng zhù jí chéng*). Beijing: China Publishing House, 1997: 220

yang in the heavens can also affect the growing and declining process in three yang (six fu organs). And yang qi in the human being would change according to the change of yang in nature.

The time for a disease to resolve has reflected that anti-pathogenic qi in the human being corresponds to the change of time in nature. Therefore, the time when tai yang disease is about to resolve is allocated during 巳 *sì* (9am to 11am), 午 *wǔ* (11am to 1pm) and 未 *wèi* (1pm to 3pm), the time when yang ming disease is about to resolve is allocated during 申 *shēn* (3pm to 5pm), 酉 *yǒu* (5pm to 7pm) and 戌 *xū* (7pm to 9pm) and the time when shao yang disease is about to resolve is allocated 寅 *yín* (3am to 5am), 卯 *mǎo* (5am to 7am) and 辰 *chén* (7am to 9am). The time during 亥 *hài* (9pm to 11pm), 子 *zǐ* (11pm to 1am) and 丑 *chǒu* (1am to 3am) is the period when yang on the earth is most weak; the time during 子 *zǐ* (11pm to 1am), 丑 *chǒu* (1am to 3am) and 寅 *yín* (3am to 5am) is the period when yang on the earth is getting stronger; the time during 丑 *chǒu* (1am to 3am), 寅 *yín* (3am to 5am) and 卯 *mǎo* (5am to 7am) is the period when yang on the earth reaches its peak. Conversely, yin on the earth is the strongest during 亥 *hài* (9pm to 11pm), 子 *zǐ* (11pm to 1am) and 丑 *chǒu* (1am to 3am); yin on the earth is moderately strong during 子 *zǐ* (11pm to 1am), 丑 *chǒu* (1am to 3am) and 寅 *yín* (3am to 5am); and yin on the earth is least strong during 丑 *chǒu* (1am to 3am), 寅 *yín* (3am to 5am) and 卯 *mǎo* (5am to 7am).

In The Yellow Emperor's Inner Classic, it is stated that tai yin bears three yin, shao yin bears two yins, and jue yin bears one yin. Yin in tai yin is the strongest, yin in shao yin is secondary to the one in tai yin, and yin in jue yin is most weak. Therefore, the time during 亥 *hài* (9pm to 11pm), 子 *zǐ* (11pm to 1am) and 丑 *chǒu* (1am to 3am) corresponds to tai yin, the time during 子 *zǐ* (11pm to 1am), 丑 *chǒu* (1am to 3am) and 寅 *yín* (3am to 5am) corresponds to shao yin, and the time during 丑 *chǒu* (1am to 3am), 寅 *yín* (3am to 5am) and 卯 *mǎo* (5am to 7am) corresponds to jue yin. And the time when tai yin disease is about to resolve is allocated during 亥 *hài* (9pm to 11pm), 子 *zǐ* (11pm to 1am) and 丑 *chǒu* (1am to 3am); the time when shao yin disease is about to resolve is allocated during 子 *zǐ* (11pm to 1am), 丑 *chǒu* (1am to 3am) and 寅 *yín* (3am to 5am) and the time when jue yin disease is about to resolve is allocated during 丑 *chǒu* (1am to 3am), 寅 *yín* (3am to 5am) and 卯 *mǎo* (5am to 7am).[16]

Figure 9.2 provides a summary of the discussion above.

16 Han Xin-Bing and He Xin-Hui. "Exploration of the mechanism and significance for the time when diseases are about to resolve in Discussion of Cold Damage." *Liaoning Journal of Traditional Chinese Medicine*, 2009 (3): 356

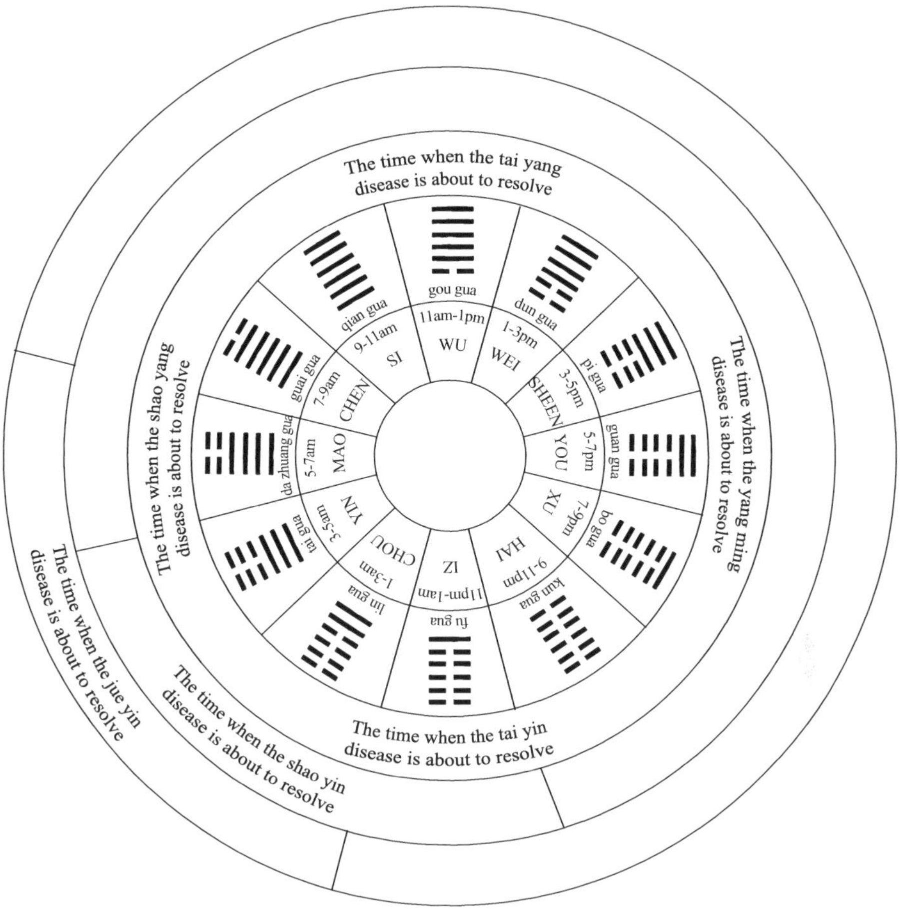

FIGURE 9.2 THE RELATIONSHIPS BETWEEN TWELVE EARTHLY BRANCHES, TWELVE DECLINING AND GROWING HEXAGRAMS AND THE RESOLVING TIME FOR DISEASES IN SIX CONFORMATIONS

The explanation by Han and He does not give an answer for the following questions:

- Why is the connection between yang disease and yin disease when they are about to resolve, especially from yang ming to tai yin and from jue yin to shao yang, in the evening and morning, respectively?
- If tai yang disease is supposed to resolve at the time when yang in the heavens is very strong, why is yin produced or descended from the heavens to the earth during this time?

To answer these questions, the theory of opening, closing and pivot should be consulted. Liu Li-Hong, a scholar from Guangxi province, first and clearly introduced this theory to explain the mechanism for tai yang to resolve during 巳 *sì* (9am to 11am), 午 *wǔ* (11am to 1pm) and 未 *wèi* (1pm to 3pm):

> Hexagrams 1 (乾 *qián*), 44 (姤 *gòu*) and 33 (遁 *dùn*) represent three periods (9am to 11am, 11am to 1pm and 1pm to 3pm, respectively). Hexagram 1 symbolizes that yang qi finally reaches the surface, hexagram 44 symbolizes that yang qi reaches its peak and hexagram 33 symbolizes full presentation of the opening function of yang qi in tai yang.[17] Each of these three has great benefit to treat tai yang disease: first, yang qi in the body reaches the surface from 9am to 11am and will help treat the exterior condition; second, the strongest yang qi from 11am to 1pm will be useful to treat the disease caused by cold; third, full presentation of the opening function of yang qi in tai yang will be beneficial for the dysfunction of opening in tai yang disease… This is why tai yang disease is about to resolve in these three periods of time.[18]

Enlightened by this thought, I answer the questions above using a combination of the theory of opening, closing and pivot, and the theory of 本氣 *běn qì* (root qi), 標氣 *biāo qì* (branch qi) and 中氣 *zhōng qì* (middle qi) in the theory of qi transformation.

As we discussed in Chapter 6, "The Theory of Qi Transformation in Six Conformations," each qi has its 本氣 *běn qì*, 標氣 *biāo qì* and 中氣 *zhōng qì*, and the change of this qi is closely related to its 中氣 *zhōng qì*. For example, qi in shao yang tends to move towards fire since its 中氣 *zhōng qì*, jue yin, belongs to wood and bears wind qi. Both wind qi and wood would be beneficial for the production of fire. (See Chapter 6 for more detailed information related to other qi.) While the closing function of jue yin refers to the process from accumulation and transformation in regard to qi movement, they are turning points for ascending and descending of qi in qi transformation. Shao yang is the pivot, which can let qi in and out and/or up and down. Interestingly, according to the relationship among the five elements, the Earthly Branches and hexagrams, 寅 *yín* (3am to 5am) and 卯 *mǎo* (5am to 7am), and hexagrams 泰卦 *tài guà* and 大壯卦 *dà zhuàng guà*, belong to wood and are shared by jue yin and shao yang. The allocation of these times and hexagrams not only

17 According to Chapter 6, "The Individual Activities and the Mutual Functioning of Yin and Yang," in *The Yellow Emperor's Inner Classic*, tai yang is in charge of opening. See Wang Bing, op. cit., p.50

18 Liu Li-Hong. *Pondering Over Chinese Medicine* (*sī kǎo zhōng yī*). Nanning: Guangxi Normal University Publishing House, 2002: 217–218

demonstrates that yang in the heavens is generated and goes up but also implies that both yin qi and yang qi have been accumulated enough for the communication and the change between yin and yang, and yang qi is ready to go up since qi in jue yin does not start at 寅 *yín* (3am to 5am) or 泰卦 *tài guà* but rather begins and accumulates starting from 丑 *chǒu* (1am to 3am) or 臨卦 *lín guà*. In other words, without help from jue yin (wind, wood and accumulation of qi), yang qi in shao yang cannot be generated and goes up. This is why shao yang is put right after jue yin and why the change from yin to yang in the morning takes place during 寅 *yín* (3am to 5am) and 卯 *mǎo* (5am to 7am), and why the connection between yang disease and yin disease in the morning when they are about to resolve occurs especially from jue yin to shao yang. Of course, when shao yang disease presents during 寅 *yín* (3am to 5am), 卯 *mǎo* (5am to 7am) and 辰 *chén* (7am to 9am), qi in shao yang in the body would not only get help from its counterpart in nature but would also be supported by qi in jue yin. Therefore, shao yang disease is likely to resolve during these periods of time.

After continually ascending in shao yang, yang would eventually reach its peak, leading to tai yang, which bears three yangs and is the strongest yang among shao yang, tai yang and yang ming. When qi reaches its peak, it cannot keep going; otherwise, it would go against natural law. This is like when a tree bears fruit, the energy of the tree should go inward and downward to the trunk and the root, leading to fall of leaves, according to Chapter 40 of Morals Classic (道德經 *dào dé jīng*), "Returning is the Motion of Dao."[19] Therefore, the movement of qi must change its direction and return. Yes, tai yang is supposed to open and qi in tai yang is supposed to be distributed to the body surface. However, it would be a big mistake to understand that this opening and distribution would keep going forever without any stop or return. Tai yang indicates that yang qi reaches its peak and it is time for it to return and descend. The opening function for tai yang implies the meaning of communicating yin and yang, i.e. qi in tai yang starts to open the door for the change from yang to yin. This is why the period of time related to tai yang is predominated by 乾卦 *qián guà*, pure yang in the heavens and on the earth. There are two hexagrams, 姤卦 *gòu guà* and 遁卦 *dùn guà*, among three hexagrams that demonstrate activity of yin qi; especially when yin qi starts to descend from the heavens onto the earth. With this descending and returning movement, the opening and

19 Sha Shao-Hai and Xu Zi-Hong, op. cit., p.79

distribution function of tai yang would be controlled. Otherwise, yang would float or even escape and tai yang would fail to perform its opening function. From this point of view, the time during 巳 *sì* (9am to 11am), 午 *wǔ* (11am to 1pm) and 未 *wèi* (1pm to 3pm) is another turning point for the change between yin and yang, particularly change from yang to yin, though this change has just started. When tai yang disease presents during 巳 *sì* (9am to 11am), 午 *wǔ* (11am to 1pm) and 未 *wèi* (1pm to 3pm), qi in tai yang functions normally, performing the best opening and distribution function to eliminate the disease, Therefore, tai yang disease is likely to resolve during these periods of time.

As time goes on, more yin qi descends from heaven and accumulates, which concords with the feature of qi transformation for yang ming, because the closing function of yang ming refers to the process of accumulation and transformation. From 申 *shēn* (3pm to 5pm), 酉 *yǒu* (5pm to 7pm) and 戌 *xū* (7pm to 9pm), which correspond to 否卦 *pǐ guà*, 觀卦 *guān guà* and剝卦 *bō guà*, one can learn that yang ming is the midway point for qi descending and qi moves from tai yang to yang ming, during which yang gradually changes from its peak to yin while yin continually descends. From these hexagrams, one might learn that qi in yang ming does more descending during the time related to yang ming since more and more yin descends from the heavens while there is still a little yang to lift in the heavens.

Why does qi in yang ming continually descend without stopping? Because its middle qi is dampness qi from tai yin, and dampness qi belongs to yin and can make dryness qi in yang ming continually go downward. As one knows, when qi in yang ming descends in the human body, the function of yang ming is normal regardless of whether the stomach and/or the large intestine is involved. When yang ming disease due to the dysfunction of descending qi in the stomach and/or the large intestine is present during 申 *shēn* (3pm to 5pm), 酉 *yǒu* (5pm to 7pm) and 戌 *xū* (7pm to 9pm), qi in yang ming of the human body gets support from qi in nature in terms of qi descending, and yang ming performs its best function in this regard. Therefore, yang ming disease is likely to resolve during this period of time regardless of heat or cold.

When one talks about the opening function of tai yin, it is natural to think that the spleen processes food, produces qi and blood and distributes them to the extremities it governs. This is just one part of the opening function of tai yin. Like yang qi moves from shao yang to tai yang, yin qi cannot go in one direction and descend without stop or returning. From

亥 *hài* (9pm to 11pm), 子 *zǐ* (11pm to 1am) and 丑 *chǒu* (1am to 3am), which correspond to 坤卦 *kūn guà*, 復卦 *fù guà* and 臨卦 *lín guà*, one can learn that tai yin would open the door for yang ming and receive yin qi from yang ming, on the one hand, and it would open the door of shao yin, letting yin qi transform into yang qi on the earth on the other hand. This is what is called "the opening refers to the beginning of qi movement."[20] Like the opening of tai yang, the opening function of tai yin also implies the communicating between yin and yang, i.e. qi in tai yin starts to open the door for receiving yin qi from yang ming and transforms it into yang qi in shao yin. Basically, according to Discussion of Cold Damage, the pathology in tai yin disease is that its qi is unable to move regardless of cold and yang deficiency or excess in the spleen, and qi of tai yin in the human body can get help from nature and do its best job in terms of opening during 亥 *hài* (9pm to 11pm), 子 *zǐ* (11pm to 1am) and 丑 *chǒu* (1am to 3am). Therefore, tai yin disease is likely to resolve during this period of time no matter what the pathology would be.

There is general agreement that the reason to state that shao yin is in charge of pivot is because it bears two yins and locates between tai yin and jue yin.

Figure 9.2 proves that shao yin indeed locates between tai yin and jue yin. However, this explanation is too vague to comprehend the exact role shao yin plays between tai yin and jue yin in regard to qi movement. According to five elements theory, tai yin belongs to earth, shao yin belongs to water and jue yin belongs to wood, and water produces wood. However, without earth, how can water be contained for the flourishing of wood? This is probably because shao yin and tai yin share two 2-hour periods and two hexagrams, which are 子 *zǐ* (11pm to 1am) and 丑 *chǒu* (1am to 3am) and 復卦 *fù guà* and 臨卦 *lín guà*. Yes, tai yin has opened the door to let yang qi generate, but this yang qi has not matured yet and it must keep growing. From 子 *zǐ* (11pm to 1am), 丑 *chǒu* (1am to 3am) and 寅 *yín* (3am to 5am), which correspond to 復卦 *fù guà*, 臨卦 *lín guà* and 泰卦 *tài guà*, one can learn that shao yin can make yang qi continually grow until it reaches its peak on the earth. Obviously, this process demonstrates that shao yin is a pivot between tai yin and jue yin. It is slow but steady and finally reaches the point where yin descends and yang ascends, and yin and yang communicate equally, which is

20 Wang Bing, op. cit., p.50

demonstrated by 泰卦 *tài guà*. This is what is called "the pivot is in charge of turning of qi elegantly."[21]

In Discussion of Cold Damage, shao yin refers to the heart and kidney, two organs that govern fire and water. Shao yin disease can be divided into heat syndrome and cold syndrome, which are related to the heart system and the kidney system, respectively, when yang (fire) and yin (water) in shao yin fail to communicate with each other. When shao yin disease due to miscommunication between fire in the heart and water in the kidney presents during 子 *zǐ* (11pm to 1am), 丑 *chǒu* (1am to 3am) and 寅 *yín* (3am to 5am), qi in shao yin of the human body gets support from qi in nature for the recovery of these communications. Therefore, shao yin disease is likely to resolve during this period of time regardless of heat or cold.

Like yang ming, the function of jue yin, which accumulates and transforms qi from tai yin and shao yin, is to close. The qi transformation of jue yin has a close relationship with shao yang, its 中氣 *zhōng qì*. From Figure 9.2, the times related to jue yin are 丑 *chǒu* (1am to 3am), 寅 *yín* (3am to 5am) and 卯 *mǎo* (5am to 7am), which correspond to 臨卦 *lín guà*, 泰卦 *tài guà* and 大壯卦 *dà zhuàng guà*. And the times related to shao yang are 寅 *yín* (3am to 5am), 卯 *mǎo* (5am to 7am) and 辰 *chén* (7am to 9am), which correspond to 泰卦 *tài guà*, 大壯卦 *dà zhuàng guà* and 夬卦 *guài guà*. They share the time related to 寅 *yín* (3am to 5am) and 卯 *mǎo* (5am to 7am) or 泰卦 *tài guà* and 大壯卦 *dà zhuàng guà*.

Yes, wood would like to grow, but without help from fire qi in shao yang, wood would not fully grow. Similarly, if jue yin does not share growing yang qi with shao yang, which is demonstrated by 泰卦 *tài guà* and 大壯卦 *dà zhuàng guà*, it would stay at 臨卦 *lín guà* where it starts and could not grow continually. The significance of jue yin to close, is to connect shao yin to shao yang by transforming qi from shao yin to shao yang. If qi only descends, yang qi would be depressed. After going through the process of closing from jue yin, yin qi accumulates and becomes stable. Just like yang ming can make yang transform into yin, jue yin can make yin transform into yang. It can receive qi from tai yin and mix this qi with qi in shao yin and finally deliver this qi to shao yang.

Based on the discussion above, jue yin must locate between shao yin and shao yang, or even three yin and three yang, make qi continually move from tai yin to shao yin, and connect qi between three yin and three

21 Ibid., p.50

yang, and serve as a turning point between yin and yang in the morning. According to Discussion of Cold Damage, the basic pathology for jue yin disease is the failure of yin and yang to connect to each other, leading to cold, heat, concurrence of cold and heat syndromes or even collapse of yin or yang. When jue yin disease, due to the failure of the communication between yin and yang, is present during 丑 *chǒu* (1am to 3am), 寅 *yín* (3am to 5am) and 卯 *mǎo* (5am to 7am), qi in jue yin of the human body gets support from qi in nature for the recovery of this communication and transformation between qi in tai yin and shao yin, three yin and three yang. Therefore, jue yin disease is likely to resolve during this period of time regardless of what it is.

Based on the analysis above, one can learn that all three yin share 丑 *chǒu* (1am to 3am), which corresponds to 臨卦 *lín guà*, the earth element, while all three yang do not share any elements, though they do contain hours that relate to earth elements such as 辰 *chén* (7am to 9am), 未 *wèi* (1pm to 3pm) and 戌 *xū* (7pm to 9pm). This is probably why all three yin closely connect to each other and there is some overlapping time for them, i.e. tai yin disease shares 子 *zǐ* (11pm to 1am) and 丑 *chǒu* (1am to 3am) with shao yin disease, while shao yin disease shares 丑 *chǒu* (1am to 3am) and 寅 *yín* (3am to 5am) with jue yin disease. In this way, the time related to three yin is much shorter than the time related to three yang. This might be an answer for why the time for the resolving in three yang diseases is longer than the time for the resolving in three yin diseases, the time for the resolving in three yang diseases is nine 2-hour periods, i.e. 18 hours, from 寅 *yín* (3am) to 戌 *xū* (9pm), while the time for resolving in three yin diseases is five 2-hour periods, i.e. 10 hours from 亥 *hài* (9pm) to 卯 *mǎo* (7am).

We have discussed the concept and mechanism for the time when diseases in six conformations are about to resolve. What role does this approach play in our daily clinical practice? This is discussed in the next section.

Significance of studying the time when diseases in six conformations are about to resolve

One thing that must be mentioned is the word "resolve," which is a literal translation for the character "解 *jiě*" in lines 9, 193, 272, 275, 291, and 328. It does not always mean the disease will automatically resolve.

Sometimes, it can mean that the disease is getting better. Sometimes, the recommended treatment is needed.

First, it can be helpful for us to predict the possibility for disease to get better or resolve. When anti-pathogenic qi is strong and/or the treatment is given in time, disorders in one of these conformations can get better or can even be cured with help from qi related to this conformation. In addition to the lines mentioned above, Zhang Ji wrote in line 30 that "when yang qi starts to recover in the middle of the night, the feet should become warm," and in line 332, he wrote for jue yin disease that "if the fever continually exists next day, the recovery can be expected in the middle of the night of the next day." Based on the principle of yin and yang, when there is time for the disease to resolve or get better, there must be time for the disease to deteriorate. Zhang Ji used a couple of lines to describe this clinical phenomenon. In line 62, he wrote that "the patient has vexation, agitation and sleeplessness during daytime and becomes peaceful at night." Obviously, vexation and agitation indicate that yang qi in shao yin still exists, though they are morbid states, while peaceful presentation reflects that yang qi in shao yin is about to be exhausted without recovery and the condition is getting worse.

Observing this phenomenon discussed in Discussion of Cold Damage, some scholars have used the term "欲劇時 *yù jù shí.*" Liu Li-Hong first put forward this term and speculated that the time for diseases to get worse in six conformation should be one opposed to the time when it is about to resolve. He wrote:

> The time when tai yang disease is about to get worse is the time opposed to 巳 *sì* (9am to 11am), 午 *wǔ* (11am to 1pm) and 未 *wèi* (1pm to 3pm), which are 亥 *hài* (9pm to 11pm), 子 *zǐ* (11pm to 1am) and 丑 *chǒu* (1am to 3am).[22]

Theoretically, this speculation is absolutely right, but it does not reflect what Zhang Ji meant in his classic. For example, in line 104, he described fever in yang ming disease as tidal fever that is getting worse during "日晡 *rì bū*," which is around 申 *shēn* (3am to 5pm), the time which corresponds to yang ming. Zhang Ji's opinion has been further explained by Zheng Shou-Quan:

> 申 *shēn* (3pm to 5pm), 酉 *yǒu* (5pm to 7pm) and 戌 *xū* (7pm to 9pm) are the times when qi in yang ming is strong. Yang ming disease can get

22 Liu Li-Hong, op. cit., p.222

> better and resolve when pathological factors in yang ming are weak, while it can get worse when pathological factors in yang ming are strong. One should observe the patient with tidal fever at "日晡 *rì bū*" to understand the mechanism for yang ming disease to resolve or get worse.[23]

In his work, Connecting Pearls for Discussion of Cold Damage (傷寒貫珠集 *shāng hán guàn zhū jí*), You Yi (also known as You Zai-Jing, 1650–1749) first pointed out that a disease in six conformations can take place at the time when it is about to resolve. He wrote:

> 申 *shēn* (3pm to 5pm), 酉 *yǒu* (5pm to 7pm) and 戌 *xū* (7pm to 9pm) are related to "日晡 *rì bū*." The tidal fever in yang ming disease takes place at "日晡 *rì bū*" while yang ming disease is also about to resolve at "日晡 *rì bū*." This indicates that 申 *shēn* (3pm to 5pm), 酉 *yǒu* (5pm to 7pm) and 戌 *xū* (7pm to 9pm) are the times for yang ming. When the disease takes place, it indicates that pathological factors are attacking yang ming. When the disease is about to resolve, it indicates that anti-pathogenic qi is recovering.[24]

In summary, the times related to each disease can not only be used to predict the possibility for this disease in six conformations to get better or resolve but can also be used as a tool to predict the deterioration of such disease, i.e. when anti-pathogenic qi overcomes pathological factors in this conformation, the related disease would get better or resolve; when pathological factors defeat anti-pathological qi in this conformation, the related disease gets worse.

These times can help to determine where a disease locates. Generally, when an illness takes place or gets worse or better at the time when a disease in six conformations is supposed to get better or resolve, it is very likely that the disease locates in such conformations, because whether or not the related disease takes place or gets worse or better depends on the fight between the anti-pathogenic qi and pathological factors in such conformation, i.e. when anti-pathogenic qi prevails, the disease gets better or resolves. Otherwise, the disease gets worse. For example, when symptoms such as tidal fever take place during 申 *shēn* (3pm to 5pm), 酉 *yǒu* (5pm to 7pm) and 戌 *xū* (7pm to 9pm), which is the time for yang ming disease to resolve, it is very likely that yang ming is involved.

---

23 Zheng Shou-Quan and Tang Bu-Qi. *Explanation for Works of Zheng Qin-An* (*zhèng qīn-ān yī shū chán shì*). Chengdu: Sichuan Publishing House, 1996: 724

24 You Yi. *Connecting Pearls for Discussion of Cold Damage* (*shāng hán guàn zhū jí*). Shanghai: Shanghai Science and Technology Publishing House, 1978: 112

Another example is that Zhang Ji presents a case in line 398 in which "the patient's pulse has returned to normal but the patient feels slight vexation in the evening." Based on slight vexation in the evening, which corresponds to the time when yang ming disease and/or tai yin disease are about to resolve, Zhang Ji found that "the qi in the stomach and spleen is still weak and unable to digest this food, which leads to slight vexation."

These times can be used as guidance for time to give the treatment. In general, it seems that Zhang Ji knew that it is better to give treatment for the disease at a time when the disease is about to be relieved. For example, for the severe case treated by Cinnamon Twig Decoction (*guì zhī tāng*) in line 12, Zhang Ji recommends that the three doses of the decoction made from the formula be finished in about half a day. Regardless of whether this half a day refers to the morning or the afternoon, it must cover either 巳 *sì* (9am to 11am) or 午 *wèi* (1pm to 3pm), which are the times when tai yang disease is about to resolve. Of course, yang qi in tai yang in nature is very strong; therefore, yang qi in tai yang in the body would get help from yang qi in nature and perform better the function of opening. In this way, it would be easier and quicker for the body to get rid of disease in tai yang.

While treating the syndrome related to tai yin disease in line 386, Zhang Ji recommends taking Regulate the Middle Pill (*lǐ zhōng wán*) three or four times during the day and two times during the night. Obviously, two times during the night must include 亥 *hài* (9pm to 11pm) or 子 *zǐ* (11pm to 1am) or 丑 *chǒu* (1am to 3am), the time when tai yin disease is about to resolve. Since the qi in tai yin in nature is very strong during this time, and the qi in tai yin of the body gets support from qi in nature during these times and does a better job of opening, it is easier and quicker for the body to resolve tai yin disease.

Based on his studies, observations and practices on the relationship between diseases in six conformations and times during the day and night, Zhang Ji presented the time when each disease in six conformations is about to resolve. Although he presented a few cases to demonstrate the significance of this approach clinically, practitioners, especially contemporary practitioners, have largely ignored this approach and have not applied it in their clinical practice. Therefore, more studies and clinical cases are needed to further prove and expand its applications.

Appendix 1

CHINESE DYNASTIES AND HISTORICAL PERIODS

Xia Dynasty		2100–1600 BC
Shang Dynasty		1600–1100 BC
Zhou Dynasty	Western Zhou	1100–770 BC
	Eastern Zhou	770–256 BC
Spring and Autumn period		770–476 BC
Warring States period		476–221 BC
Qin Dynasty		221–206 BC
Han Dynasty	Western Han	206 BC to 24 AD
	Eastern Han	24–220 AD
Three Kingdoms period		220–265 AD
Western Jin		265–316 AD
Eastern Jin		316–420 AD
Northern and Southern Dynasties		420–581 AD
Sui Dynasty		581–618 AD
Tang Dynasty		618–907 AD
Five Dynasties period		907–960 AD
Song Dynasty	Northern Song	960–1127 AD
	Southern Song	1127–1279 AD
Yuan Dynasty		1279–1368 AD
Ming Dynasty		1368–1644 AD
Qing Dynasty		1644–1911 AD
Republic of China		1911–1949 AD
People's Republic of China		1949 to present

Appendix 2

AUTHORS OF CHINESE MEDICINE BOOKS

Given name	Honorific name	Alias	Dates (AD)
Ban Gu	Ban Meng-Jian		32–92
Cai Lu-Xian			c. 1937
Cao Bing-Zhang	Cao Chi-Dian		1878–1956
Cao Jia-Da	Cao Ying-Fu		1866–1937
Chao Yuan-Fang			550–630
Chen Bo-Tan	Chen Wen-Wei	Chen Ying-Qi	1863–1938
Chen Cun-Ren	Chen Cheng-Yuan		1908–1990
Chen Liang-Shi			c. 1661
Chen Meng-Lei	Chen Ze-Zhen	Chen Sheng-Zhai	1650–1741
Chen Nian-Zu	Chen Xiu-Yuan		c. 1753–1823
Chen Ping-Bo			Unknown
Chen Rui-Chun			1936–2008
Chen Shi-Wen			c. 1110
Chen Yi-Ren			1924–2004
Cheng Dan-An	Cheng Qi-Tong	Cheng Qiu-Wu	1899–1957
Cheng Guo-Pen	Cheng Zhong-Ling		1662–1735
Cheng Lin	Cheng Yun-Lai		c. 1674
Cheng Shi-De			1919–2009
Cheng Wu-Ji			1063–1156
Cheng Ying-Mao	Cheng Jiao-Qian		c. 1669
Cheng Zhao-Huan			1944–2012
Cheng Zhi	Cheng Fu-Sheng		c. 1669
Dai Tian-Zhang	Dai Lin-Jiao		c. 1660
Deng Shao-Xian	Deng Xu-Cheng		1898–1971
Du Si-Jing	Du Jing-Fu		1235–1320
Fang Yao-Zhong			1921–1995

Fang You-Zhi	Fang Zhong-Xing		1523–1593
Gao Xue-Shan	Gao Han-Zhi		c. 1871
Ge Hong	Ge Ya-Chuan		c. 284–364
Guo Yong	Guo Zi-He		1106–1187
He Bing-Yuan	He Lian-Chen		1861–1929
He Xiu-Shan			c. 1800
He Zhi-Xiong			1913–1983
Huang Fu-Mi	Huang Xuan-Yan		215–282
Huang Qian	Huang Zhu-Zhai	Huang Wei-Han	1886–1960
Huang Yuan-Yu	Huang Kun-Zai		1705–1750
Jin Li-Meng			c. 1445
Jin Shou-Shan			1921–1983
Ke Qin	Ke Yun-Bo		c. 1669
Koretada Nakanishi			1724–1803
Koso Kitamura			1804–1876
Kyushin Yumoto			1876–1947
Li Gao	Li Ming-Zhi	Li Dong-Yuan	1180–1251
Li Ke-Shao			1910–1996
Li Pei-Sheng			1914–2009
Li Shi-Zhen	Li Dong-Bi		1518–1593
Li Yan-Shi			c. 1957
Li Yin-Lan			c. 1957
Liao Hou-Ze	Lang Qin-Sheng		1923–1998
Ling Yi-Kui			1922–1992
Liu Du-Zhou			1917–2003
Liu Wan-Su	Liu Shou-Zhen	Liu He-Jian	c. 1110
Liu Xi	Liu Cheng-Guo		c. 167
Lu Mao-Xiu	Lu Jiu-Zhi		c. 1886
Lu Pen-Nian	Lu Yuan-Lei		1894–1955
Lu Yu-Chen	Lu Zhu-Zhi		1876–1963
Lu Zi-Yi	Lu Zi-Yao		1599–1664
Lu Zu-Chang			c. 1160
Luo Mei	Luo Dan-Sheng	Luo Dong-Yi	1662–1722
Lü Zhen-Ming	Lü Jian-Xun	Lü Cha-Cun	1796–1852
Ma Shi	Ma Zhong-zhua	Ma Xuan-Tai	c. 1600
Meng Cheng-Yi	Meng Xing-Zhou		c. 1777
Motohiro Tamba	Motohiro Taki		1755–1810
Motokata Tamba	Motokata Taki		1795–1857
Motosugu Tamba	Motosugu Taki		1789–1827

Given name	Honorific name	Alias	Dates (AD)
Pang An-Shi	Pang An-Chang		1042–1099
Pei Shen		Pei Shen-Zhi	1917–1989
Pu Fu-Zhou	Pu Qi-Yu		1888–1975
Qian Huang	Qian Tian-Lai		c. 1707
Qin Bo-Wei	Qin Zhi-Ji	Qian-Zhai	1901–1970
Qin Huang-Shi	Qin Zhi-Zhen		c. 1714
Qiu Qing-Yuan	Qiu Ji-Sheng		1879–1948
Ran Jing-Dian	Ran Jian-Hong	Ran Xue-Feng	1879–1963
Ren Ying-Qiu			1914–1984
Ruan Yuan	Ruan Bo-Yuan		1764–1849
Shen Feng-Hui	Shen Dan-Cai		c. 1801
Shen Jin-Ao	Shen Qian-Lu		1701–1775
Shen Lin-Xi			c. 1874
Shen Ming-Zong	Shen Mu-Nan		c. 1684
Shen Wen-Peng	Shen Yao-Feng		Unknown
Shi Zhen-Sheng			1930–1998
Shu Zhao	Shu Chi-Yuan	Shen Zhai Xue Ren	c. 1739
Sozan Shirozu			1713–1784
Sun Ding-Yi			c. 1899
Sun Si-Miao			581–682
Tang Bu-Qi			1917–2004
Tang Li-Shan	Tang Da-Lie		c. 1792
Tang Zong-Hai	Tang Rong-Chuan		1846–1897
Tao Hong-Jing	Tao Tong-Ming		456–536
Tao Hua	Tao Shang-Wen	Tao Jie-An	1369–1463
Todo Yoshimasu			1702–1773
Wan Quan	Wan Mi-Zhai		1499–1582
Wan You-Sheng			1917–2003
Wang Ang	Wang Ren-An	Wang Heng	1615–1694
Wang Bing	Qi Xuan-Zi		710–804
Wang Hao-Gu	Wang Jin-Zhi	Wang Hai-Zang	c. 1264
Wang Hu	Wang Ling-You	Qing Xi Zi	c. 1680
Wang Ken-Tang	Wang Yu-Tai	Wang Sun-An	1549–1613
Wang Lu	Wang An-Dao	Qi Sou	1132–1391
Wang Su			195–254
Wang Tai-Lin	Wang Xu-Gao	Wang Zai-Xing	1798–1862
Wang Tao			670–755
Wang Xi	Wang Shu-He		201–280

Wang Xue-Tai			1925–2008
Wang Zi-Jie	Wang Jin-San		c. 1658
Wei Li-Tong	Wei Geng-Yu	Wei Nian-Ting	c. 1721
Wu Kun	Wu Shan-Fu		1551–1620
Wu Qian	Wu Ji		1689–1748
Wu Ren-Ju	Wu Ling-Ya		c. 1702
Wu Tang	Wu Ju-Tong		1758–1836
Wu Yi-Luo	Wu Zun-Cheng		1704–1766
Wu You-Xing	Wu You-Ke		1582–1652
Wu Zhen	Wu Kun-An		c. 1796
Wu Zhong-Quan	Wu Pei-Heng		1888–1971
Xing Xi-Bo			1906–1977
Xu Chi	Xu Wu-Cheng		c. 1722
Xu Da-Chun	Xu Ling-Tai		1693–1771
Xu Hong	Xu Zong-Dao		c. 1424
Xu Mian-Zhai	Xu Qin-Xun		1900–1982
Xu Rong-Zhai	Xu Guo-Chun		1911–1982
Xu Shen	Xu Shu-Zhong		c. 100
Xu Shu-Wei	Xu Zhi-Ke		1076–1154
Yamada Seichin			1749–1787
Yang Shang-Shan			c. 650
Yang Xuan	Yang Li-Shan	Yang Yu-Heng	c. 1754
Ye Gui	Ye Tian-Shi		1666–1745
Yi Yin	Yi Zhi		c. 1630 BC
Yodo Odai			1799–1871
You Yi	You Zai-Jing		1650–1749
Yu Chang	Yu Jia-Yan		1585–1644
Yu Chang-Rong			1919–2003
Yu Wu-Yan	Yu Yu		1900–1963
Yu Zhao-Yuan	Yu Gen-Chu		1734–1799
Yue Mei-Zhong	Yue Zhong-Xiu	Chu Yun	1900–1982
Yun Shu-Jue	Yun Tie-Qiao		1878–1935
Zhang Bing-Lin	Zhang Tai-Yan		1869–1936
Zhang Jie-Bin	Zhang Jing-Yue		1563–1640
Zhang Lu	Zhang Lu-Yu	Shi Wan Lao Ren	1617–1699
Zhang Nan	Zhang Xu-Gu		c. 1825
Zhang Sui-Chen	Zhang Qing-Zi		1589–1668
Zhang Xi-Chun	Zhang Shou-Fu		1860–1933
Zhang Xi-Ju	Zhang Ling-Shao		c. 1644

Given name	Honorific name	Alias	Dates (AD)
Zhang Yuan-Su	Zhang Jie-Gu		c. 1131
Zhang Zhi-Cong	Zhang Yin-An		1616–1674
Zhao En-Jian			1926–1999
Zhao Kai-Mei	Zhao Xuan-Du	Qing Chang Lao Ren	1563–1624
Zhao Li-Xun			1934–1996
Zheng Chong-Guang	Zheng Zai-Xin	Zheng Su-Fu	1638–1716
Zheng Shou-Quan	Zheng Qin-An		1824–1911
Zhou Yang-Jun	Zhou Yu-Zai		c. 1671
Zhu Gong	Zhu Yi-Zhong		1050–1125
Zhu Wei-Ju	Ao Shuang Xuan Zhu		1884–1951
Zhu Zhen-Heng	Zhu Dan-Xi		1281–1358
Zou Han-Huang	Zou Zhong-Chen		c. 1840
Zou Shu	Zou Run-An		1790–1844
Zuo Ji-Yun			1891–1942

BIBLIOGRAPHY

Anonymous. *Materia Medica by Shen Nong* (*shén nóng běn cǎo jīng*) 神農本草經. Beijing: Scientific and Technological Literature Publishing House, 1996

Anonymous. *Dictionary in Kang Xi Era* (*kāng xī zì diǎn*) 康熙字典. Chengdu, Chengdu Ancient Book Store, 1980

Anonymous. *Super Book* (*shàng shū*) 尚書. Beijing: China Publishing House, 1980

Anonymous. *Spiritual Pivot* (*líng shū jīng*) 靈樞經. Beijing: People's Health Publishing House, 1963

Anonymous. *Keys to Choose Points for Acupuncture and Moxibustion from Bright Hall* (*míng táng kǒng xué zhēn jiǔ zhì yaò*) 明堂孔穴針灸治要. There is general agreement that this book was published prior to Discussion of Cold Damage (year unknown)

Business Publishing House (ed.) *Three Books on Discussion of Cold Damage* (*shāng hán lùn zhù sān zhǒng*) 傷寒論注三種. Beijing: Business Publishing House, 1957

Cao Jia-Da. *Records for Clinical Application of Classic Formulas* (*jīng fāng shí yàn lù*) 經方實驗錄. Shanghai: Shanghai Science and Technology Publishing House, 1979

Cao Jia-Da. *The Combined Book of Exploring Real Meaning for Discussion of Cold Damage and Essentials and Formula Discussions from the Golden Cabinet* (*cáo shì shāng hán jīn guì fā wēi hé kān*) 曹氏傷寒金匱發微合刊. Shanghai: Shanghai Health Publishing House, 1956

Cai Lu-Xian. *Collections of Chinese Medical Literature* (*zhōng guó yī yào huì hǎi*) 中國醫藥匯海. Shanghai: Chinese Publishing House, 1941

Chao Yuan Fang, textually researched and annotated by Ding Guang-Di et al. *Annotation and Commentary for Discussion of the Origins of Symptoms of Diseases* (*jiào zhù zhū bìng yuán hòu lùn*) 校注諸病源候論. Beijing: People's Health Publishing House, 1991

Chen Bo-Tan (*guì zhī èr má huáng yī tāng*). *I Have Read Discussion of Cold Damage* (*dù guò shāng hán lùn*) 讀過傷寒論. Beijing: People's Health Publishing House, 1954

Chen Bo-Tao. *Formulas from Zhang Zhong-Jing and Their Clinical Applications* (*zhòng-jǐng fāng yǔ lín chuáng*) 仲景方與臨床. Beijing: Chinese Medical Scientific and Technological Publishing House, 1991

Chen Cun-Ren. *Collections of Chinese and Japanese Medical Literature* (*huáng hàn yì xué cóng shū*) 皇漢醫學叢書. Shanghai: Publishing House of Shanghai College of Traditional Chinese Medicine, 1993

Chen Liang-Shi. *Annotation on Six Conformations in Discussion of Cold Damage* (*shāng hán lùn liù jīng lùn zhù*) 傷寒論六經論注. In Teaching and Research Section of Nanjing College of Traditional Chinese Medicine (eds) *Translation and Explanation for Discussion of Cold Damage* (*shāng hán lùn yì shì*) 傷寒論譯釋. Shanghai: Shanghai Science and Technology Publishing House, 1980

Chen Meng-Lei et al. (eds) *Complete Records for All Medical Literature* (*yī bù quán lù*) 醫部全錄. Beijing: People's Health Publishing House, 1959

Chen Ming et al. *Key Points of Clinical Practice for Cold Damage by Liu Du-Zhou* (*liú dù-zhōu shāng hán lín zhèng zhǐ yào*) 劉渡舟傷寒臨證指要. Beijing: Learning Garden Publishing House, 1998

Chen Ming and Zhang Yin-Sheng. *Selection of Cases Studies by Famous Doctors Who Specialized in Discussion of Cold Damage* (*shāng hán míng yī yàn àn jīng xuán*) 傷寒名醫驗案精選. Beijing: Learning Garden Publishing House, 1998

Chen Nian-Zu. *Section Two of New Annotation and Collation for Books by Chen Xiu-Yuan* (*xīn jiào zhù chén xiū-yuán yī shū dì èr jí*) 新校注陳修園醫書第二集. Fuzhou: Fujian Scientific and Technological Publishing House, 2003

Chen Nian-Zu. *Song of the True Formulas for Discussion of Cold Damage* (*shāng hán zhēn fāng gē kuò*) 傷寒真方歌括. Fuzhou: Fujian Scientific and Technological Publishing House, 1985

Chen Nian-Zu. *Song of the Formulas from Zhang Zhong-Jing* (*cháng shā fāng gē kuò*) 長沙方歌括. Shanghai: Shanghai Science and Technology Publishing House, 1963

Chen Ping-Bo. *Reading Discussion of Cold Damage* (*shāng hán lùn dú*). In Shen Feng-Hui (ed.) *Guide to the Study of Discussion of Cold Damage* (*shāng hán pǔ*) 傷寒譜. Jiading: Big and Middle Hall, 1803

Chen Rui-Chun. *Study of Discussion of Cold Damage by Chen Rui-Chun* (*chén ruì-chūn lùn shāng hán*) 陳瑞春論傷寒. Beijing: China Publishing House of Traditional Chinese Medicine, 1996

Chen Shi-Wen et al. (eds) *Imperial Grace Formulary of Tai Ping Era* (*tài píng huì míng hé jì jú fāng*) 太平惠民和劑局方. Beijing: People's Health Publishing House, 1959

Chen Yi-Ren *Search for the Truth for Discussion of Cold Damage* (*shāng hán lùn qǐu shì*) 傷寒論求是. Shanghai: Shanghai Science and Technology Publishing House, 2008

Chen Yi-Ren. "Initial discussion for 'One cannot study Discussion of Cold Damage without understanding root qi, brand qi and middle qi in six qi'." *Jiangsu Journal of Traditional Chinese Medicine*, 1981 (5): 25

Cheng Dan-An. *New Explanation for Discussion of Cold Damage* (*shāng hán lùn xīn zhù*) 傷寒論新注. Nanjing: Jiangsu People's Publishing House, 1956

Chengdu College of Traditional Chinese Medicine. *Textbook for Discussion of Cold Damage* (*shāng hán lùn jiáng yì*) 傷寒論講義. Shanghai: Shanghai Scientific and Technological Publishing House, 1964

Cheng Guo-Pen. *Medical Comprehension* (*yī xué xīn wù*) 醫學心悟. Tianjin: Tianjin Science and Technology Publishing House, 1999

Cheng Shi-De et al. *Selected Explanations for Basic Question* (*sù wèn zhù shì huì cuì*) 素問註釋匯粹. Beijing: People's Health Publishing House, 1982

Cheng Wu-Ji. *Annotating and Explaining Discussion of Cold Damage* (*zhù jiě shāng hán lùn*) 註解傷寒論. Beijing: People's Health Publishing House, 1978

Cheng Wu-Ji. *Understanding the Truth for Discussion of Cold Damage* (*shāng hán míng lǐ lùn*) 傷寒明理論. Shanghai: Business Publishing House, 1955

Cheng Ying-Mao. *True Classification and Analysis for Lines in Discussion of Cold Damage and Supplementary After-Reading Discussion of Cold Damage* (*shāng hán lùn hòu tiǎo biàn, dú shāng hán lùn zhuì yú*) 傷寒論後條辨・讀傷寒論贅餘. Beijing: China Publishing House of Traditional Chinese Medicine, 2009

Cheng Zhao-Huan et al. *Comprehension in the Heart for Discussion of Cold Damage* (*shāng hán xīn wù*) 傷寒心悟. Beijing: Learning Gardening Publishing House, 1989

Cheng Zhi. *Commentary on Classic Discussion of Cold Damage* (*shāng hán jīng zhù*) 傷寒經注. In Guan Qing-Zeng et al. (eds) *Ancient and Contemporary Study for Discussion of Cold Damage* (*shāng hán lùn gǔ jīn yán jiū*) 傷寒論古今研究. Shenyang: Liaoning Scientific and Technological Publishing House, 1994

Chinese Academy of Traditional Chinese Medicine et al. *Concise Dictionary for Traditional Chinese Medicine* (*jiǎn míng zhōng yī dà cí diǎn*) 簡明大中醫辭典. Beijing: People's Health Publishing House, 1979

Chinese Academy of Traditional Chinese Medicine. *Collection of Case Studies by Yue Mei-Zhong* (*yuè méi zhōng yī àn jí*) 岳美中醫案集. Beijing: People's Health Publishing House, 1978

Chinese Academy of Traditional Chinese Medicine. *Dr. Pu Fu-Zhou's Clinical Experiences* (*pú fǔ-zhōu yì liáo jīng yàn*) 蒲輔周醫療經驗. Beijing: People's Health Publishing House, 1976

Craig Mitchell et al. *Shāng Hán Lùn On Cold Damage*. Brookline: Paradigm Publications, 1999

Dai Tian-Zhang. *Clear Differentiation for Warm-Pathogen and Pestilential Diseases* (*wēn yì míng biàn*) 瘟疫明辨. Shanghai: Shanghai Science and Technology Publishing House, 1959

Deng Tie-Tao. *Diagnostic Science in Chinese Medicine* (*zhōng yī zhěn duàn xué*) 中醫診斷學. Shanghai: Shanghai Science and Technology Publishing House, 1984

Dong Xiu and Fang Xian. *Wonderful Formula* (*qí xiào liáng fāng*) 奇效良方. Beijing: Business Publishing House, 1959

Du Si-Jing (ed.) *Outstanding Medicine to Benefit Life* (*jì shēng bá cuì*) 濟生拔粹. Shanghai: Business Publishing House, 1938

Du Yu-Mao. "Exploration of several issues related to Zhang Ji's life." *Journal of Shanxi College of Traditional Chinese Medicine*, 1982 (2): 38

Editorial Committee of Sea of Chinese Character. *Sea of Chinese Character* (*cí hǎi*) 辭海. Shanghai: Shanghai Dictionary Publishing House, 1979

Editorial Department of Business Publishing House. *Origin of Chinese Characters* (*cí yuán*) 辭源. Beijing: Business Publishing House, 1980

Editorial Panel for Medical Works by Physicians of Wu Area (ed.) *Medical Works by Physicians of Wu Era* (*wú zhōng yì jí*) 吳中醫集. Nanjing: Jiangsu Science and Technology Publishing House, 1993

Fang Xian-Ling. *Historical Events for Jin Dynasty* (*jìn shū*) 晉書. Changsha: Yue Lu Publishing House, 1997

Fang Yao-Zhong et al. *Practical Internal Medicine in Chinese Medicine* (*shí yòng zhōng yī nèi kē xué*) 實用中醫內科學. Shanghai: Shanghai Science and Technology Publishing House, 1985

Fang You-Zhi. "Treatise on Discussion of Cold Damage" (*shāng hán lùn tǐao biàn*) 傷寒論條辨. In Business Publishing House (ed.) *Three Books on Discussion of Cold Damage* (*shāng hán lùn zhù sān zhǒng*) 傷寒論注三種. Beijing: Business Publishing House, 1957

Feng Shi-Lun et al. *Passing Down Truth for a Classic Formula* (*jīng fāng chuán zhēn*) 經方傳真. Beijing: China Publishing House of Traditional Chinese Medicine, 1994

Fu You-Feng "Textual research for the concept of shang han." *Helongjiang Journal of Traditional Chinese Medicine*, 1987 (2): 6–8

Gan Zu-Wang. *Three Works by Gan Zu-Wang* (*gān zǔ wàng yī xué sān shū*) 干祖望醫學三書. Jinan: Shandong Science and Technology Publishing House, 2002

Gao Da-Lun. *Study on Qi Cultivation: Book on Bamboo Slips Dug from Tombs in Han Dynasty at Zhang Jia Mountain* (*zhāng jiā shān hàn jián yǐn shū yán jiū*) 張家山漢簡引書研究. Chengdu: Bashu Publishing House, 1995

Gao Da-Lun. *Annotation and Explanation on Pulse Book on Bamboo Slips Dug from Tombs in Han Dynasty at Zhang Jia Mountain* (*zhāng jiā shān hàn jiǎn mài shū jiào shì*) 張家山漢簡脈書校釋. Chengdu: Bashu Publishing House, 1992

Gao Xue-Shan. *Clarification for Writing on the Esteemed Discussion of Cold Damage* (*shāng hán shàng lùn biàn sì*) 傷寒尚論辨似. Beijing: People's Health Publishing House, 1958

Greta Young Jie De and Robin Marchment. *Shāng hán lùn Explained* (傷寒論講解與臨床心得). Amsterdam: Elsevier, Churchill Livingstone, 2009

Guan Qing-Zeng et al. *Ancient and Contemporary Study for Discussion of Cold Damage* (*shāng hán lùn gǔ jīn yán jiū*) 傷寒論古今研究. Shenyang: Liaoning Scientific and Technological Publishing House, 1994

Guangzhou College of Traditional Chinese Medicine and China Academy of Traditional Chinese Medicine. *Dictionary for Chinese Medicine* (*zhōng yī dà cí diǎn*) 中醫大辭典. Beijing: People's Health Publishing House, 1979

Guo Yong. *Replenishment for Discussion of Cold Damage* (*shāng hán bǔ wáng lùn*) 傷寒補亡論. Shanghai: Shanghai Science and Technology Publishing House, 1959

Guo Zhong-Guo. "Preliminary exploration of the meaning of Tai Lu and Yao Lu." *Forum for Doctors to Practice Chinese Medicine*, 2001 (1): 52

Guo Zi-Guang. "Exploration of the principle of differentiation and treatment in Discussion of Cold Damage." *Journal of Chengdu College of Traditional Chinese Medicine*, 1979 (1): 2

Guo Zi-Guang and Feng Xian-Xun. *New Classification of Formulas and Syndromes in Discussion of Cold Damage* (*shāng hán lùn tāng zhèng xīn biān*) 傷寒論湯證新編. Shanghai: Shanghai Health Publishing House, 1983

Guohui Liu. *Warm Pathogen Diseases: A Clinical Guide* (*wēn bìng lín chuáng zhǐ nán*) 溫病臨床指南. Seattle: Eastland Press, 2001

Han Xiang-Ling et al. "The disharmony between the nutritive qi and the defensive qi, and Cinnamon Twig Decoction (*guì zhī tāng*)." *Tianjin Journal of Traditional Chinese Medicine*, 2000 (6): 35

Han Zhao-Qi. *Commentary on Historical Records* (*shǐ jì píng zhù běn*) 史記評註本. Changsha: Yue Lu Press, 2004

Hao Ri-Jin. *Literature Study for Theoretical Source and Development of Qi Transformation in Six Conformations in Discussion of Cold Damage*. Hubei College of Traditional Chinese Medicine, 2008

Hao Wan-Shan. "On establishing discipline of Discussion of Cold Damage and its content." *Journal of Beijing University of Traditional Chinese Medicine*, 1995 (11): 28

Hao Yin-Qing. "Searching for the root of the theory of qi transformation in six conformations of Discussion of Cold Damage." *Shanxi Journal of Traditional Chinese Medicine*, 1994 (4): 52

He Bing-Yuan. *Revised and Expanded Discussion of Warm-Pathogen Disease* (*chóng dìng guáng wēn rè lùn*) 重訂廣溫熱論. Beijing: People's Health Publishing House, 1961

He Xin-Hui. "Exploration of the syndrome of the disharmony between the nutritive qi and the defensive qi." *Forum for Chinese Medical Doctors*, 1998 (1): 4

He Yun-He. "Brief explanation for six conformations." *Fujian Journal of Traditional Chinese Medicine* 1957 (1): 1

He Zhi-Xiong. "Exploration of the essence of six conformations in Discussion of Cold Damage." *New Chinese Medicine*, 1983 (2): 6

He Zhi-Xiong. *Selected Explanations for Discussion of Cold Damage and Answer for Question Related* (*shāng hán lùn xuán shì hé tí dá*) 傷寒論選釋和題答. Guangzhou: Guangdong Shanghai Science and Technology Publishing House, 1981

Huang Fu-Mi. *Acupuncture Jia and Yi Classic* (*zhēn jiǔ jiǎ yǐ jīng*) 針灸甲乙經. Shanghai: Business Publishing House, 1955

Huang Huang. *Fifty Herbs and Syndromes by Zhang Zhong-Jing* (*zhāng zhòng-jǐng wǔ shí wèi yào zhèng*) 張仲景五十味藥證. Beijing: Health Publishing House, 1998

Huang Qian. "What I have learned from studying Discussion of Cold Damage and Miscellaneous Diseases by Zhang Zhong-Jing." *Shanghai Journal of Traditional Chinese Medicine*, 1955 (7): 24

Huang Qian. *Collection of Commentaries for Discussion of Cold Damage and Miscellaneous Diseases* (*shāng hán zá bìng lùn jí zhù*) 傷寒雜病論集注. Nanjing: Central Chinese Medicine Hall, 1925

Huang Wen-Dong. "My ideas on six conformations differentiation and treatments in Discussion of Cold Damage." *Shanghai Journal of Traditional Chinese Medicine*, 1955 (11): 24

Huang Yuan-Yu. *Explanation for Difficult Questions in Discussion of Cold Damage* (*shāng hán xuán jiě*) 傷寒懸解. In Li Yu-Bin (ed.) *Study of Discussion of Cold Damage by Huang Yuan-Yu* (*huáng yuán-yù dú shāng hán*) 黃元禦讀傷寒. Beijing: People's Military Medical Press, 2010

Hubei College of Traditional Chinese Medicine. *Selected Reading from Discussion of Cold Damage* (*shāng hán lùn xuǎn dù*) 傷寒論選讀. Shanghai: Shanghai Scientific and Technological Publishing House, 1979

Hu Guo-Chen. *Collection of the Works of Famous Physicians in Tang, Song, Jin and Yuan Dynasty* (*táng sòng jīn yuán míng yī quán shū dà chéng*) 唐宋金元名醫全書大成. Beijing: China Chinese Medical Publishing House, 2006

Jia-Fu Feng and Jane English. *Tao Te Ching*. New York: Vintage Books, 1972

Jiang Chun-Hua. *Understanding the Meaning of Discussion of Cold Damage* (*shāng hán lùn shì yì*) 傷寒論識義. Shanghai: Shanghai Health Publishing house, 1985

Jiang Chun-Hua. "Discussion of several issues on six conformations in Discussion of Cold Damage." *Shanghai Journal of Traditional Chinese Medicine*, 1962 (8): 17

Jiang Jian-Guo. *Explanation for Difficult Points in Discussion of Cold Damage* (*shāng hán lùn shì nán*) 傷寒論釋難. Shanghai: The Publishing House of Shanghai University of Traditional Chinese Medicine, 2007

Jiang Jian-Guo and Li Shu-Pei. *Analysis of Difficult Questions in Discussion of Cold Damage* (*shāng hán xī yí*) 傷寒析疑. Beijing: Scientific and Technological Documents Publishing House, 1999

Jiangsu Research Institute of Traditional Chinese Medicine. *Explanation for the Formulas in Discussion of Cold Damage* (*shāng hán lùn fāng jiě*) 傷寒論方解. Nanjing: Jiangsu Science and Technology Publishing House, 1978

Jiang You-Li. "On 'The defensive qi comes from the lower burner.'" Journal of Traditional Chinese Medicine, 1981 (12): 13

Jiang You-Li. *Taoist Culture and Chinese Medicine* (*dào jiā wén huà yǔ zhōng yī xué*) 道家文化與中醫學. Fuzhou: Fu Jian Science and Technology Publishing House, 1997

Jin Li-Meng et al. *Collection of Medical Formulas According to Their Different Types* (*yī fāng lèi jù*) 醫方類聚. Beijing: People's Health Publishing House, 1957

Jin Shou-Shan. *Selected Medical Discussions from Jin Shou-Shan* (*jīn shòu-shān yī lùn xuán jí*) 金壽山醫論選集. Beijing: People's Health Publishing House, 1983

Jing San-Long and Shao Zhi-Qian. *Buddhism Parables* (*bǎi yù jīng*) 百喻經. Xian: Tai Bai Art Publishing House, 2005

Ke Qin. *Commentary on Surviving with Discussion of Cold Damage* (*shāng hán lái sū jí, shāng hán lùn zhù*) 傷寒來蘇集・傷寒論注. Shanghai: Shanghai Science and Technology Publishing House, 1978

Ke Qin. *Discussion of Special Topic in Surviving with Cold Damage* (*shāng hán lái sū jí, shāng hán lùn yì*) 傷寒來蘇集・傷寒論翼. Shanghai: Shanghai Science and Technology Publishing House, 1978

Ke Qin. *Surviving with Discussion of Cold Damage* (*shāng hán lái sū jí*) 傷寒來蘇集. Shanghai: Shanghai Science and Technology Publishing House, 1978

Koretada Nakanishi. *Study on Discussion of Cold Damage* (*shāng hán lùn zhī yán jiū*) 傷寒論之研究. Beijing: People's Health Publishing House, 1957

Li Fang et al. *Book Review by Emperor in Tai Ping era* (*tài píng yù lán*) 太平御覽. Beijing: Chinese Publishing House, 1960

Li Gao. *Secret Formulas in Orchid Room* (*lán shì mì cáng*) 蘭室秘藏. In Ye Chuan et al. (eds) *Collection of Famous Works from Four Scholars in Jin-Yuan Era* (*jīn yuán sì dà jiā míng zhù jí chéng*) 金元四大家名著集成. Beijing: China Chinese Medicine Publishing House, 1995

Li Han-Zhang et al. *History of Hunan Province* (*hú nán tōng zhì*) 湖南通誌. Changsha: Pavilion of Respect for Classics in Learning Palace, 1885

Li Hang-Zhou. *Exploration for Balanced View of Qi Transformation Reflected by Resolving Time for Diseases in Six Conformation in Discussion of Cold Damage (shāng hán lùn liù jīng bìng yù jiě shí suǒ àn hán qì huà píng héng guān tān jiū).* Beijing: Beijing University of Chinese Medicine, 2011

Li Jing et al. *Study for the Formulas, Syndromes and Herbs in Discussion of Cold Damage (shāng hán lùn fāng zhèng yào yán jiū)* 傷寒論方證藥研究. Haerbing: Heilongjiang Scientific and Technological Publishing House, 1992

Li Ke-Shao. *Explanation of Confusing Points in Discussion of Cold Damage (shāng hán jiě huò lùn)* 傷寒解惑論. Shandong: Shandong Scientific and Technological Publishing House, 1978

Li Ke-Shao et al. *Translation and Explanation for Discussion of Cold Damage (shāng hán lùn yǔ shì)* 傷寒論語釋. Shandong: Shandong Scientific and Technological Publishing House, 1982

Li Le-Yi. *Five Hundred Cases for Changes to Chinese Characters* (revised edition) *(hàn zì yán biàn wǔ bǎi lì)* 漢字演變五百例. Beijing: Publishing House of Beijing Language University, 2002

Li Pei-Sheng et al. *Teaching Reference Books for Traditional Chinese Medical Colleges: Discussion of Cold Damage (gāo děng zhōng yī yuàn xiào jiào xué cān káo shū: shāng hán lùn)* 高等中醫院校教學參考書:傷寒論. Beijing: People's Health Publishing House, 1987

Li Shi-Zhen. *Detailed Outline of the Materia Medica (běn cǎo gāng mù)* 本草綱目. Beijing: People's Health Publishing House, 1981

Li Shun-Bao. *Complete Collection for Versions of Discussion of Cold Damage (shāng hán lùn bǎn běn dà quán)* 傷寒論版本大全. Beijing: Learning Garden Publishing House, 2001

Li Wen-Bo. *General Explanation for the Book of Changes (yì jīng tōng jiě)* 易經通解. Beijing: China Publishing House of Contributing to Public, 2008

Li Wen-Rui. *Differentiation and Treatment Related to Formulas and Syndrome in Discussion of Cold Damage (shāng hán lùn tāng zhèng lùn zhì)* 傷寒論湯證論治. Beijing: Publishing House for People's Army Medical Doctor, 1989

Li Xin-Ji. *Thorough Explanation for Discussion of Cold Damage (shāng hán lùn tōng shì)* 傷寒論通釋. Beijing: Beijing: People's Health Publishing House, 2003

Li Xin-Ji. *Explanation for Difficult Points in Discussion of Cold Damage (shāng hán lùn yí nán jiě dú)* 傷寒論疑難解讀. Beijing: Beijing: People's Health Publishing House, 1998

Li Yan-Shi. *Itemized Explanation for Discussion of Cold Damage and Essentials and Formula Discussions from the Golden Cabinet (shāng hán jīn guì tiǎo shì)* 傷寒金匱條釋. Beijing: People's Health Publishing House, 1957

Li Yin-Lan. *Explanation Line by Line for Discussion of Cold Damage (shāng hán lùn tiǎo xì)* 傷寒論條析. Beijing: People's Health Publishing House, 1963

Li Yu-Bin. *Study Discussion of Cold Damage by Huang Yuan-Yu (huáng yuán-yù dú shāng hán)* 黃元禦讀傷寒. Beijing: Peoples' Military Medial Press, 2010

Liang Hua-Long. "Origin and application of the theory of opening, closing and pivot in six conformations." *Henan Journal of Traditional Chinese Medicine*, 1998 (2): 5

Liao Hou-Ze. *Explanation for the Syndromes Recorded in Discussion of Cold Damage and Essentials from Golden Cabinet* (*shāng hán jīn guì huì zhèng quán jiě*) 傷寒金匱匯證詮解. Beijing: Ancient Chinese Medical Literatures Publishing House, 1996

Liaoning College of Traditional Chinese Medicine. *Ancient Literatures in Medicine* (*yī gǔ wén*) 醫古文. Shenyang: Liaoning Scientific and Technological Publishing House, 1986

Lin Qian-Liang and Wang Gui-Miao. *Collection of Studies for Herbs in Classical Formula* (*jīng fāng zhōng yào yán jiū jí chéng*) 經方中藥研究集成. Beijing: Ancient Chinese Medical Literature Publishing House, 1992

Lin Yi-Kui et al. *Chinese Medical Herbs* (*zhōng yào xué*) 中藥學. Shanghai: Shanghai Science and Technology Publishing House, 1984

Liu Du-Zhou. "The theory of qi transformation in Discussion of Cold Damage." *New Chinese Medicine*, 1983 (2): 4

Liu Du-Zhou. "Discussion of several issues in Discussion of Cold Damage." *Journal of New Medicine*, 1978 (1): 18

Liu Du-Zhou and Fu Shi-Yuan. *Explanation for Discussion of Cold Damage* (*shāng hán lùn quán jiě*) 傷寒論詮解. Tianjin: Tianjin Scientific and Technological Publishing House, 1983

Liu Du-Zhou, Nie Hui-Min and Fu Shi-Yuan. *Synopsis for Discussion of Cold Damage* (*shāng hán qiè yào*) 傷寒挈要. Beijing: People's Health Publishing House, 1983

Liu Du-Zhou et al. *Textual Research and Annotation for Discussion of Cold Damage* (*shāng hán lùn jiào zhù*) 傷寒論校注. Beijing: People's Health Publishing House, 1991

Liu Li-Hong. *Pondering Over Chinese Medicine* (*sī kǎo zhōng yī*) 思考中醫. Nanning: Guang Xi Normal University Publishing House, 2002

Liu Shao-Wu. "Informally exploring that six conformations should be viewed as six diseases." *New Chinese Medicine*, 1979 (4): 12

Liu Wan-Su. *Direct Study for Cold Damage* (*shāng hán zhí gé*) 傷寒直格. In *Formulas from Yang Ren-Zhai Plus Four Other Books* (*rén zhāi zhí zhǐ fāng wài sì zhǒng*). Shanghai: Shanghai Ancient Literature Publishing House, 1991

Liu Wan-Su. *Formulas from the Discussion Illuminating the The Yellow Emperor's Basic Question* (*huáng dì sù wèn xuān míng lùn fāng*) 黄帝素問宣明論方. In *Formulas from Yang Ren-Zhai Plus Four Other Books* (*rén zhāi zhí zhǐ fāng wài sì zhǒng*) 仁齋直指外四種. Shanghai: Shanghai Ancient Literature Publishing House, 1991

Liu Yong-Min. "A study of Classical Methods to Make Formulas and Rhymed Formula for Keys to Employ Herbs According to Zang-fu Organs: Discussing the great influence of early Taoist culture on traditional Chinese medical science." *Dunhuang Research*, 2010 (3): 60

Liu Yu-Jian. *Numbers and Doctrine of Book of Changes During West and East Han Dynasty* (*liáng hàn xiàng shù yì xué yán jiū*) 兩漢像數易學研究. Nanning: Guangxi Education Publishing House, 1995

Liu Zhen-Ming et al. *Basics for Ancient Medical Literatures* (*yī gǔ wén jī chǔ*) 醫古文基礎. Beijing: People's Health Publishing House, 1980

Lu Mao-Xiu. *Medical Works in Shi Bu House* (*shì bǔ zhāi yī shū*) 世補齋醫書. Shaoxing: Shan Zuo Press, 1886

Lu Pen-Nian. *Current Explanation for Discussion of Cold Damage* (*shāng hán lùn jīn shì*) 傷寒論今釋. Beijing: Learning Garden Publishing House, 2008

Lu Zi-Yi. *Copy and Comment That Can Help in Deeply Understanding Discussion of Cold Damage by Zhong-Jing* (*zhòng-jǐng shāng hán lùn shū chāo jīn pī*) 仲景傷寒論書鈔金錍. In Nie Hui-Min et al. (eds) *Collection of Explanations on Discussion of Cold Damage* (*shāng hán lùn jí jiě*) 傷寒論集解. Beijing: Learning Garden Publishing House, 2001

Luo Mei. *Broad Discussion of The Yellow Emperor's Inner Classic* (*nèi jíng bó yì*) 內經博議. In Qiu Qing-Yuan (ed.) *Collection of Rare Chinese Medical Books* (*zhēn běn yī shū jí chéng*) 珍本醫書集成. Shanghai: Shanghai Science and Technology Publishing House, 1985

Lü Zhen-Ming. *Search for the Source of Discussion of Cold Damage* (*shāng hán xún yuán*) 傷寒尋源. Changchun: Continent Publishing House, 1942

Ma Ji-Xing and Li Xue-Qin. *Fifty-two Diseases and Their Formulas in Books Written on Silk from Tombs in Han Dynasty at Ma Wang Dui* (*má wáng duī hàn mù bó shū, wǔ shí èr bìng fāng*) 馬王堆漢墓帛書・五十二病方. In *The Panel to Recover Books Written on Silk from Tombs in Han Dynasty at Ma Wang Dui*. Beijing: Publishing House of Cultural Relics, 1979

Ma Shi. *Exploration of the Deep Meaning for Syndrome and Commentary for Basic Question of The Yellow Emperor's Inner Classic* (*huáng dì nèi jīng sù wèn zhù zhèng fā wēi*) 黃帝內經素問注證發微. In Cheng Meng-Lei et al. (eds) *Complete Records for All Medical Literature* (*yī bù quán lù*) 醫部全錄. Beijing: People's Health Publishing House, 1959

Ma Yi-Chao, Jiang Jian-Guo and Lu Xiao-Ming. "Discussion of several issues related to formulas of Bupleurum decoctions, their syndromes and harmonization." *Journal of Shandong University of Traditional Chinese Medicine*, 1979 (1): 21

Meng Cheng-Yi. *Points of Essence in Discussion of Cold Damage* (*shāng hán diǎn jīng*) 傷寒點精. In Guan Qing-Zeng et al. (eds) *Ancient and Contemporary Study for Discussion of Cold Damage* (*shāng hán lùn gǔ jīn yán jiū*) 傷寒論古今研究. Shenyang: Liaoning Scientific and Technological Publishing House, 1994

Motokata Tamba. *Description of Meaning for Discussion of Cold Damage* (*shāng hán shù yì*) 傷寒述義. Beijing: People's Health Publishing House, 1955

Nanjing College of Traditional Chinese Medicine. *Annotation and Explanation for Difficult Questions* (*nàn jīng jiào shì*) 難經校釋. Beijing: People's Health Publishing House, 1979

Nie Hui-Min. *Study of Discussion of Cold Damage by Nie Hui-Min* (*niè shì shāng hán xué*) 聶氏傷寒學. Beijing: Learning Garden Publishing House, 2005

Nie Hui-Min. "On 'Harmonization' in Discussion of Cold Damage." *Journal of Chinese Medicine*, 2002 (17): 4,199

Nie Hui-Min. *Discussion of Cold Damage and Its Clinical Application* (*shāng hán lùn yǔ lín zhèng*) 傷寒論與臨證. Beijing: People's Health Publishing House, 1993

Nie Hui-Min. *Analysis Meaning for Discussion of Cold Damage* (*shāng hán lùn xī yì*) 傷寒論析義. Beijing: Ancient Chinese Medical Literature Publishing House, 1987

Nie Hui-Min et al. (eds) *Collection of Explanations on Discussion of Cold Damage* (*shāng hán lùn jí jiě*) 傷寒論集解. Beijing: Learning Garden Publishing House, 2001

Nie Hui-Min et al. *Selection of Explanations for Classical Formulas* (*jīng fāng fāng lùn huì yào*) 經方方論匯要. Changsha: Hunan Science and Technology Publishing House, 1999

Nie Hui-Min et al. *Textbook for Discussion of Cold Damage* (*shāng hán lùn jiáng yì*) 傷寒論講義. Beijing: Learning Gardening Publishing House, 1996

Pang An-Shi. *General Discussion for the Discussion of Cold Damage* (*shāng hán zǒng bìng lùn*) 傷寒總病論. In Tian Si-Sheng et al. (eds) *Complete Medical Works from Zhu Gong and Pang An-Shi* (*zhū gōng páng ān-shí yī xué quán shū*) 朱肱龐安時醫學全書. Beijing: China Chinese Medical Publishing House, 2006

Paul Procter et al. *Longman Dictionary of Contemporary English*. London: Pitman Press, 1978

Pei Shen. *Identification of Syndromes Treated by Discussion of Cold Damage* (*shāng hán fāng zhèng shí*) 傷寒方證識. Lanzhou: Gansu Science and Technology Publishing House, 1987

Pei Yong-Qing. *Fifty Discussions for Clinical Application of Discussion of Cold Damage* (*shāng hán lùn lín chuáng yìng yòng wǔ shí lùn*) 傷寒論臨床應用五十論. Beijing: Learning Garden Publishing House, 1995

Qian Chao-Chen. *Thorough Examination of All Literature Related to Discussion of Cold Damage* (*shāng hán lùn wén xiàn tōng kǎo*) 傷寒論文獻通考. Beijing: Learning Gardening Publishing House, 1993

Qian Huang. *Trace to Source for Discussion of Cold Damage* (*shāng hán sù yuán jí*) 傷寒溯源集. Shanghai: Shanghai Health Publishing House, 1957

Qin Bo-Wei. *Medical Lecture in Modest House* (*qiān zhāi yī xué jiǎng gǎo*) 謙齋醫學講稿. Shanghai: Shanghai Science and Technology Publishing House 1964

Qin Huang-Shi. *Full Understanding of Discussion of Cold Damage* (*shāng hán dà bái*) 傷寒大白. Beijing: People's Health Publishing House, 1982

Qiu Qing-Yuan (ed.) *Collection of Rare Chinese Medical Books* (*zhēn běn yī shū jí chéng*) 珍本醫書集成. Shanghai: Shanghai Science and Technology Publishing House, 1985

Ran Jing-Dian. *Comments on Discussion of Cold Damage* (*rǎn zhù shāng hán lùn*) 冉注傷寒論. Beijing: Science and Technology Literature Publishing House, 1982

Ren Ying-Qiu. *Collection of the Papers of Ren Ying-Qiu* (*rèn yìng-qiū wén jí*) 任應秋文集. Beijing: People's Army Physician Publishing House, 2009

Ren Ying-Qiu. *Classified Explanation for Differentiation and Treatment in Discussion of Cold Damage* (*shāng hán lùn zhèng zhì lèi quán*) 傷寒論證治類詮. Beijing: Science and Health Publishing House, 1959

Ren Ying-Qiu et al. *Various Schools in Chinese Medicine* (*zhōng yī gè jiā xué shuō*) 中醫各家學說. Shanghai: Shanghai Scientific and Technological Publishing House, 1980

Ruan Yuan. *Commentary on Thirteen Classics* (*shí sān jīng zhù shū*) 十三經注疏. Beijing: China Publishing house, 1980

Sha Shao-Hai. *Primary Explanation for Hexagram in the Book of Changes* (*yì guà qiǎn shì*) 易卦淺釋. Guiyang: Guizhou People Publishing House, 1987

Sha Shao-Hai and Xu Zi-Hong. *Complete Translation of Lao Zi* (*lǎo zǐ quán yì*) 老子全譯. Guiyang: Guizhou People's Publishing House, 1989

Shang Chi-Chang et al. *Application Guidance for Herbal Combination in Classical Formula* (*jīng fāng pèi wǔ yòng yào zhǐ nán*) 經方配伍用藥指南. Beijing: China Publishing House of Traditional Chinese Medicine, 1998

Shanghai Ancient Literature Publishing House. *Formulas from Yang Ren-Zhai Plus Four Other Books* (*rén zhāi zhí zhǐ fāng wài sì zhǒng*) 仁齋直指外四種. Shanghai: Shanghai Ancient Literature Publishing House, 1983

Shen Jin-Ao. *Outline for Discussion of Cold Damage* (*shāng hán lùn gāng mù*) 傷寒論綱目. Beijing: Learning Garden Publishing House, 2009

Shen Lin-Xi. *Collection of Classifications for Discussion of Cold Damage* (*shāng hán fēn lèi jí chéng*) 傷寒分類集成. In Guan Qing-Zeng et al. (eds) *Ancient and Contemporary Study for Discussion of Cold Damage* (*shāng hán lùn gǔ jīn yán jiū*) 傷寒論古今研究. Shenyang: Liaoning Scientific and Technological Publishing House, 1994

Shen Ming-Zong. *Differentiation and Treatment for Six Conformations in Discussion of Cold Damage* (*shāng hán liù jīng biàn zhèng zhì fǎ*) 傷寒六經辨證治法. Shanghai: Shanghai Health Publishing House, 1957

Shen Wen-Peng. *Reading Discussion of Cold Damage* (*shāng hán lùn dú*) 傷寒論讀. In Li Pei-Sheng et al. (eds) *Teaching Reference Books for Traditional Chinese Medical Colleges: Discussion of Cold Damage* (*gāo děng zhōng yī yuàn xiào jiào xué cān káo shū: shāng hán lùn*) 高等中醫院校教學參考書:傷寒論. Beijing: People's Health Publishing House, 1987

Shi Zhen-Sheng. *Collaborating the Lines for Construing Discussion of Cold Damage* (*shāng hán lùn chuàn jiě*) 傷寒論串解. Beijing: Chinese Medical Ancient Literature Publishing House, 1987

Shi Zheng-Chu "Discussion of the relationship between 'The Defensive Qi Comes from the Lower Burner' and 'The Defensive Qi Comes from the Upper Burner'." *The Journal of Wen Zhou Medical College*, 1982 (2): 79

Shu Zhao. *Collection of Commentaries for Discussion of Cold Damage by Mr. Shu* (*shū shì shāng hán lùn jí zhù*) 舒氏傷寒論集注. Beijing: Chinese Ancient Medical Literature Publishing House, 1994

Sozan Shirozu. *Discussion of Cold Damage Taught by Sozan Shirozu* (*shāng hán lùn liú shì zhuàn*) 傷寒論劉氏傳. In Jiang Chun-Hua (ed.) *Understanding the Meaning of Discussion of Cold Damage* (*shāng hán lùn shì yì*) 傷寒論釋義. Shanghai: Shanghai Health Publishing house, 1985

Sun Ding-Yi. *Syntactic and Semantic Analysis of Discussion of Cold Damage* (*shāng hán zá bìng lùn zhāng jù*) 傷寒論雜病論章句. In Guan Qing-Zeng et al. (eds) *Ancient and Contemporary Study for Discussion of Cold Damage* (*shāng hán lùn gǔ jīn yán jiū*) 傷寒論古今研究. Shenyang: Liaoning Scientific and Technological Publishing House, 1994

Sun Si-Miao. *Supplement to Thousand Ducat Formulas* (*qiān jín yì fāng*) 千金翼方. Beijing: People's Health Publishing House, 1955

Sun Si-Miao. *Thousand Ducat Formulas for Emergent Cases* (*bèi jí qiā jīn yào fāng*) 備急千金要方. Beijing: People's Health Publishing House, 1982

Tang Li-Shan. *Collection of Papers of Physicians of Wu Area* (*wú yī huì jiǎng*) 吳醫匯講. Shanghai: Shanghai Science and Technology Publishing House. 1983

Tang Zong-Hai. *On Blood Disorders* (*xuè zhèng lùn*) 血證論. Shanghai: Shanghai People's Publishing House, 1977

Tang Zong-Hai. *Correction for Preliminary Commentary for Discussion of Cold Damage* (*shāng hán lùn qiān zhù bǔ zhèng*) 傷寒論淺注補正. In *Five Types of Medical Works in Relation to the Connection Between Chinese Medicine and Western Medicine* (*zhōng xī huì tōng yī xué wǔ zhòng*) 中西匯通醫學五種. Shanghai: Publishing House of Selling Thousands Books, 1908

Tao Hong-Jing. *Collected Commentary for Materia Medica By Shen Nong* (*běn cǎo jīng jí zhù*) 本草經集注. Beijing: People's Health Publishing House, 1978

Tao Hua, textually studied by Huang Jin-Ming and Fu Xi-Qin. *Six Books for Discussion of Cold Damage* (*shāng hán liù shū*) 傷寒六書. Beijing: People's Health Publishing House, 1990

Teaching and Research Section for Discussion of Cold Damage, Jiangsu School of Traditional Chinese Medicine. *Explanation for Discussion of Cold Damage* (*shāng hán lùn shì yì*) 傷寒論釋譯. Nanjing: Jiangsu People's Publishing House, 1958

Teaching and Research Section of Nanjing College of Traditional Chinese Medicine. *Translation and Explanation for Discussion of Cold Damage* (*shāng hán lùn yì shì*) 傷寒論譯釋. Shanghai: Shanghai Science and Technology Publishing House, 1980

Teaching Section of Discussion of Cold Damage and Warm Pathogen Disease at Shanghai College of Traditional Chinese Medicine. *Discussion of Cold Damage* (*shāng hán lùn*) 傷寒論. Shanghai: Shanghai Science and Technology Publishing House, 1983

Tian Si-Sheng et al. *Complete Medical Works from Zhu Gong and Pang An-Shi* (*zhū gōng páng ān-shí yī xué quán shū*) 朱肱龐安時醫學全書. In *Collection of the Works of Famous Physicians in Tang, Song, Jin and Yuan Dynasty* (*táng sòng jīn yuán míng yī quán shū dà chéng*) 唐宋金元名醫全書大成. Beijing: China Chinese Medical Publishing House, 2006

Wan Quan. *Selected Important Approaches from Discussion of Cold Damage in the Medical Works Passed Down from Wan's Family* (*wàn shì jiā chuán shāng hán zhāi jǐn*) 萬氏家傳傷寒摘錦. Wuhan: Hubei Science and Technology Publishing House, 1984

Wan Xiao-Gang. "Brief History of School of Study of Febrile Diseases and Its Development." In Xiong Man-Qi et al. (eds) *Discussion of Cold Damage in a Series of Advanced Books for Chinese Medicine* (*zhōng yī yào xué gāo jí cóng shū: shāng hán lùn*) 中醫藥學高級叢書傷寒論. Beijing: People's Health Publishing House, 2000

Wan You-Sheng. *Key Points to Learn in Discussion of Cold Damage* (*shāng hán lùn zhī yào*) 傷寒論知要. Nanchang: Jiangxi People's Publishing House, 1982

Wan You-Sheng. "On unification of discussion of Cold Damage and warm pathogen diseases." *Yunnan Journal of Traditional Chinese Medicine*, 1981 (1): 1

Wan You-Sheng. "On unification of six conformations in Discussion of Cold Damage, four levels and three burners differentiations in warm pathogen diseases." *Chinese Medicine in Jiangxi*, 1980 (4): 7

Wan You-Sheng. "On the essence of three yin and three yang in Discussion of Cold Damage." *Jiangsu Journal of Traditional Chinese Medicine*, 1980 (4): 35

Wan You-Sheng. "Discussion on transverse view in Discussion of Cold Damage and vertical view in warm pathogen disease." *Chinese Medicine in Jiangxi*, 1957 (1): 52

Wang Ang. *Collected Explanations for Medical Formulas* (*yī fāng jí jiě*) 醫方集解. Shanghai: Shanghai Science and Technology Publishing House, 1959

Wang Bing. *Basic Questions of The Yellow Emperor's Inner Classic* (*huáng dì nèi jīng sù wèn*) 黄帝內經素問. Beijing: People's Health Publishing House, 1963

Wang Hao-Gu. *Herbs for Making Formulas* (*tāng yè běn cǎo*) 湯液本草. Beijing: People's Health Publishing House, 1956

Wang Hao-Gu. *These Things Are Hard to Know* (*cǐ shì nán zhī*) 此事難知. In Du Si-Jing (eds) *Outstanding Medicine to Benefit Life* (*jì shēng bá cuì*) 濟生拔粹. Shanghai: Business Publishing House, 1938

Wang Hu. *Commentary on Differentiation in Discussion of Cold Damage* (*shāng hán lùn biàn zhèng guáng zhù*) 傷寒論辯證廣注. Shanghai: Shanghai Health Publishing House, 1958

Wang Ji-Min et al. *Translation and Comments for Brief Historical Stories of States* (*guó yǔ yì zhù*) 國語譯註. Guangzhou: Hundreds Flower Island Literature and Arts Publishing House, 1992

Wang Ke-Qin. "Discussion of Cold Damage in Japan." *Heilongjiang Journal of Traditional Chinese Medicine*, 1985 (1): 53

Wang Ke-Qiong. *Standards for Applying Classic Formula* (*jíng fāng shǐ yòng biāo zhǔn*) 經方使用標準. Lanzhou: Gansu Science and Technology Publishing House, 1990

Wang Ken-Tang. *Indispensable Tools of Pattern Treatments* (*zhèng zhì zhǔn shéng*) 證治準繩. Shanghai: Shanghai Science and Technology Publishing House, 1959

Wang Lu. *Discourse on Tracing Back to the Medical Classics* (*yī jīng sù huí jí*) 醫經溯洄集. Nanjing: Jiangsu Science and Technology Publishing House, 1984

Wang Qi et al. *Lecture and Explanation for Discussion of Cold Damage* (*shāng hán lùn jiǎng jiě*) 傷寒論講解. Zhengzhou, Henan Scientific and Technological Publishing House, 1988

Wang Qi et al. *Application of Classic Formulas* (*jīng fāng yìng yòng*) 經方應用. Yinchuan, Ningxia People's Publishing House, 1981

Wang Qi et al. *Modern Explanation for Basic Question of The Yellow Emperor's Inner Classic* (*sù wèn jīn shì*) 素問今釋 Guiyang: Guizhou People Publishing House, 1981

Wang Qing-Guo and Wang Zhen. "Forty-one opinions about study on six conformations for Discussion of Cold Damage." *Journal of Beijing University of Traditional Chinese Medicine* 1997, (20): 4

Wang Shi-Min. "Exploration of the relationship among Rhymed Formula for Keys to Employ Herbs According to Zang-fu Organs, Classical Methods to Make Formulas and Discussion of Cold Damage and Miscellaneous Diseases." *Journal of Traditional Chinese Medicine*, 1998 (11): 694

Wang Tai-Lin. *Six Medical Books from Wang Xu-Gao* (*wáng xù gāo yī shū liù zhǒng*) 王旭高醫書六種. Shanghai: Shanghai Science and Technology Publishing House, 1978

Wang Tao. *Arcane Essentials from the Imperial Library* (*wài tái mì yào*) 外台秘要. Shanghai: Shanghai Ancient Literature Publishing House, 1991

Wang Xi. Pul*ses Classic* (*mài jīng*) 脈經. Beijing: People's Health Publishing House, 1985

Wang Xian Qian. *Supplement for Commentary of Explanation of Names* (*shì míng shū zhèng bǔ*) 釋名疏證補. Shanghai: Shanghai Ancient Literatures Publishing House, 1984

Wang Xue-Tai. *Textual Research, Commentary and Annotation for Rhymed Formula for Keys to Employ Herbs According to Zang-fu Organs* (*fǔ xíng jué zàng fǔ yòng yào fǎ yào jiào zhù*) 輔行訣臟腑用藥法要校注. Beijing: People's Military Medical Press, 2008

Wang Zhan-Xi. *Clinical Application of Discussion of Cold Damage* (*shāng hán lùn lín chuáng yìng yòng*) 傷寒論臨床應用. Beijing: Scientific and Technological Literature Publishing House, 1990

Wang Zi-Jie. *Selection and Commentary for Ancient Formulas in Red Flower Garden* (*jiàng xuě yuán gǔ fāng xuán zhù*) 絳雪園古方選注. Shanghai: Shanghai Science and Technology Publishing House, 1982

Wei Li-Tong, annotated by Liu Cong-Ming et al. *Original Meaning in Discussion of Cold Damage* (*shāng hán lùn běn yì*) 傷寒論本義. Beijing: Ancient Chinese Medical Literature Publishing House, 2008

Wen Chang-Lu. "Section one of review and commentary for theoretical study of Discussion of Cold Damage in recent hundred years." *Henan Journal of Traditional Chinese Medicine*, 2007 (3): 1

Wen Chang-Lu et al. *Collection of Studies for Works Written by Zhang Zhong-Jing* (*zhāng zhòng-jǐng yán jiū jí chéng*) 張仲景研究集成. Beijing. Chinese Medical Ancient Literature Publishing House, 2004

Wu Kun. *Commentary by Mr. Wu on Basic Questions of The Yellow Emperor's Inner Classic* (*huáng dì nèi jīng sù wèn wú zhù*) 黃帝內經吳注. In Cheng Shi-De et al. (eds) *Selected Explanations for Basic Questions* (*sù wèn zhù shì huì cuì*) 素問註釋匯粹. Beijing: People's Health Publishing House, 1982

Wu Qian et al. *Annotation and Explanation for Cold Damage in Golden Mirror of the Medical Tradition* (*yī zōng jìn jiàn, dìng zhèng shāng hán lùn zhù*) 醫宗金鑑・訂正傷寒論注. Beijing: People's Health Publishing House, 1973

Wu Ren-Ju. *Inherit the Past and Usher in the Future for Medicine* (*yī zōng chéng qǐ*) 醫宗承啟. In Guan Qing-Zeng et al. *Ancient and Contemporary Study for Discussion of Cold Damage* (*shāng hán lùn gǔ jīn yán jiū*) 傷寒論古今研究. Shenyang: Liaoning Scientific and Technological Publishing House, 1994

Wu Tang. *Systematic Differentiation of Warm Disease* (*wēn bìng tiǎo biàn*) 溫病條辨. Beijing: People's Health Publishing House, 1963

Wu Yi-Luo. *Classified Channels in Discussion of Cold Damage* (*shāng hán fēn jīng*) 傷寒分經. Ganshui: Benefit Hall, 1766

Wu You-Xing. *Discussion of Warm Epidemics* (*wēn yì lùn*) 溫疫論. Changchun: Liaoning Science and Technology Publishing House, 1997

Wu Zhen. *Complete Understanding for Cold Damage* (*shāng hán zhǐ zhǎng*) 傷寒指掌. Shanghai: Science and Technology Publishing House, 1959

Xi Zheng-Long. "Section one of School of Studying Febrile Diseases and School of Studying Discussion of Cold Damage." *Shangdong Journal of Traditional Chinese Medicine*, 1991 (6): 22–23

Xi Zheng-Long. "Section two of School of Studying Febrile Diseases and School of Studying Discussion of Cold Damage." *Shangdong Journal of Traditional Chinese Medicine*, 1992 (1): 20

Xing Xi-Bo et al. *Clinical Practice Record for Discussion of Cold Damage* (*shāng hán lùn lín chuáng shí yàn lù*) 傷寒論臨床實驗錄. Tianjin: Tianjin Science and Technology Publishing House, 1984

Xiong Man-Qi et al. *Discussion of Cold Damage in a Series of Advanced Books for Chinese Medicine* (*zhōng yī yào xué gāo jí cóng shū: shāng hán lùn*) 中國醫學高級叢書傷寒論. Beijing: People's Health Publishing House, 2000

Xu Chi. *Collection of Commentaries for Discussion of Cold Damage* (*shāng hán lùn jí zhù*) 傷寒論集注. In Editorial Panel for Medical Works by Physicians of Wu Era (ed.) *Medical Works by Physicians of Wu Area* (*wú zhōng yì jí*) 吳中醫集. Nanjing: Jiangsu Science and Technology Publishing House, 1993

Xu Da-Chun. *Classification of Formulas in Discussion of Cold Damage* (*shāng hán lùn lèi fāng*) 傷寒論類方. Beijing: People's Health Publishing House, 1984

Xu Hong. *Commentary for Formulas in Golden Mirror and Interior Platform* (*jīn jìng nèi tái fāng yì*) 金鏡內台方議. Nanjing: Jiangsu Science and Technology Press, 1985

Xu Mian-Zhai. *Medical Discussion in Endeavor House* (*miǎn zhāi yī huà*) 勉齋醫話. In Guan Qing-Zeng et al. *Ancient and Contemporary Study for Discussion of Cold Damage* (*shāng hán lùn gǔ jīn yán jiū*) 傷寒論古今研究. Shenyang: Liaoning Scientific and Technological Publishing House, 1994

Xu Shen. *Explanation for Chinese Characters* (*shuō wén jiě zì*) 說文解字. Beijing: Chinese Publishing House, 1963

Xu Shu-Wei. *Formulas of Universal Benefit from My Practice* (*pǔ jǐ běn shì fāng*) 普濟本事方. Shanghai: Shanghai Science and Technology Publishing House, 1959

Xue Zhen-Bin. "Preliminary exploration of the idea that tai yang is in charge of the nutritive qi and defensive qi." *Shanxi Journal of Traditional Chinese Medicine*, 1985 (10): 434

Xu Zhi-Gang. *Complete Explanation for the Analects of Confucius* (*lùn yǔ tōng shì*) 論語通釋. Beijing: People Literatures Publishing House, 1997

Yan Hong-Chen et al. *Analyzing Key Points in Discussion of Cold Damage* (*shāng hán lùn xī yào*) 傷寒論析要. Changchun: Jilin People's Publishing House, 1984

Yang Dian-Xing. "Exploring how the defensive qi originates from the lower burner." *Sichuan Journal of Traditional Chinese Medicine*, 1989 (3): 2

Yang Hua-Sen et al. *Concise Dictionary for Traditional Chinese Medicine* (*jiǎn míng zhōng yī zì diǎn*) 簡明中醫字典. Guiyang: Guizhou People's Publishing House, 1985

Yang Shang-Shan. *Simplicity of The Yellow Emperor's Inner Classic* (*huáng dì nèi jīng tài sú*) 黃帝內經太素. Beijing: People's Health Publishing House, 1955

Yang Tian-Yu. *Comments and Explanation for Book of Rites* (*lǐ jí yì zhù*) 禮記譯註. Shanghai: Shanghai Ancient Literature Publishing House, 2004

Yang Xuan. *Systematic Differentiation of Cold Damage and Warm Disease* (*shāng hán wēn yì tiǎo biàn*) 傷寒瘟疫條辨. Beijing: China Chinese Medicine Publishing House, 2002

Ye Chuan et al. (eds) *Collection of Famous Works from Four Scholars of the Jin-Yuan Era* (*jīn yuán sì dà jiā míng zhù jí chéng*) 金元四大家名著集成. Beijing: China Chinese Medicine Publishing House, 1995

Ye Gui. *Discussion of Warm-Heat Disorders* (*wēn rè lùn*) 溫熱論. In Tang Li-Shan (ed.) *Collection of Papers from Physicians of Wu Area* (*wú yī huì jiǎng*) 吳醫匯講. Shanghai: Shanghai Science and Technology Publishing House, 1983

Ye Gui. *Case Histories from the Compass of Clinical Patterns* (*lín zhèng zhǐ nán yī àn*) 臨證指南醫案. Shanghai: Shanghai Science and Technology Publishing House, 1959

Yi Yin. *Classical Methods to Make Formulas* (*tāng yè jīng fǎ*) 湯液經法. Excerpted in Wang Xue-Tai (ed.) *Textual Research, Commentary and Annotation for Rhymed Formula for Keys to Employ Herbs According to Zang-fu Organs* (*fǔ xíng jué zàng fǔ yòng yào fǎ yào jiào zhù*) 輔行訣臟腑用藥法要校注. Beijing: People's Military Medical Press, 2008

Yi Zhi-Biao et al. *Study on Rhymed Formula for Keys to Employ Herbs According to Zang-fu Organs* (*fǔ xíng jué zàng fǔ yòng yào fǎ yào yán jiū*) 輔行訣臟腑用藥法要. Beijing: Learning Garden Publishing House, 2009

Yin Jian et al. *Contemporary Research and Clinical Application for Chinese Herbs* (*zhōng yào xiàn dài yán jiū yǔ lín chuáng yìng yòng*) 中藥現代研究與臨床應用. Beijing: Chinese Ancient Medical Literature Publishing House, 1995

Yodo Odai. *Comprehensive Explanation for Classified Formulas* (*lèi jù fāng guáng yì*) 類聚方廣義. In Lu Pen-Nian (ed.) *Current Explanation for Discussion of Cold Damage* (*shāng hán lùn jīn shì*) 傷寒論今釋. Beijing: Learning Garden Publishing House, 2008

You Yi. *Connecting Pearls for Discussion of Cold Damage* (*shāng hán guàn zhū jí*) 傷寒貫珠集. Shanghai: Shanghai Science and Technology Publishing House, 1978

Yu Bo-Hai et al. *Collection of Famous Books on Discussion of Cold Damage, Essentials and Formula Discussions from the Golden Cabinet and Warm Disease* (*shāng hán jīn guì wēn bìng mīng zhù jí chéng*) 傷寒金匱溫病名著集成. Beijing: China Publishing House, 1997

Yu Chang. *Attachment for Writing on the Esteemed Discussion* (*shàng lùn hòu piān*) 尚論後篇. In Zhang Hai-Peng and Chen Rui-Hua (eds) *Textual Research and Annotation for Commentary for Discussion of Cold Damage by Ten Scholars* (*shāng hán lùn zhù shí rén shù*) 傷寒論注十人書. Learning Garden Publishing House, 2009

Yu Chang. *Writing on the Esteemed Discussion* (*shàng lùn piān*) 尚論篇. In Yu Bo-Hai et al. (eds) *Collection of Famous Books on Discussion of Cold Damage, Essentials and Formula Discussions from the Golden Cabinet and Warm Disease* (*shāng hán jīn guì wēn bìng mīng zhù jí chéng*) 傷寒金匱溫病名著集成. Beijing: China Publishing House, 1997

Yu Chang. *Precepts for Physicians* (*yī mén fă lü*) 醫門法律. Shanghai: Shanghai Science and Technology Publishing House, 1983

Yu Chang-Rong. *Selection of Key Points and Analysis for Discussion of Cold Damage* (*shāng hán lùn huì yào fēn xī*) 傷寒論匯要分析. Fuzhou: Fujian Science and Technology Publishing House, 1985

Yu Wu-Yan. *New Explanation for Discussion of Cold Damage* (*shāng hán lùn xīn yì*) 傷寒論新義. Shanghai: Publishing House of Selling Thousands Books, 1953

Yu Zhao-Yuan. *Revised Popular Guide to the Discussion of Cold Damage* (*chóng dìng tōng sú shāng hán lùn*) 重訂通俗傷寒論. Hangzhou: New Medicine Press, 1956

Yun Shu-Jue. *Study on Discussion of Cold Damage* (*shāng hán lùn yán jiū*) 傷寒論研究. In Yun Shu-Jue (ed.) *Study on Discussion of Cold Damage and Records for Speeches Related to Clinical Practice* (*shāng hán lùn yán jiū yŭ lín zhèng yán jiăng lù*) 傷寒論研究與臨證演講錄. Beijing: Learning Garden Publishing House, 2007

Yun Shu-Jue. "On six conformations in Discussion of Cold Damage." *Literatures for Chinese Medicine*, 1936 (1): 134

Yun Shu-Jue. *Commentary for Collection of Explanations for Discussion of Cold Damage* (*shāng hán lùn jí yì àn*) 傷寒論輯義按. In *Medicinal Covers for Medical Works* (*yào ān yī xué cóng shū*) 藥盦醫學叢書. Shanghai: Business Publishing House, 1934

Yun Shu-Jue. *Medicinal Covers for Medical Works* (*yào ān yī xué cóng shū*) 藥盦醫學叢書. Shanghai: Business Publishing House, 1934

Zhang Bing-Lin. *Medical Idea by Zhang Tai-Yan* (*zhāng tài-yān yī lùn*) 章太炎醫論. Beijing: People's Health Publishing House, 1957

Zhang Deng-Ben. "Answers to questions regarding 'The Defensive Qi Comes from the Lower Burner'." *Shanxi Journal of Traditional Chinese Medicine*, 1981 (6): 41

Zhang Deng-Ben and Sun Li-Jun. "Applications of the theory of biao, ben and zhong qi in differentiation and treatment for diseases in six conformations in Discussion of Cold Damage." *Journal of Shanxi College of Traditional Chinese Medicine*, 2002 (9): 1

Zhang Hai-Peng and Chen Rui-Hua. *Textual Research and Annotation for Commentary for Discussion of Cold Damage by Ten Scholars* (*shāng hán lùn zhù shí rén shù*) 傷寒論注十人書. Learning Garden Publishing House, 2009

Zhang Heng-Liu et al. *Explanation and Clinical Application for Discussion of Cold Damage* (*shāng hán lùn jiě dú yŭ lín chuáng yìng yòng*) 傷寒論解讀與臨床應用. Shanghai: Publishing House of Shanghai University of Traditional Chinese Medicine, 2006

Zhang Ji. *Essentials and Formula Discussions from the Golden Cabinet* (*jīn gùi yào lüè fāng lùn*) 金匱要略方論. Beijing: People's Health Publishing House, 1964

Zhang Ji. *Classic of the Golden Coffer and Jade Sheath* (*jīn guì yù hán jīng*) 金匱玉函經. Beijing: People's Health Publishing House, 1955

Zhang Jia-Li. *Selected Reading for Essentials and Formula Discussions from the Golden Cabinet* (*jīn gùi yāo lüè xuán dú*) 金匱要略選讀. Chinese Medicine Publishing House, 1999

Zhang Jie-Bin. *Appendices to the Classified Classic* (*lèi jīng fù yì*) 類經附翼. Beijing: People's Health Publishing House, 1982

Zhang Jie-Bin. *Illustration of the Classified Classic* (*lèi jīng tú yì*) 類經圖翼. Beijing: People's Health Publishing House, 1982

Zhang Jie-Bin. *Classified Classic* (*lèi jīng*) 類經. Beijing: People's Health Publishing House, 1980

Zhang Lu. *Continuation for Discussion of Cold Damage* (*shāng hán zuăn lùn*) 傷寒纘論. In Zhang Min-Qing et al. (eds) *Complete Medical Works by Zhang Lu* (*zhāng lù yī xué quán shū*) 張璐醫學全書. Beijing: Chinese Medical Publishing House, 2004

Zhang Lu. *Comprehending Medicine by Zhang* (*zhāng shì yī tōng*) 張氏醫通. Beijing: China Publishing House of Traditional Chinese Medicine, 1995

Zhang Min-Qing et al. *Complete Medical Works by Zhang Lu* (*zhāng lù yī xué quán shū*) 張璐醫學全書. Beijing: Chinese Medical Publishing House, 2004

Zhang Nan. *Alert Misunderstanding in Medical Gate* (*yī mén bàng hē*) 醫門棒喝. Licheng: Three Friends Benefit Studio, 1909

Zhang Nan. *Original Ideas in Discussion of Cold Damage* (*shāng hán lùn běn zhǐ*) 傷寒論本旨. In *Alert Misunderstanding in Medical Gate* (*yī mén bàng hē èr jí*) 醫門棒喝. Licheng: Three Friends Benefit Studio, 1909

Zhang Xi-Chun. *Records of Heart-felt Experience in Medicine with Reference to the West* (*yī xué zhōng zhōng cān xī lù*) 醫學衷中參西錄. Shijiazhuang: Hebei People's Publishing House, 1974

Zhang Xi-Ju. *Direct Explanation for Discussion of Cold Damage* (*shāng hán lùn zhí jiě*) 傷寒論直解. Qiantang: Three Extras Hall, 1712

Zhang Yuan-Su, annotated by Ren Ying-Qiu. *Origins of Medicine* (*yī xué qǐ yuán*) 醫學啟源. Beijing: People's Health Publishing House, 1978

Zhang Zheng-Yao and Xin Bo. "Textual research for the publishing time of 'Fifty-two Diseases and Their Formulas Written on Silk'." *Journal of History for Cultural Relics*, 2007 (6): 9

Zhang Zheng-Zhao. *Back to Truth for Discussion of Cold Damage* (*shāng hán lùn guī zhēn*) 傷寒論歸真. Changsha: Hunan Science and Technology Publishing House, 1993

Zhang Zhi-Cong. *Ancestor Stamp for Discussion of Cold Damage* (*shāng hán lùn zōng yìn*) 傷寒論宗印. In Zheng Lin et al. (eds) *Complete Medical Works by Zhang Zhi-Cong* (*zhāng zhì-cōng yī xué quán shū*) 張志聰醫學全書. Beijing: China Publishing House of Traditional Chinese Medicine, 2005

Zhang Zhi-Cong. *Collection of Commentaries for Discussion of Cold Damage* (*shāng hán lùn jí zhù*) 傷寒論集注. In Zheng Lin et al. (eds) *Complete Medical Works by Zhang Zhi-Cong* (*zhāng zhì-cōng yī xué quán shū*) 張志聰醫學全書. Beijing: China Publishing House of Traditional Chinese Medicine, 2005

Zhang Zhi-Cong. *Collection of Commentaries for Spiritual Pivot of The Yellow Emperor's Inner Classic* (*líng shū jīng jí zhù*) 靈樞經集注. In Zheng Lin et al. (eds) *Complete Medical Works by Zhang Zhi-Cong* (*zhāng zhì-cōng yī xué quán shū*) 張志聰醫學全書. Beijing: China Publishing House of Traditional Chinese Medicine, 2005

Zhang Zhi-Min. *The Methods to Apply the Formulas in Discussion of Cold Damage* (*shāng hán lùn fāng yùn yòng fǎ*) 傷寒論方運用法. Hangzhou, Zhejiang Science and Technology Publishing House, 1984

Zhang Zhi-Min. "Primary exploration of the features and significance of classifying syndromes according to six diseases in Discussion of Cold Damage." *Zhejiang Journal of Traditional Chinese Medicine*, 1980 (1): 21

Zhao En-Jian. *Study on Discussion of Cold Damage* (*shāng hán lùn yán jiū*) 傷寒論研究. Tianjin: Tianjin Science and Technology Publishing House, 1987

Zhao Li-Xun et al. *Annotation and Commentary for Complete Medical Works by Jing-Yue* (*jiào zhù jǐng yuè quán shū*) 校注景岳全書. Beijing: People's Health Publishing House, 1991

Zheng Chong-Guang. *Differentiation of the Syndromes in Discussion of Cold Damage* (*shāng hán lùn zhèng biàn*) 傷寒論證辨. In Guan Qing-Zeng et al. (eds) *Ancient and Contemporary Study for Discussion of Cold Damage* (*shāng hán lùn gǔ jīn yán jiū*) 傷寒論古今研究. Shenyang: Liaoning Scientific and Technological Publishing House, 1994

Zheng Lin et al. *Complete Medical Works by Zhang Zhi-Cong* (*zhāng zhì-cōng yī xué quán shū*) 張志聰醫學全書. Beijing: China Publishing House of Traditional Chinese Medicine, 2005

Zheng Shou-Quan and Tang Bu-Qi. *Explanation for Works of Zheng Qin-An* (*zhèng qīn-ān yī shū chán shì*) 鄭欽安醫書闡釋. Chengdu: Sichuan Publishing House, 1996

Zhou Yang-Jun. *Three Annotations for Discussion of Cold Damage* (*shāng hán lùn sān zhù*) 傷寒論三注. Huiji: Hall of the Pine Heart, 1736

Zhou Zhen-Fu. *Translation and Commentary for Book of Changes* (*zhōu yì yì zhù*) 周易譯注. Hongkong: Chinese Publishing House, 2000

Zhu Gong. *The Book to Safeguard Life Based on Classifying Patterns* (*lèi zhèng huó rén shū*) 類證活人書. In *Complete Medical Works of Zhu Gong and Pang An-Shi* (*zhū gōng páng ān-shí yī xué quán shū*) 朱肱龐安時醫學全書. In Tian Si-Sheng et al. (eds) *Collection of Works of Famous Physicians from the Tang, Song, Jin and Yuan dynasties* (*táng sòng jīn yuán míng yī quán shū dà chéng*) 唐宋金元名醫全書大成. Beijing: China Chinese Medical Publishing House, 2006

Zhu Wei-Ju. *Answers to Difficult Questions for Discussion of Cold Damage* (*shāng hán zhì nán*) 傷寒質難. Shanghai: People's Bookstores, 1950

Zhu You-Wu. *Annotating and Commentating Song Dynasty Version of Discussion of Cold Damage* (*sòng běn shāng hán lùn jiào zhù*) 宋本傷寒論校注. Changsha: Hunan Scientific and Technological Publishing House, 1982

Zhu Zhang-Zhi et al. *Clinical Application and Study for Classical Formulas* (*jīng fāng lín chuáng yùn yòng yǔ yán jiū*) 經方臨床運用與研究. Guangzhu: Guangdong Economical Publishing House, 1997

Zhu Zhen-Heng. *Teaching of* (*Zhu*) *Dan-Xi* (*dān xī xīn fǎ*) 丹溪心法. Beijing: China Publishing House of Traditional Chinese Medicine, 2008

Zou Han-Huang. *Brief Explanation for Discussion of Cold Damage and Miscellaneous Diseases* (*shāng hán zá bìng lùn jiān*) 傷寒雜病論箋. In Guan Qing-Zeng et al. (eds) *Ancient and Contemporary Study for Discussion of Cold Damage* (*shāng hán lùn gŭ jīn yán jiū*) 傷寒論古今研究. Shenyang: Liaoning Scientific and Technological Publishing House, 1994

Zou Shu. *Exploration and Commentary for Materia Medica by Shen Nong* (*běn jīng shū zhèng*) 本經疏證. Shanghai: Shanghai Science and Technology Publishing House, 1957

Zuo Ji-Yun. *Collections and References of Classified Formulas and Case Studies Related to Discussion of Cold Damage* (*shāng hán lùn lè fāng fă àn huì cān*) 傷寒論類方法案匯參. Tianjin: Tianjin Scientific and Technological Publishing House, 2000

SUBJECT INDEX

abdominal fullness 102
abdominal pain 102
abdominal palpation 65
abnormal progression 60
acrid herbs 67
  in fire spirit school 66
acupuncture method 61, 62, 92
acute febrile diseases 47
adapting method 61
alchemy
  Daoist roots 32
  influence on Zhang Ji 33
alternating chills and fever 172
  in blood chamber invasion 193
annotations
  1949 to present 68–73
  Discussion of Cold Damage 45
  of Discussion of Cold Damage 51–52
  of theories, treatment approaches, formulas 48
anti-pathogenic qi 90, 94
  damage to 134
  in jue yin disease 91
  prevailing times 235
  strength of 96
as above, so below 169
astringing method 92
automatic recovery 40, 42
autumn 119, 120

balance 178
bamboo slips
  collecting disconnected 51
  original 48
Beijing University of Traditional Chinese Medicine 46, 70
benevolence 30
bitter taste 144–145
  in shao yang disease 179
black warrior formula 35, 38
bleeding 40
blood amassment syndromes 151
blood chamber invasion 193
blood vessels 83
blood-amassment syndrome 98
bluegreen dragon formula 35, 38
body surface 199
body surface symptoms, in shao yang disease 173
branch qi 106, 107, 108
  correspondences to zang-fu organs 124
  resolving time and 228

Bureau of Textual Research and Correction for Medical Literature 51

case studies
  by Australian scholars 73
  elucidating Discussion of Cold Damage using 68
Changsha county 39
  Zhang Ji as commissioner 24
channel borders 89
channel syndromes 52
  in yang ming disease 138
channel theory 95
channels 86, 94
  and zang-fu organ function 95
  for disease pattern differentiation 88
chapter additions, by Wang Xi 56
character construction 158
Chengdu College of Traditional Chinese Medicine 86, 150, 188
chest
  as pathway for defensive qi circulation 194
  in yang ming disease 99
  progression from tai yang to 196
chest-binding syndromes 23, 98, 151
China Academy of Traditional Chinese Medicine 80
Chinese civil war 65
Chinese medical journals 76
Chinese medicine
  historical systematization 27
  importance of Discussion of Cold Damage to 44
  importance of six conformations 79
  integrating with Western medicine 45
  legalization by PRC, 69
  prehistoric bases 27
Chinese philosophers 30
chong
  disease progression to 175, 176
  origin in kidney and uterus 193
  progression from tai yang to 197
  tai yang qi and 193
classification, in Confucianism 31
classifying disease method 61
clear differentiating method 61
clear heat method 62

clearing, harmonization by 165
closing function 129, 131, 150, 151
  in jue yin 228, 232
  in yang ming disease 100, 150, 152, 230
cold 18
  as yin pathological factor 202
  aversion to 89
  effects of mild 57
  in urinary bladder and conception vessel 23
  injury to nutritive qi by 52, 54, 55
  lurking, in winter 55
  predominance in shang han syndrome 200, 202
  warm pathogen disease due to 55
cold accumulation, in organs 22–23
cold and heat, differentiating 74
cold attack 17, 88
cold damage, school of 44–48
cold hands/feet 42
cold invasion 18
cold qi 112, 114, 118, 119, 121
  counteracting by maximum yang 113
  in tai yang disease 140
  in winter 120
  interaction with heat qi 120
  tai yang and 111
cold-damp syndromes 142
cold-toxin 47
communication theory 69
complexity of channels, *liù jīng* as 85–87
conception vessel 23
Confucianism
  as ruling ideology in Zhang Ji's time 39
  benevolence in 30
  classification of people in 31
  duty in 30
  filial piety in 30
  historical-political ascendance 29
  influence on Zhang Ji 29–43
  Zhang Ji's fondness for 30
Confucius
  quotations by Zhang Ji 30
  Zhang Ji's interest in 24
constrained spleen 142
contagion 20, 21, 22
cosmology 110
cu pulse 43

cultural landscape
Confucianism and Daoism influences 29–43
Zhang Ji's time 27–28, 28–29
Cultural Revolution 69
culture, as product of society 27
cybernetics 69

damp 18
in shao yang disease 101
damp qi 114, 119, 120, 142, 143, 146
and dryness qi 120
balancing dryness qi with 99, 100
in tai yin 102
tai yin and 111
damp-warm disease 17
Daoism
case study involving Zhang Ji 31–32
formula names and 35
gods worshipped in 38
indirect references by Zhang Ji 31
influence on Zhang Ji 29–43, 32, 38
nature principles in 40
political uprisings influenced by 39
revival in Eastern Han Dynasty 39
role in Eastern Han Dynasty literature 28
Western Han Dynasty context 28
Daoist names, political reasons to avoid 38
decoctions
administering 75
finishing 215
defensive and nutritive qi 86, 97
injury by wind-cold 52
defensive qi 185
as turbid 186
circadian circulation 188
circulation outside of vessels 186, 195
circulation routes 206
deficiency state 189, 208
disharmony with nutritive qi 22, 29
dispersion by lung 193, 207
dispersion in upper burner 189
engenderment from food 195
generation of 97
harmonizing through heart 207
injury by mild cold 57
injury by wind 51, 54, 55
lower burner origination 189, 192
middle burner origination 189
movement from kidney to bladder 193
movement from kidney to spleen 193
movement from kidney to surface 188
nourishment in middle burner 189
origination 185–191
pivot function and 193
production and distribution routes 193–194
production on body surface 206
reinforcing 207
relationship to kidney 188
relationship to three burners and urinary bladder 188
routes of circulation 194
shao yang role in 177
stagnation 193, 200, 201
supporting with Aconiti Radix Lateralis 207
unreasonable strength 200, 201, 203
weakness with nutritive qi harmony 200
yang nature 198
deficiency and excess 86
differentiating 74
deteriorated syndromes 22
deterioration time 234
predictive uses 235
diagnosis 75
diagnostic methods
eight 61
line rearrangement according to 55, 61
diarrhea
in tai yang disease 98
in tai yin disease 102
differentiation and treatment approaches 53, 200
nutritive and defensive qi theory and 190
principles 73–75
sub-school emphasizing 46
Wang Xi's contributions 49
wind *versus* cold injury 57
differentiation methods, Li Pei-Sheng 74
differentiation systems 27
role of disapproval in 42
direction of movement 229
harmonization and 184
pivot role 232
yang and yin qi 229–230
disapproval 41
role in disease differentiation 42
disease complications 149
disease deterioration 234
disease duration 51, 80
disease layers 88–90
disease location 96
depth and superficiality 89
liù jīng and 88–90, 89
predictive uses of resolving times 235
disease onset 49
disease pattern differentiation
channels for 88
liù jīng and 88
disease progression 41, 49
causes in tai yang disease 196–197
debates on 78
from tai yang qi 194
from tai yang to shao yin 188–189
from tai yin disease 102
from three yang to three yin 178
in jue yin disease 147
in shao yin disease 147
in tai yang disease 98–99, 151
in tai yin disease 146
in yang ming disease 100, 143
sentence of showing manifestation and 42
tai yang to shao yang 164
tai yang to shao yin 141
to jue yin 104, 105
to shao yin 103
to yin channels 214
using three yin and three yang 94
disease quality 96
in yang ming disease 100
disease regression 41
sentence of showing manifestation and 42
disease resolution
per six conformations 76
prediction of 40
disease stages 90–91
diseases
externally contracted 19–20
relevance of *shāng hán* to 18–19
disharmony, between nutritive and defensive qi 29
dissipating method 165
harmonization by 165
dizziness 144
in shao yang disease 145, 179
door hinge
pivot as 169–170
shao yang as 183
dry mouth, in shao yang disease 179
dry throat 144
in shao yang disease 145
drying, harmonization by 165
dryness 18, 39
dryness qi 112, 114, 119, 120, 125, 136
balancing with damp qi 100, 102
control of damp qi by 116
in yang ming 99
yang ming and 111
duty 30

early studies 48–50
earth 125
earthly branches belonging to 222
earth element
number five significance 222–223
role in resolving times 222–223
role in three yin 233
Earthly Branches 210
see also Twelve Earthly Branches
Eastern Han Dynasty 21, 28, 46, 51
alchemy in 32
Eastern Jin 237
economic conditions 27
eight diagnostic parameters 73, 74
harmonization among 165

emperor names, taboo against use in formulas 38
essence 55
evil qi 134
exogenous pathological factors 97
qi deficiency and 217
exterior and interior, differentiating 74
externally contracted diseases 22, 25
caused by cold toxin 47
causes 17–18
five types 17
herbal formulas in pre-Zhang Ji texts 34
relevance of *shāng hán* to 19–20
resolving times 209, 224
stages to classify 90–91

febrile disease 17
febrile diseases, relevance of *shāng hán* to 19–20
feeble pulse, yang deficiency and 42
fever, slight in shao yang disease 173
filial piety 30
fire 39
earthly branches belonging to 222
fire god Lu 67
fire god Zheng 67
fire qi 111, 112, 114, 118, 144
and wind qi 119
fire spirit school 65, 66–67, 77
fire stagnation, in shao yang disease 101
fire-water communication 103
firing methods, as wrong treatment 60
five, numerological significance 222–223
Five Celestial Movements 91
five constellation movement and six qi 108
Five Dynasties 237
Discussion of Cold Damage studies 48–50
scholarly contributions 51
five elements 123
and Twelve Earthly Branches 222
historical development 27
school of 45
five stages 90
flare-up fire
from shao yang 101
in shao yang disease 144
flavor, as herbal quality 180
floating pulse 89, 199
floating yang 200
flying snake formula 35
foot jue yin 85, 136
foot shao yang 85, 178
foot shao yin 85
foot tai yang 85, 136
foot tai yin 85, 136
foot yang ming 85
formula collection school 45
formula names, assigning to syndromes 58–59
four-god decoctions 39
four-level differentiation 66, 76
fu syndromes 54
in yang ming disease 138

gall bladder 104
as extraordinary fu organ 170
shao yang and 100
geographic regions, categorizing formulas by 45
Great Harmony Hall (*tài hé diàn*) 156
Guangzhou College of Traditional Chinese Medicine 80

hand shao yang 136
hairs, tai yang channel and 83
half exterior and half interior 52, 90, 101, 155
absence from Zhang Ji's writings 155, 182
introduction by Cheng Wu-Ji 155
Han Dynasty
Chinese medical advances 27
Zhang Ji's summary of medical achievements 27
hand and foot channels 81
hand shao yang 136, 178
hand shao yin 136
hand tai yang 136
hand yang ming 136
hand-copied versions, Discussion of Cold Damage 70
harmonization 157, 179
among Eight Diagnostic Parameters 165
and direction of movement 184
as treatment approach 159, 163
different methods of 165
first introduction as treatment approach 163
for abnormalities 165
for shao yang disease 163, 167, 178
in jue yin disease 167
introduction of concept 163
Ming Dynasty conception 165
narrow and broad senses 166
nutritive and defensive qi 205
overexpansion of concept 166–167
second cooking method 182
through sweating 205
harmonizing method 62, 92
harmony
as abnormality 161
as formula administration method 162
as formula preparation method 163
as notes of music 158
as return to normal 161
concept of 156
describing clinical manifestations 162
in Chinese culture and philosophy 156–157
in Discussion of Cold Damage 155
in pathology descriptions 161
in Zhang Ji's writings 29
physiological meaning 161
use by Zhang Ji 161
headache 89
heart
fire in 97
in shao yin disease 232
progression from tai yang to 196
shao yin and 103
three yang and 83
yang deficiency due to wrong treatment 192
heart fire 104
heat 18
heat and cold syndrome, in jue yin disease 105
heat qi 112, 114, 118, 119, 125
from shao yin 97
in shao yin disease 146
shao yin and 103, 111
herbal formulas
adaptation to four-level differentiation 66
assignment to syndromes 55
chief herbs and naming conventions 38
classification by function 45
comparison of Cinnamon Twig with Ephedra 20
comparisons between Zhang Ji and source texts 36–37
correlating names with syndromes 58
Daoist naming conventions 35, 39
flavor and nature 180
for harmonizing shao yang 164
hot and cold natures 80
in shao yin disease 147
in tai yang disease progression 141
in tai yin disease 146
line rearrangement by 58, 78
naming conventions 38
origin of Zhang Ji's 32–33
pairing with corresponding syndromes 75
relationship to syndromes 58, 59, 74, 78
six-gods formulas 35
source texts for Zhang Ji 38
two dan formulas 35
warm and cold natures 51
herbs
flavor and temperature 204
large dosage in fire spirit school 67
recorded in Discussion of Cold Damage 244–246
sour flavor 206
historical authors 238–243
hook old formula 35
hot herbs 67
Hubei College of Traditional Chinese Medicine 95
huo luan disease 70

injury, by pathological factors 19
inquiry 75
inscription on bone 157
integrative medicine school 45, 63
intensive studies period 50–65
interior excess heat, in yang ming disease 100
internal disorders 23, 25
  in tai yang disease 97
  Ming Dynasty contritutions 57
  treating with Zhang Ji's formulas 22
interspaces
  and shao yang 82
  in body tissues 173–174
  progression from tai yang to 196
interstices 174
  nutritive and defensive qi among 199
  relationship to zang-fu and three burners 175, 176
  shao yang channel and 83
inward movement, in yang ming 100

Japan
  literature on Discussion of Cold Damage 64–65
  scholarship from 68, 69
  war against invasion by 65
Jiangsu School of Traditional Chinese Medicine 84
Jin Dynasty 48–50
jue yin 21, 87, 92, 116, 117
  and jue yin disease 104–105
  area of extent 83
  as one yin 112, 115, 177
  as turning point between yin and yang 233
  as weakest yin 104
  closing function 129, 131, 228, 232
  disease progression 152
  failure to close 152
  inward-moving qi in 104
  mechanism of qi transformation 127
  pivot function 167
  resolving time 211
  role in direction of qi movement 232
  tissue correspondences 83
  wind qi and 111, 125
  yang qi generation with help from 229
jue yin disease 90, 104–105
  anti-pathogenic qi in 91
  direct attack 105
  progression from shao yin 104
  qi obstruction in 104
  qi stagnation in 105
  qi transformation in 147–154
  resolving time 209, 210, 212, 226, 233
  Shanghai College scholarship 70

kidney
  as root of defensive qi 192–193
  in shao yin disease 232
  origination of defensive qi in 188
  progression from tai yang to 197
  relationship to interstices and three burners 176
  shao yin and 103
kidney yang
  defensive qi production by 97
  tonifying to benefit defensive qi 192, 193
king fire 105, 118, 125, 136
Korea, literature on Discussion of Cold Damage 64

large intestine, progression from tai yang disease 197
life gate fire 97
line rearrangement 46, 59
  according to diagnostic/treatment methods 61
  by Ke Qin 58
  by syndrome and formula relationships 74–75
  by treatment approaches 49, 50
  by Yu Chang 55
  during Eastern Han and Five Dynasties periods 51
  scholarly contributions 48
  scholarly debates on 78
  Wang Xi's contributions 49
  Yu Chang's observations 54
liver 100
  jue yin and 104
lower burner
  defensive qi origination in 185, 186, 187, 189
  symptoms in shao yang disease 172
lung
  and tai yin 102
  dispersion of defensive qi by 189
  progression from tai yang to 196
lung qi, descending with Armenicae Semen Amarum 204

macrocosm 110
mediating method 61
medical ethics 30
medicine, as product of society 27
menstruation, catching cold during 193
metal 125
  earthly branches belonging to 222
midday-midnight relationships 224
middle burner 100
  nutritive qi circulation in 186
  origination of defensive qi in 189
  support for defensive qi in 189
  symptoms in shao yang disease 172
middle qi 106–107, 108
  for three yin and three yang 111
  interaction with root qi 118–121
  resolving time and 228

Ming Dynasty 46, 237
  harmonization concept in 165
  internal medicine scholarship 57
ministerial fire 100, 104, 105, 114, 119, 125, 133, 136, 145, 151
mistake correction 45
moistening, harmonization as 163
moxibustion method 62, 92
multiple studies 1949 to present 69
muscles
  yang ming channel and 83
  yang ming correspondences 82
mutual dependence 40
mutual transformation 40

Nanjing College of Traditional Chinese Medicine 70, 74, 107
  textual research by 69
nape stiffness 89
national textbook
  line classifications in 71
  translation into English 73
natural order 29
nature principles, in Zhang Ji's writings 40
neck, in tai yang disease 199
Northern and Southern Dynasties 25, 237
  introduction of Western medicine during 63
  seminal texts written 33
Northern Song Dynasty 25, 237
nutritive and defensive qi 86, 96, 185
  ancient theory 185–186
  complete obstruction 201, 205
  disharmony between 97, 201
  formulas treating disharmony 59
  four types of disharmony 200
  harmonizing 159, 163, 168, 185
  herb differentiation 185
  herbs for obstruction 192
  invasion by wind-cold 54, 55
  meeting inside vessels 198
  mutually supportive relationship 198
  normal relationship 198
  origination from heart and lung 192
  production and circulation 186
  relationship between 195–208
  shang han syndrome 202
  tai yang and 83, 208
  treatments for 195–208
  weakness of 200
  Zhang Ji's use of terminology 190
  zhong feng syndrome 201
nutritive qi 185
  as clear qi 186
  circulation in vessels 186, 195
  disharmony with defensive qi 22, 29
  effects of severe wind 57
  injury by cold 54, 55 52
  leakage *versus* deficiency 200–201
  obstruction by sour flavor 206

relationship to blood 191
stagnation 200
weakness 200, 203
yin nature 198

observation 75
one yang 112, 115, 119, 128
generation in heavens 219
generation on earth 218
remaining in heavens 220
remaining on earth 220
shao yang as 177, 225
one yin 104, 112, 113, 115, 118, 127
generation in heavens 220
generation on earth 219
jue yin as 177
remaining on earth 218
opening, closing, and pivot 98, 133, 135, 150, 153
for three yin and three yang 129
in yang ming disease 100
resolving time and 227–228
shao yang role 101
shao yin role 103
tai yang role 98
tai yin role 102
theory of 108
opening and closing
in shao yang 178–179
role of orifices in 183
opening function 129, 150, 151
in tai yin 102, 230
tai yang and 97, 150
tai yin 230–231
oracle bones 157
orifices
and shao yang 178
as pivots 179, 183
outline 54

palpation 75
panting 43
pathological factors 20
injury by 19
invasion with open interstices 175
progression in shao yang disease 91
progression to chong and uterus 175
warring with anti-pathogenic qi 171–172
pathology
as disapproval for normal physiology 41
line classification by 71
pattern differentiation
based on six conformations 80
liù jīng as 88–96, 89, 94
Pavlov's higher nervous activity theory 69
peasant uprisings 28, 29
and deprecation of Daoism 39
People's Republic of Chine 237
legalization of Chinese medicine by 69
pericardium 100
jue yin and 104
philosophy, culture and 27
phlegm
due to water accumulation 141
in shao yang disease 101
phonetic complex 157
physiological structure and function 87, 94
pi syndromes 98
pivot
as door hinge 169, 170
between three yin and three yang 177
dysfunction of shao yang 172
harmonizing, of shao yang 164
jue yin as 167
role in direction of qi movement 232
shao yang as 101, 183
shao yin as 231
supporting defensive qi via 207
three burners as 175
pivot function 129, 130, 150, 151
in shao yang 150, 151, 152, 153, 178
orifices and 179
recovering using herbs 181
vertical qi movement by 173
Zhang Ji's mention of 173
pores
closed with cold predominant 201
open with wind predominant 200
releasing wind-cold through 204
prediction, using resolving times 234
private copies
end of tradition 51
secrecy and 48–49
prognosis 74
line reordering according to 49
promote urination method 62
promote vomiting method 62
pulses 142
for tai yang 89
purging 40, 92, 144, 165
harmonization as 162, 165
improper promotion of 102, 196–197
in yang diseases 167
mistaken promotion of 60
purging method 62

qi
blood, and water 65
from food transformation 186
processed from food 195
theory of 27
qi and blood deficiency, open interstices with 175
qi movement of the five elements 109
qi stagnation
in jue yin 104
in jue yin disease 105
in shao yang disease 101
qi transformation 85, 86, 87, 91, 94, 95, 96, 108, 121
among three pairs of qi 123
clinical significance 140–154
contributions of sub-school 64
debates on 78, 106–108
disorders in six conformations 64
excess and deficiency in 137
explaining with six conformations 63
for shao yang 125
for tai yin 125
historical review of theory 108–117
importance to theory of three yin/three yang 107
in bladder and small intestine 98
in jue yin disease 147–154, 232
in shao yang disease 144–145
in shao yin disease 146–147
in six channels 132
in six conformations 149
in tai yang disease 140–142
in tai yin disease 146
in yang ming 99
in yang ming disease 142–144
lack of contemporary understanding 153
liù jīng and 85–87
mechanisms 127–128
root and branch relationships 116
school of 107, 132–140, 153, 154
shao yang as pivot 228
shao yin and 103
sub-school of 63
theory of 76, 77, 131, 133, 139
yang pathological factors to yin 102
qi transformation theory 95
Qin Dynasty 237
Chinese medical advances during 27
Qing Dynasty 237
intensive studies during 50
scholarly trends 65–66

recovering method 61
red bird formula 35, 38
regular treatment method 61
release exterior method 62
release interior method 62
relieving exterior, harmonization by 165
Republic of China 46, 237
resolving time
allocations by conformation 211
clinical application 233–236
facts 211–213
fever in yang ming disease 235
five-element correspondences 222
for diseases in six conformations 209–210
jue yin disease 210, 226, 233
lack of contemporary interest in 236
longer in three yang diseases 233
mechanism of 216–232
order of progress 213
predictive uses 234

resolving time *cont.*
sequence from yang to yin disease 213
shao yang disease 210, 213, 226
shao yin disease 210, 226, 232
six conformations 211, 212
tai yang disease 209, 214, 215, 217, 226, 236
tai yin disease 210, 226, 231
theory 213–215
three two-hour periods 215
treatment guidance using 236
Twelve Earthly Branches allocations 211
yang ming disease 209, 226, 235
reverse thought 40
rice porridge 192
river map 223
root and branch 111, 116
root qi 106, 107, 108
correspondences to zang-fu organs 124
for three yin and three yang 111
interaction with middle qi 118–121
resolving time and 228

scholarly contributions 48, 49, 78
by Wang Xi 56
early studies 50
scholarly disagreements 78
school of applying ancient formulas 64
school of applying both ancient formulas and contemporary formulas 64
school of cold damage 44–48
school of Discussion of Cold Damage 83
unification with warm pathogen disease school 76–78
school of studying Discussion of Cold Damage 44–48
at Shaoxing area 66
classics school 45
compilations and annotations 45
fire spirit school 65, 66–67
formula collections 45
formula function classification 45
formulas by geographic regions 45
four periods 48
integrative medicine school 45
intensive studies period 50–65
Japanese schools 64
mistake correction school 45
new studying approaches 65–69
scholarly contributions 48
school of strengthening yang 66–67
skeptics school 46
sub-school of integrative medicine 63
warming and clearing methods 45
warming and tonifying approach 45
yang tonification school 45
school of supporting yang 148
seasons
and six qi 114–115
and three yin/three yang 114–115
second cooking method 182
self-healing ability 40
sentence of showing manifestation 41
Shang Dynasty 237
shang han syndrome 21, 22, 200, 203, 205
body location 203
disharmony of nutritive and protective qi in 202
with cold predominant 202
Shanghai College of Traditional Chinese Medicine 69–70
shao yang 21, 87, 92, 116, 117, 119
adjusting disharmony with stomach 182
and fire qi 122
and shao yang disease 100–101
area of extent 83
as door hinge 183
as middle qi for jue yin 111
as one yang 112, 115, 177
as pivot 169, 177, 182, 228
as pivot *versus* door hinge 171
as weakest yang 177
door hinge function 169–170
dysfunction of pivot 172
fire qi and 125
harmonizing pivot of 164
in Discussion of Cold Damage 155
interspaces and 82
mechanism of qi transformation 128
Minor Bupleurum Decoction for 164
pivot function 129, 153, 178
progression from tai yang to 196
qi fluorishing time 213
qi maturation time 223
qi movement towards fire 228
recovering pivot function 101, 181
relationship to jue yin 100
resolving time 211
role of orifices 178
symbolic meaning of pivot 178–179
tai yang qi and 193
shao yang channel
location 101
tissue correspondences 83
shao yang disease 90, 100–101, 133
alternating chills and fever in 172
body surface symptoms 173
classification of symptoms and signs 172–173
fire stagnation in 101
harmonization as treatment approach 163, 178
lower burner symptoms 172
middle burner symptoms 172
outline for 179
progression and regression in 91
qi stagnation as 101
qi transformation in 144–145
resolving time 209, 210, 212, 226
Shanghai College scholarship 70
single herbs in 177–178
sinusitis and allergy in 179
slight fever in 173
symptoms and signs 171
treatment approaches 145, 167
upper burner symptoms 172
water retention in 101
shao yin 21, 42, 87, 92, 116, 117, 118, 119
and heat qi 122
and shao yin disease 103–104
area of extent 83
as middle qi for tai yang 111
as pivot between tai yin and jue yin 231
as two yins 112, 115, 177
direct attack by cold 103
dysfunction 152
heat qi from 97, 111, 125
mechanism of qi transformation 128
pivot function 129
qi maturation time 223
qi movement role 231
relationship to tai yang 96, 103
resolving time 211
tissue correspondences 83
shao yin disease 41, 90, 103–104
heat and cold syndromes 232
qi transformation in 146–147
resolving time 209, 210, 212, 226, 232
Shanghai College scholarship 70
sinusitis, and pivot function 179
six anatomical systems 60
liù jīng as 82–84
six channels 81
as anachronism 92
liù jīng as 81–82
six conformations 73–74, 75, 76, 79–81, 108, 148, 154
controversy over 72
debates on 78
deterioration times in 234
differentiation by 60, 67
difficulty in understanding 79
disease resolution according to 76
disorders of qi transformation in 64
explaining qi transformation using 63
importance to studying Discussion of Cold Damage 51
resolving time for diseases 209–210, 211
tai yang qi in 191–195
treatment differentiation by 57
six conformations differentiation 94–95, 96
six conformations diseases 79–81, 94, 96–105
jue yin and jue yin disease 104–105

shao yang and shao yang disease 100–101
shao yin and shao yin disease 103–104
tai yang and tai yang disease 96–99
tai yin and tai yin disease 102
yang ming and yang ming disease 99–100
six diseases 92–96, 93
as pathological concept 92
six qi 45, 84, 91, 132
and three yin and three yang 114–115
as root 116
generation by qi movement of five elements 109
in heavens and human body 134, 135
pairings 116
theory of 108
three yin/yang and 110
zang-fu correspondences 125
six stages, introduction of term 91
six-gods formulas 35
skin
and tai yang 82
effects in shang han syndrome 202
tai yang channel and 83
skin diseases 25
small intestine 139
progression from tai yang to 197
tai yang and 96
smelling 75
social conditions 27
Song Dynasty 46, 49, 237
Bureau of Textual Research and Correction for Medical Literature 51
intensive studies during 50
Shanghai College scholarship 70
sub-school of qi transformation in 63
source qi 90
convergence via interstices 174–175
distribution by three burners 174
Southern Song Dynasty 237
special topics 76–78
scholarly contributions 48
spleen
damp qi and 99
progression from tai yang to 196, 197
role in yang ming disease 142
tai yin and 102
tonifying qi herbally 182
Spring and Autumn period 28, 237
harmony principle during 158
stages concept 95
stagnant heat syndromes 141
stomach
dryness qi and 99
harmonization of qi 162
progression from tai yang to 197
sub-schools 46
qi transformation 63, 64
Sui Dynasty 64, 237
summer heat 18
sunrise, variation by season 224
sunset, variation by season 224
sweating 43
absence of 206
action of Cinnamomi Ramulus 203–204
before and after Cinnamon Twig Decoction 205
cautions for promotion of 142
during menstruation 203
improper promotion of 102, 143, 196–197
mistaken promotion of 60
promotion of 40, 85, 92, 141, 162, 164, 165, 167
spontaneous 201, 204, 207, 208
spontaneous *versus* promotion of 205
stopping by harmonization 204–205
tai yang opening/closing role 98
sweating disorder 22
spontaneous 29
symptoms and signs differentiation 52, 58, 62, 89
syndrome differentiation, in Ming Dynasty 57
syndromes
correlating with formula names 58
groupings into six stages 91–92
importance according to Ke Qin 58
line rearrangement according to 55
liù jīng as 91–96
pairing formulas with corresponding 75
relationship to formulas and herbs 58, 74, 78
six groups o92f

tai yang 21, 87, 90, 91, 92, 116, 117, 138, 178
and cold qi 122
and tai yang disease 96–99
area covered by 83
as fence 190
as first layer to be attacked 190
as longest channel 190
as middle qi for shao yin 111
as strongest yang 97
as three yangs 112, 115, 177
broader meaning 191
circadian peak 217
cold and water in 91
cold qi and 111, 125
failure to open 98
mechanism of qi transformation 127
opening function 97, 129, 130, 133, 151
outward movement of 97
relationship to shao yin 96
resolving time 211, 225, 230
skin and 82
symptoms, signs, pulses 89
three yangs in 229
transmuted syndromes in 98
treatment principles 141
tai yang channel
tissue correspondences 83
versus tai yang 190
tai yang disease 22, 42, 52, 85, 90, 92, 93, 96–99
classification approaches 54
cold or hot 97
disease progression 99
due to nutritive and defensive qi disharmony 199
formula names for 58
locations relative to body surface 202, 203
manifestations 141
possible progressions 194
progression 98–99
progression and treatments 196–197
progression to chong and uterus 193
qi transformation clinical applications 140–142
resolving time 23, 209, 212, 214, 215, 217, 226, 236
Shanghai College scholarship 69–70
treatments related to heat 98
urination problems and diarrhea in 98
wrong treatment 102
tai yang qi 191
chong and 193
disorder of production and distribution 196–197
heart and lung relationships 192
in six conformations 191–195
nutritive and defensive qi as 199, 208
production and distribution 194
shao yang and 193
uterus and 193
tai yin 21, 87, 92, 116, 117
and damp qi 122
and tai yin disease 102
area of extent 83
as branch for damp qi 112
as middle qi for yang ming 111
as strongest yin 102
as three yins 11, 177
damp qi and 111, 125
mechanism of qi transformation 128
opening function 129, 131, 134, 151, 230, 231
relationship to yang ming 102
resolving time 211
tai yin disease 90, 102
qi transformation in 146
resolving time 209, 210, 212, 223, 226
Shanghai College scholarship 70
Tang Dynasty 46, 237
sequestering of Zhang Ji's formulas during 49

teaching methods, for Discussion of Cold Damage 76
tendons, jue yin channel and 83
text authenticity 53
textual research 69–73
by Nanjing College of Traditional Chinese Medicine 69
Lin Yi's contributions 51
scholarly contributions 48
three, numerological significance 221
three burners
as fu organ 174
as pivot 175
distribution of source qi by 174
kidney correspondence with 174
relationship to interstices and zang-fu 175, 176
role of interstices in 174–175
role of tai yang in 192
water passages and 174
three burners differentiation 76
Three Kingdoms period 48, 237
three outlines doctrine 56
three yang diseases 92, 133
channel and fu syndromes 137–138
three yangs 21, 84, 85, 87, 94, 96, 112, 113, 115, 121, 127, 225, 229
above-waist areas and 82
generation in heavens 219
generation on earth 218
hiding on earth 220
liù jīng and 84–85, 85–87, 86, 93
shao yang weakness among 101
tai yang as 177
three yin and three yang 72, 109
as branch 116
flow of qi in 177
mechanism of qi transformation 127
mutual interactions 134
opening, closing, and pivot functions 129
qi transformation theory and 107
root, branch, and middle qi for 111
six qi and 110
three yin diseases 92, 133
three yins 21, 84, 85, 87, 94, 96, 115, 120, 128, 177
below-waist areas and 83
generation on earth 220
liù jīng and 84–85, 86, 93
shao yin as pivot 103
tidal fever 235
in yang ming disease 234
tight pulse
in shao yin disease 41
sequential meanings 42
tissue correspondences, six channels 83
tonifying method 92, 165
harmonization by 165
top secret tradition 48–49
toxicity, as disease cause 65
translation
1949 to present 69–73
from ancient to modern Chinese 71–72
transmuted syndromes 98, 151
treatment approaches
based on six conformations 57
eight 61
for half exterior and half interior 155
harmonization 159, 162
line reordering according to 49, 55, 61
liù jīng and 94
selection of 75
shao yang disease 145
special topics 76
ten 62
treatment principles 52
treatment systems 2
trigrams 217
see also Twelve Declining and Growing Hexagrams
true and false manifestations 74
twelve channels 124, 132, 136
borders 89
Twelve Declining and Growing Hexagrams 216, 218–221, 224, 228
combining with Earthly Branches 217
relationship to earthly branches 227
yin and yang changes revealed in 221
Twelve Earthly Branches 210, 228
combined with hexagrams 217
five element correspondences 222
relationship to hexagrams 227
resolving times and 227
significance for human body 216
time allocations 211
two dan formulas 35
two qi relationships 121
two yangs 112, 113, 115, 120, 127, 225
generation in heavens 219
generation on earth 218
remaining in heavens 220
remaining on earth 219
yang ming as 177, 225
two yins 103, 112, 113, 115, 118, 128
generation in heavens 220
generation on earth 220
remaining on earth 218
shao yin as 177

unusual method 61
upper and lower, differentiating 74
upper burner
defensive qi origination in 185, 186–187
dispersion of defensive qi in 189
upper burner symptoms, in shao yang disease 172
urgent and trivial conditions, differentiating 74
urinary bladder 85
cold in 23
heart fire descending to 139
progression from tai yang disease to 197
relationship to interstices and three burners 176
tai yang and 96
urination, promotion of 40
urination problems, in tai yang disease 98
uterus
progression from tai yang to 197
relationship to interstices and three burners 176
tai yang qi and 193

versions, Discussion of Cold Damage 44
vexation, in evening 236
visceral bind disorder 2
vomiting
improper promotion of 102, 196–197
mistaken promotion of 60
promotion of 40, 92, 165

warm interior method 62
warm pathogen disease 17, 66
annotating Discussion of Cold Damage using 55
harmonization method for 165, 166
school of 83
warm pathogen disease school, unification with school of Discussion of Cold Damage 76
warming and clearing methods 45, 92, 165
harmonization by 165
Warring States period 28, 237
harmony principle during 159
water 39
earthly branches belonging to 222
water accumulation syndromes 141, 151
water passages 174
water retention, in shao yang disease 101
water-accumulation syndrome 98
weather changes 113, 116
production of branch qi in 121–126
six qi and 111
Western countries, circulation of Discussion of Cold Damage in 73
Western Han Dynasty
alchemy in 32
harmonization approach during 159
socioeconomic conditions 28
Western Jin 237
Western medicine
integrating with Chinese medicine 45
introduction to China 63

white tiger formula 35, 38
wind 17, 39
  as yang pathological factor 202
  attack of nose and throat by 207
  due to qi stagnation 105
  effects on nutritive qi 57
  injury to defensive qi by 52, 54, 55
  invasion due to defensive qi deficiency 189
  predominance in zhong feng syndrome 200, 201
wind qi 112, 114
  interaction with fire qi 118
  jue yin and 111
wind stroke 17
wind-cold invasion 22, 200
  and obstruction of nutritive and defensive qi 192
  injury to defensive and nutritive qi by 52, 55
  of nutritive and defensive qi 54
  with cold predominant 202
  with wind predominant 201
winter 120
women, *shāng hán* in 21
women's disorders 25
  applying Zhang Ji's formula to 23
  source texts for Zhang Ji 32
wood 125
  earthly branches belonging to 222
wrong treatment 43, 50
  disease progression due to 196–197
  in tai yang disease 192
  tai yin disease and 102

Xia Dynasty 237

yang
  avoiding damage to 142
  controlling role over yin 67
  hiding on earth 220
  origination in upper burner 187
  peak time between heaven and earth 219
  peak time in heavens 219, 220
  peak time on earth 219
yang channels
  onset and progression 51, 80
  tai yang dominance among 88
yang classification 177
yang collapse 105
yang deficiency 98
  feeble pulse and 42
  in spleen 142
  with cold accumulation in organs 22–23
yang ming 21, 87, 91, 92, 116, 117, 178
  and fire qi 122
  and yang ming disease 99–100
  as middle qi for tai yin 111
  as midway point for qi descending 230
  as two yangs 112, 115, 177
  closing function 100, 129, 130, 131
  direction of qi movement 230
  dry and metal in 91
  dryness qi and 111, 125
  mechanism of qi transformation 127
  muscle and 82
  qi maturation time 223
  qi transformation for 137
  relationship to tai yin 99
  resolving time 211
  treatment methods 167
yang ming channel, tissue correspondences 83
yang ming disease 52, 90, 92, 93, 99–100
  channel syndromes in 138
  connection to tai yin 227
  interior excess heat 100
  progression to tai yin disease 100
  qi transformation in 142–144
  resolving time 209, 212, 226, 235
  Shanghai College scholarship 70
yang qi
  and fire spirit school 66–67
  clear 188
  peak and directional change 229
  recovery during night 221, 234
  school of strengthening 66–67
  sectarian bias 77
yang tonification school 45
yang within yin 216
yin and yang
  and circadian rhythms 217
  combinations in root and branch relationships 117
  condition at different times 216
  differentiating 74
  direction of qi movement 229–230
  failure to connect in jue yin disease 233
  function and circulation 177
  hexagrams revealing changes of 221
  historical development 27
  turning points in direction 230
  weather change and 121
yin and yang qi, quantity of 96
yin channels, disease onset and progression 51, 80
yin classification 177
yin qi
  in heavens and on earth 221
  peak and descent time 229
yin within yang 216
yin yang yi disease 21
  Shanghai College scholarship 70
Yuan Dynasty 237
  Discussion of Cold Damage studies 50

zang-fu organs 85, 86, 87, 94, 95
  correspondences to qi transformation 124
  discerning normal functions of 41
  liù jīng as 85–87
  relationship to interstices and three burners 175
  Zhang Ji's failure to use 96
zhong feng syndrome 21, 22, 200, 201, 203
  body location 203
  effects on muscle and skin 202
  with wind predominant 201
Zhou Dynasty 237

AUTHOR INDEX

Ao Shuang Xuan Zhu 67

Ban Gu 28
Ban Meng-Jian 28

Cao Bing-Zhang 66
Cao Chi-Dian 66
Cao Jia-Da 63, 68
Cao Ying-Fu 63
Chen Bo-Tan 116
Chen Nian-Zu 56, 63, 106, 137
Chen Shi-Wen 207
Chen Xiu-Yuan 56, 63, 106, 107
Chen Yi-Ren 73
Cheng Guo-Pen 165
Cheng Jiao-Qian 89
five elements and Twelve Earthly Branches 222
Cheng Wu-Ji 25, 26, 46, 50, 52, 53, 54, 57, 62, 155, 163, 164
on yin and yang times 216–217
Cheng Ying-Mao 89
five elements and Twelve Earthly Branches 222
on tai yang disease 199
Cheng Zhong-Ling 165
Chun Yu-Yi 38
Confucius 28, 159
authorship 31

Dai Lin-Jiao 165
Dai Tian-Zhang 165
Deng Shao-Xian 150
Deng Xu-Cheng 150
Dong Zhong-Shu 29
Du Du 24

Fan Ye 24
Fang Jiang-Jun 34
Fang You-Zhi 50, 53, 54, 55, 56, 61, 81, 88
combining nutritive and defensive qi 190
Fang Zhong-Xing 53
Feng Shi-Lun 50
Feng Ye 73
Fu You-Feng 20

Gao Bao-Heng 26
Ge Zhi-Chuan 34
Guo Yong 85
Guo Zi-Guang 73, 90
Guo Zi-He 85

Hao Wan-Shan 71–72
He Bing-Yuan 6, 166
He Lian-Chen 66, 166
He Xiu-Shan 66
He Yong 30
He Yun-He 92
He Zhi-Xiong 87
Hu Xi-Shu 73
Hu Xi-Xu 73
Hua Tuo 24, 29
Hua Yuan-Hua 34
Huang Fu Xuan Yan 34
Huang Fu-Mi 33, 34, 38
on defensive qi origins 187
Huang Kun-Zai 63, 136
Huang Qian 17
Huang Wen-Dong 91, 92
Huang Yuan-Yu 63, 136
Huang Zhong-Li 53
Huang Zhu-Zhai 17

Jiang Chun-Hua 86
Jiang Qiu-shi 80

Ke Qin 50, 58, 59, 60–61, 82, 88, 164, 178, 179
contributions 60
on tai yang qi and heart/lung 192
Ke Yun-Bo 58, 82, 164, 178
Koso Kitamura 64

Lao Zi 28, 40, 41, 158
number three significance 221
Li Dan 158, 221
Li Dong-Bi 85
Li Er 158, 221
Li Ke-Shao 72, 86
Li Pei-Sheng 73, 74
Lin Yi 24, 25, 26, 51, 52, 57, 69, 70
Liu Che 29
Liu Du-Zhou 70, 73, 87, 145
Liu Li-Hong 234
Liu Wan-Su 53
Lü Cha-Cun 18
Lü Jian-Xun 18, 62
Lu Pen-Nian 68, 91
Lu Yu-Chen 67
Lu Yuan-Lei 63, 68, 91
Lü Zhen-Ming 18, 62
Lu Zhu-Zhi 67
Lu Zi-Yao 63, 133, 135
Lu Zi-Yi 133, 135
Lu Zu-Chang 63, 133

Luo Mei 117
Luo Xi-Wen 73

Ma Yi-Chao 167, 168
Marchment, Robin 73
Mencius 18, 19
Mitchell, Craig 73, 80
Motohiro Taki 68
Motohiro Tamba 64, 68
Motokata Taki 64
Motokata Tamba 64

Nakanishi Koretada 18
Nie Hui-Min 73, 166

Pang An-Chang 47
Pang An-Shi 47

Qi Xuan-Zi 91, 122, 129, 170
Qian Huang 50, 57, 60, 215
contributions 61
on resolving times 213, 217
Qian Tian-Lai 57
on resolving times 213

Ren Ying-Qiu 18, 46, 62, 71
influence on research 47

Shen Jin-Ao 62
Shen Qian-Lu 62
Sozan Shirozu 64
Sun Qi 26
Sun Si-Miao 48, 50, 54, 58
on defensive qi origins 186
on resolving times 213

Tang Bu-Qi 67
Tang Da-Lie 61
Tang Li-Shan 61
Tang Rong-Chuan 63, 64
Tang Zong-Hai 63, 64, 138
Tao Hong-Jing 34, 35, 38, 50
Tao Tong-Ming 34
Todo Yoshimasu 64

Wan You-Sheng 76
Wang Ang 207
Wang Bing 91, 129, 150, 170, 177
Wang Hong-Han 63
Wang Hu 81, 88
Wang Hui-Yuan 63

Wang Ling-You 81, 88
Wang Lu 53
Wang Ren-An 207
Wang Shu-He 25, 49, 53, 54, 55, 56
Wang Tao
  on defensive qi origins 186
Wang Xi 25, 26, 46, 49, 50, 53, 54, 56
  addition of chapters by 56, 57
  debate over errors 55
Want Ling-You 88
Wei Si 34
Wei Xun 24
Wiseman, Nigel 73
Wu Kun 129
Wu Kun-An 66
Wu Ling-Ya 62
Wu Pei-Heng 67
Wu Pu 34
Wu Ren-Ju 62
Wu Shan-Fu 129
Wu Zhen 66
Wu Zhong-Quan 67

Xiong Man-Qi 73, 87
Xu Da-Chun 50, 59
  on sweating before and after Cinnamon Twig Decoction 205
Xu Guo-Chun 66
Xu Ling-Tai 59
Xu Rong-Zhai 66
Xu Shen 157
Xu Shu-Zhong 157
Xun Zi 28

Yang Shang-Shan 186
Ye Gui 66
Ye Tian-Shi 66
You Yi 50, 57, 61
  disease deterioration times 235
You Zai-Jing 57, 89
Yu Chang 54, 56, 61, 76
  line reordering by 55
  on resolution times 225
Yu Chang-Rong 73
Yu Gen-Chu 66
Yu Jia-Yan 54
  on resolution times 225
Yu Zhao-Yuan 66
Yun Shu-Jue 63, 68, 79, 89
Yun Tie-Qiao 63, 79, 89
Yung Jie De, Greta 73

Zhang Bing-Lin 107
Zhang Bo-Zu 24
Zhang Heng-Liu 28
Zhang Ji 17, 18, 46, 57, 58, 74, 82, 89, 93, 94, 100, 143, 144, 146, 147, 149, 155, 160, 162, 163, 168, 171, 173, 174, 175, 178, 180, 183, 214
  academic approaches 44
  advocacy of Confucian medical ethic 30
  antiquated language 71
  biographical details 24
  classic texts referred to by 52
  combining nutritive and defensive qi 190
  companion books by 23
  defensive qi generation strategy 206
  differentiation skills 200
  dropped chapters 54
  influence of Confuciansim 30
  lack of contemporary fame 29
  nutritive and defensive qi theory 191
  on defensive qi origins 192
  on qi changes 224, 234
  on resolving times 209, 217, 236
  source texts 34
  strategies for working with defensive qi 206–207
  study of Yellow Emperor's Inner Classic 189
  summation of Han medical achievements by 27
  textual work on 51
  two formulas for nutritive/defensive qi 203–204
  two-hour resolution periods 212
  use of four-god decoctions 39
  use of *Yellow Emperor's Inner Classic* 20
  works summary 26
  yin and yang changes 221
Zhang Jia-Li 175
Zhang Jia-Shan 30
Zhang Jie-Bin 123, 130, 137, 165, 170
Zhang Jing-Yue 123, 130, 165, 170
Zhang Ling-Shao 65, 138
Zhang Qing-Zi 56
Zhang Sui-Chen 56
Zhang Tai-Yan 107
Zhang Xi-Ju 63, 138
Zhang Yin-An 63, 134, 143, 144, 148
Zhang Zheng-Zhao 21, 96
Zhang Zhi-Cong 56, 63, 107, 134, 143, 144, 148
  on Cinnamon Twig Decoction 204
  on defensive qi origins 186
Zhang Zhi-Ming 93
Zhang Zhong-Jing 24, 44, 72, 81, 88, 92, 136
Zhao En-Jian 108
Zhao Kai-Mei 69, 70
Zhao Yi-Kong 195
Zheng Qin-An 67, 148
Zheng Shou-Quan 67, 148
Zhi Fa-Shi 34
Zhu Dan-Xi 207
  spontaneous sweating treatment 208
Zhu Gong 51, 80, 88
Zhu Wei-Ju 67, 90
Zhu Y88i-Zhong
Zhu Yi-Zhong 51, 80, 88
Zhu Zhen-Heng 297
Zhuang Zhou 171
Zhuang Zi 28, 171
Zhuang Zi-Xiu 171
Zuo Ji-Yun 45, 63
Zuo Qiu-Ming 158

CLASSIC TEXTS INDEX

500 Cases for Changes to Chinese Characters (漢字演變五百例 *hàn zì yán biàn wŭ băi lì*) 157

Acupuncture Jia and Yi Classic (針灸甲乙經 *zhēn jiŭ jiă yĭ jīng*) 24, 31, 33, 91
 defensive qi origins 187
Analects of Confucius (論語 *lùn yŭ*) 159
Annotating and Explaining Discussion of Cold Damage (註解傷寒論 *zhù jiě shāng hăn lùn*) 25, 26, 52
 introduction of half exterior and half interior in 155
 shao yang disease concept 163–164
Annotation and Commentary for Complete Medical Works by Jing-Yue (校注景岳全書 *jiào zhù jĭng-yuè quán shū*) 165
Answers to Difficult Questions for Discussion of Cold Damage (傷寒質難 *shāng hán zhì nàn*) 90

Bamboo Slips in the Han Dynasty Dug from Zhang Jia-Shan (張家山漢簡 *zhāng jiā shān hàn jiăn*) 30
Basic Questions (素問 *sù wèn*) 17, 19, 20, 91, 92, 113, 132
 defensive qi origins 187
 disease resolution times 209, 225
 five elements qi movement in 109–111
 qi interactions in 122
 shao yang pivot concept 169, 170
 theory of qi transformation in 108
 three burners in 174
 three yin and three yang in 131
 yang classifications 177
 yin and yang changes 216
Beginning and Source of Medicine (醫學原始 *yī xué yuán shĭ*) 63
Book of Changes (周易繫辭下 *zhōu yì*) 31
 disease resolution times and 217–221
Book of Rites (禮記 *lĭ jì*)
 concept of harmony 159
Book Reviewed by the Emperor of the Tai Ping Era (太平禦覽 *tài píng yù lán*) 29–30
Book to Safeguard Life Based on Classifying Patterns (類證活人書 *lèi zhèng huó rén shū*) 80
Brief Historical Stories for States (國語 *guó yŭ*) 158

Classic of the Golden Coffer and Jade Sheath, The (金匱玉函經 *jīn gùi yù hán jīng*) 25, 26, 51, 70
Classical Methods to Make Formulas (湯液經法 *tāng yè jīng fă*) 33, 34, 35, 38, 39, 50
Classification of Formulas in Discussion of Cold Damage (傷寒論類方 *shāng hán lùn lèi fāng*) 59
Clear Differentiation for Warm-Pathogen and Pestilential Diseases (溫疫明辨 *wēn yĭ míng biàn*) 165
Collection of Commentaries for Cold Damage (傷寒論集注 *shāng hán lùn jí zhù*) 134
Collections and References of Classified Formulas and Case Studies Related to Discussion of Cold Damage (傷寒論類方法案匯參 *shāng hăn lùn lè fāng fă àn huì cān*) 45
Commentaries for Spiritual Pivot of the Yellow Emperor's Inner Classic (靈樞經集注 *líng shū jīng jí zhù*) 186
Commentary on Differentiation in Discussion of Cold Damage (傷寒論辨證廣注 *shāng hán lùn biàn zhèng guăng zhù*) 81
Comments on Editorial Elaboration for Discussion of Cold Damage (傷寒論輯義按 *shāng hán lùn jí yì àn*) 63, 68
Complete Classification of Syndromes and Their Treatments in Discussion of Cold Damage (傷寒論證治類詮 *shāng hán lùn zhèng zhì lèi quán*) 62–63
Completed Book by Zhong-Jing (仲景全書 *zhòng-jĭng quán shū*) 69, 70
Completely Understanding Cold Damage (傷寒指掌 *shāng hán zhĭ zhàng*) 66
Comprehensive Explanation for Syndromes and Formulas in Six Conformations (六經方證通解 *liù jīng fāng zhèng tōng jiě*) 63
Connecting Pearls for Discussion of Cold Damage (傷寒貫珠集 *shāng hán guàn zhū jí*) 57, 61, 89
 disease onset and resolution times 235
Correction for Preliminary Commentary for Discussion of Cold Damage (傷寒論淺注補正 *shāng hán lùn qiān zhù bŭ zhèng*) 63
Current Explanation for Discussion of Cold Damage (傷寒論今釋 *shāng hán lùn jīn shì*) 63, 68, 107

Detailed Outline of the Materia Medica (本草綱目 *bĕn căo gāng mù*) 85
Detailed Outlines for Discussion of Cold Damage (傷寒論綱目 *shāng hán lùn gāng mù*) 62
Dictionary for Chinese Medicine (中醫大辭典 *zhōng yī dà cí diàn*) 106
Difficult Questions (難經 *nàn jīng*) 17, 20, 28, 52
 interstices concept 173
 three burners concept 174
Discussion of Cold Damage (傷寒論 *shāng hăn lùn*) 17, 19, 20, 21, 22, 23, 25, 29, 44, 53, 79, 81, 91, 94, 134, 195, 200
 absence of pivot character in 171
 absence of six channels in 92, 93
 adaptation of earlier formulas in 34, 35
 adaptation of harmony concept in 162
 additions by Wang Xi 54
 adoption of formulas from 66
 applications of qi transformation theory 140–154
 case studies 68
 Chang Wu-Ji's analysis 62

Cheng Wu-Ji's disease resolution commentary 216–217
Cheng Wu-Ji's harmony concept 163
circulation abroad 64
citation of Confucius 30
comparison of formulas in 36–37
confusion over harmonization concept 167
Daoist influences 40
debate about qi transformation in 106–108
defensive and nutritive qi issues 185, 189
defensive qi route 193
descriptions of time 214
differentiation and treatments in 153–154
disease deterioration times 234
disease progression in 143
disease resolution times 215
earliest publication date 51–52
Fang You-Zhi on 82
half exterior and half interior in 155, 183
handwritten copies 26
harmony character in 161
herbs recorded in 244–246
historical formula precedents in 35
importance of yin and yang change in 135
internal disorders 97
Jiang Chun-Hua on 86
jue yin disease progression in 147–148
line classification 59
Liu Du-Zhou on 87
medical ethics in 31
methods of working with defensive qi 206–207
national textbook 71
opening, closing and pivot theory in 150
pathology in tai yin disease 231
preface 33
qi transformation in 107, 116, 139
Qian Huang's contribution 6061
relationship to Sun Si-Miao's work 213
role of Minor Bupleurum Decoction 179
scholarly contributions 78
school of qi transformation in 132–140
sentence of showing manifestation 42
shao yang disease symptoms in 173
shao yang disease transformation in 145
shao yang disease treatment 178
shao yin disease onset 103
shao yin disease syndromes 232
six conformations in 80, 96
sources of formulas in 38
tai yang disease 199
tai yang qi in six conformations in 191–195
tai yang, heart, and lung 197
tai yin disorders 102
three burners as pivot 175
three yang disease classification in 138
versions 51
versions in Japan 63, 65
Wang Xi's contribution 56
yang ming disease progression 100
Yu Chang's rearrangement 55
Zhu Gong on 88

Discussion of Cold Damage and Miscellaneous Diseases (傷寒雜病論 *shāng hán zá bìng lùn*) 24–25, 26
Discussion of Cold Damage Annotated by Zhang Qing-Zi (張卿子傷寒論 *zhāng qīng-zǐ shāng hán lùn*) 56
Discussion of Cold Damage in a Series of Advanced Books for Chinese Medicine (中醫藥學高級叢書傷寒論 *zhōng yī yào xué gāo jí cóng shū: shāng hán lùn*) 87
Discussion of Special Topic on Surviving with Cold Damage (傷寒來蘇集, 傷寒論翼 *shāng hán lái sū jí, shāng hán lùn yì*) 59, 82
shao yang disease symptoms 179

Editorial Elaboration for Discussion of Cold Damage (傷寒論輯義 *shāng hán lùn jí yì*) 68
Essentials and Formula Discussions from the Golden Cabinet (金匱要略方論 *jīn guì yào lüè fāng lùn*) 25, 51
defensive qi issues 189
handwritten copies 26
interstices and three burners 174
three burners as pivot 175
Explanation for Chinese Characters (說文解字 *shuō wén jiě zì*) 157
pivot character 169
Explanation for Difficult Questions in Discussion of Cold Damage (傷寒懸解 *shāng hán xúan jiě*) 136
Explanation of Confusing Points in Discussion of Cold Damage (傷寒解惑論 *sháng háng jiě huò lùn*) 72
Exploring Real Meaning for Discussion of Cold Damage (傷寒發微 *shāng hán fā wēi*) 65, 68

Fifty-two Diseases and Their Formulas (五十二病方 *wǔ shí èr bìng fāng*) 159
Flexible Medical Methods (醫法圓通 *yī fǎ yuán tōng*) 67
Formulas by Zhang Zhong-Jing (張仲景方 *zhāng zhòng-Jǐng fāng*) 25, 26, 49, 60

Historical Book for the Han Dynasty (漢書 *hàn shū*) 28
History of the Later Han Dynasty (後漢書 *hòu hàn shū*) 24

Inherit the Past and Usher in the Future for Medicine (醫宗承啟 *yī zōng chéng qǐ*) 62

Key Points to Learn from Discussion of Cold Damage (傷寒知要 *shāng hán zhī yào*) 76
Key Points to Study Discussion of Cold Damage (傷寒大要 *shāng hán dà yào*) 45, 65
Keys to Choose Points for Acupuncture and Moxibustion from Bright Hall (明堂孔穴針灸治要 *míng táng kǒng xué zhēn jiǔ zhì yaò*) 187

Materia Medica by Shen Nong (神農本草經 *shén nóng běn cǎo jīng*) 28
Bupleuri Radix nature 180, 181
Medical Comprehension (醫學心悟 *yī xué xīn wù*) 165
Morals Classic (道德經 *dào dé jīng*) 28, 40, 41, 158
qi directional changes 229
shao yang pivot theory in 167

New Classification of Formulas and Syndromes in Discussion of Cold Damage (傷寒論湯證新編 *shāng hán lùn tāng zhèng xīn biān*) 75

Origin of Chinese Characters (辭源 *cí yuán*) 111, 186

Passing Down Truth for a Classic Formula (經方傳真 *jīng fāng chuán zhēn*) 73
Popular Guide to the Discussion of Cold Damage (通俗傷寒論 *tōng sú shāng hán lùn*) 66
Pulse Book, A (脈書 *mài shū*)
pivot concept 170
Pulse Classic (脈經 *mài jīng*) 49, 50

Records for Clinical Application of Classic Formulas (經方實驗錄 *jīng fāng shí yàn lù*) 68
Replenishment for Discussion of Cold Damage (傷寒補亡論 *shāng hán bǔ wáng lùn*) 85

Revised and Expanded Discussion of Warm-Pathogen Disease (重訂廣瘟熱論 *chóng dìng guáng wēn rè lùn*) 166
Rhymed Formula for Keys to Employ Herbs According to Zang-fu Organs (輔行訣臟腑用藥法要 *fù xíng jué zàng fǔ yòng yào fǎ yào*) 33, 34, 60
comparisons with Zhang Ji formulas 36–37

Search the Source for Discussion of Cold Damage (傷寒尋源 *shāng hán xún yuán*) 18
Search the Truth for Discussion of Cold Damage (傷寒論求是 *shāng hán lùn qiú shì*) 74
Searching the Source for Discussion of Cold Damage (*shāng hán xún yuán*) 62
Shang Han Lun Explained (傷寒論講解與臨床心得 shāng hán lùn jiǎng jiě yǔ lín chuáng xīn dé) 73
Shang Han Lun: On Cold Damage 73
Spiritual Pivot (靈樞 *líng shū*) 91
defensive qi circulation 195
defensive qi circulation route 200
defensive qi origins 187
nutritive and defensive qi theory 186
opening, closing and pivot in 129, 132
shao yang pivot concept 169
three burners and interstices 174
three yin and three yang in 131
Study for the Classic of the Golden Coffer and Jade Sheath (金匱玉函經研究 *jīn gùi yù hán jīng yán jiū* 70
Study on Discussion of Cold Damage (傷寒之研究 *shāng hán zhī yán jiū*) 18
Superficial Comments on Discussion of Cold Damage (傷寒論淺注 *shāng hán lùn qián zhù*) 106
Supplement to Thousand Ducat Formulas (千金翼方 *qiān jīn yì fāng*) 50, 213
disease resolving times 215
Surviving with Discussion of Cold Damage (傷寒來蘇集 *shāng hán lái sū jí*) 58

Teaching of (Zhu) Dan-Xi (丹溪心法 *dān xī xīn fǎ*) 207
Teaching Reference Books for Traditional Chinese Medical Colleges: Discussion of Cold Damage (高等中醫院校教學參考書:傷寒論 *gāo děng zhōng yī yuàn xiào jiāo xué cān kǎo shū: shāng hán lùn*) 71
Textual Research and Annotation for Discussion of Cold Damage (傷寒論校注 *shāng hán lùn jiào zhù*) 70, 71
Thousand Ducat Formulas for Emergent Cases (千金翼方 *qiān jīn yì fāng*) 50
Translation and Explanation for Discussion of Cold Damage (傷寒論譯釋 *shāng hán lùn yì shì*) 69
Translation for Discussion of Cold Damage with Contemporary Chinese (白話傷寒論 *bái huà shāng hán lùn)* 72
Treatise on Discussion of Cold Damage (傷寒論條辨 *shāng hán lùn tiáo biàn*) 54
on tai yang qi 190
True Classification and Analysis for Lines in Discussion of Cold Damage and Supplementary After-Reading Discussion of Cold Damage (傷寒論後條辨·讀傷寒論贅餘 *shāng hán lùn hòu tiáo biàn, dú shāng hán lùn zhuì yú*) 88–89, 199
Truth Teaching in Medicine (醫理真傳 *yī lǐ zhēn chuán*) 67
Understanding the Truth for Discussion of Cold Damage (傷寒明理論 *shāng hán míng lǐ lùn*) 52
harmonization concept 164

Yellow Emperor's Inner Classic (黃帝內經 *huáng dì nèi jīng*) 27–28, 30, 39, 52, 86, 88, 93, 96, 109, 113, 133, 191
as reference for Zhang Ji 163
clinical applications 140
cosmology and macrocosm in 110
defensive qi circulation 195, 206
defensive qi origins 187, 188
disease onset and resolution times 224, 225
disease resolution times 209
harmony character in 159, 160, 161, 162
interstices concept 173
nutritive and defensive qi theory 185
opening, closing and pivot in 132
pivot concept 101
qi interactions in 122
qi transformation in 123, 131, 137
shao yang pivot concept 169, 170
shao yin and tai yang qi transformation in 126
tai yin qi transformation in 125
theory of qi transformation in 108–117
three burners as pivot 175
three burners concept 174
three yin and three yang in 112, 129, 225, 226
yang classifications 177
Zhang Ji's study of 94, 189

HERB AND FORMULA INDEX

Aconite Accessory Root Decoction (*fù zǐ tāng*) 147
Aconiti Radix Lateralis (*fù zǐ*) 37, 66, 67, 98, 192, 207
Alismatis Rhizoma (*zé xiè*) 142
Appropriate Decoction (*dǐ dàng tāng*) 197
Appropriate Pill (*dǐ dàng wán*) 197
Armenicae Semen Amarum (*xìng rén*) 162, 205, 207, 297
Ass-Hide Gelatin Decoction (*huáng lián ē jāo tāng*) 39
Astragali Radix (*huáng qí*) 192, 207, 208
Atractylodis Macrocephalae Rhizoma (*bái zhú*) 142, 207

Black Warrior Decoction 38
Bluegreen Dragon Decoction (*qīng lóng tāng*) 39
Bupleuri Radix (*chái hú*) 179, 180, 181, 182, 207
Bupleurum Decoction (*chái hú zhèng*) 58, 74, 167

Cinnamomi Cortex (*ròu guì*) 66, 67
Cinnamomi Ramulus (*guì zhī*) 36, 66, 98, 142, 204, 205, 207, 208
Cinnamon Twig and Ginseng Decoction (*guì zhī rén shēn tāng*) 196
Cinnamon Twig and Licorice Decoction (*guì zhī gān cǎo tāng*) 141, 196
Cinnamon Twig Decoction (*guì zhǐ tang*) 22, 35, 36, 38, 50, 55, 57, 58, 59, 85, 98, 151, 162, 163, 169, 184, 185, 192, 203, 204, 205, 208, 215, 236
  harmonization using 168
  opening tai yang with 133
  treating wind-cold with 141
Cinnamon Twig Decoction minus Cinnamon Twig plus Poria and White Atractylodes (*guì zhī qù guì jiā fú líng bái zhú tāng*) 141
Cinnamon Twig Decoction minus Peony (*guì zhī qù sháo yào tāng*) 196
Cinnamon Twig Decoction minus Peony plus Aconite Accessory Root (*guì zhī qù sháo yào jiā fù zǐ tāng*) 196
Cinnamon Twig Decoction plus Pueraria (*guì zhī jiā gé gēn tāng*) 98, 151
Cinnamon Twig plus Aconite Accessory Root Decoction (*guì zhī jiā fù zǐ tāng*) 141
Codonopsis Radix (*dǎng shēn*) 192
Combination of Half Cinnamon Twig Decoction (*guì zhī tāng*) and Half Ephedra Decoction (*guì zhī má huáng gè bàn tāng*) 98
Combination of Two Parts Cinnamon Twig Decoction and One Part Ephedra Decoction (*guì zhī èr má huáng yī tāng*) 98
Coptidis Rhizoma (*huáng lián*) 36
Coptis and Ass-Hide Gelatin Decoction (*huáng lián ē jiāo tāng*) 35, 36, 38, 147, 152

Decoction to Drain the Epigastrium (*xiè xīn tāng*) 35, 37, 38
Dry Ginger (*gān jiāng*) 66
Dry Ginger and Aconite Accessory Root Decoction (*gān jiāng fù zǐ tāng*) 141

Ephedra Decoction (*má huáng tāng*) 35, 38, 50, 55, 57, 58, 85, 98, 151, 185, 205
  treating wind-cold with 141
Ephedra, Apricot Kernel, Licorice and Gypsum Decoction (*má huáng xìng rén gān cǎo shí gāo tāng*) 141
Ephedra, Asarum, and Aconite Accessory Root Decoction (*má huáng xì xīn fù zǐ tāng*) 149
Ephedrae Herba (*má huáng*) 85, 205, 207
Evodia Decoction (*wú zhū yú tāng*) 100

Five-Ingredient Powder with Poria (*wù líng sǎn*) 141, 142, 197
Fresh Ginger Decoction to Drain the Epigastrium (*shēng jiāng xiè xīn tāng*) 197
Frigid Extremities Decoction (*sì nì tāng*) 141, 146, 147, 152, 167, 197

Gardenia and Prepared Soybean Decoction (*zhī zǐ chǐ táng*) 152, 196
Ginseng Radix (*rén shēn*) 36, 37, 182
Glycyrrhizae Radix (*gān cǎo*) 37
Glycyrrhizae Radix Preparata (*zhì gān cǎo*) 182, 204, 205, 207
Gypsum fibrosum (*shí gāo*) 37

Half Cinnamon Twig and Half Ephedra Decoction (*guì zhī má huáng gè bàn tāng*) 151

Jade Windscreen Powder (*yù píng fēng sǎn*) 207
Jujubae Fructus (*dà zǎo*) 192, 204, 206, 207

Lepidii/Descurainiae Semen (*tíng lì zǐ*) 37, 162
Licorice Decoction to Drain the Epigastrium (*gān cǎo xiè xīn tāng*) 197
Lophatherum and Gypsum Decoction (*zhú yè shí gāo tāng*) 37

Major Black Warrior Decoction (*dà xuán wǔ tāng*) 37
Major Bluegreen Dragon Decoction (*dà qīng long tāng*) 35, 36, 38, 50, 55, 58–59, 142, 149, 196
Major Decoction [for pathogens] Stuck in the Chest (*dà xiàn xiōng tāng*) 196
Major Flying Snake Decoction (*dà téng shé tāng*) 37
Major Hook Old Decoction (*dà gōu chén tāng*) 37
Major Order the Qi Decoction (*dà chéng qì tāng*) 37, 144
Major Red Bird Decoction (*dà zhū què tāng*) 36
Major White Tiger Decoction (*dà bái hǔ tāng*) 37
Major Yang Dan Decoction (*dà yáng dàn tāng*) 36
Major Yin Dan Decoction (*dà yīn dàn tāng*) 36
Maor Bluegreen Dragon Decoction (*dà qīng lóng tāng*) 141
Minor Black Warrior Decoction (*xiǎo xuán wǔ tāng*) 37

Minor Bluegreen Dragon Decoction (*xiǎo qīng lóng tāng*) 35, 36, 50, 141, 196
Minor Bupleurum Decoction (*xiǎo chái hú tāng*) 35, 36, 38, 153, 156, 163, 171, 173, 175, 181, 196, 197
harmonizing exterior and interior with 164
recovering pivot function via 174, 181
Minor Decoction [for pathogens] Stuck in the Chest (*xiǎo xiàn xiǎo xiàn*) 196
Minor Flying Snake Decoction (*xiǎo téng shé tāng*) 37
Minor Hook Old Decoction (*xiǎo gōu chén tāng*) 37
Minor Order the Qi Decoction (*xiǎo chéng qì tāng*) 144, 163
Minor Red Bird Decoction (*xiǎo zhū què tāng*) 36
Minor White Tiger Decoction (*xiǎo bái hǔ tāng*) 37
Minor Yang Dan Decoction (*xiǎo yáng dàn tāng*) 35, 36
Minor Yin Dan Decoction (*xiǎo yīn dàn tāng*) 36

Natrii Sulfas (*máng xiāo*) 37, 162
Nelumbinis Folium (*hé yè*) 180
Nelumbinis Semen (*lián zǐ*) 180
Newly Augmented Cinnamon Twig Decoction with the Addition of One Liang Each of Peony and Fresh Ginger and Three Liang of Ginseng (*guì zhī jiā sháo yà shēng jiāng gè yì liǎng rén shēn sān liǎng xīn jiā tāng*) 36

Order the Qi Decoction (*chéng qì tāng*) 152

Paeoniae Radix Alba (*bái sháo*) 36, 204, 205–206, 207
Peach Pit Decoction to Order the Qi (*táo hé chéng qì tāng*) 197
Pinellia Decoction to Drain the Epigastrium (*bàn xià xiè xīn tāng*) 37, 197
Pinellia Pill 39
Pinelliae Rhizoma (*bàn xià*) 37, 181, 182
Polyporus (*zhū líng*) 142
Poria (*fú líng*) 142
Poria, Cinnamon Twig, Atractylodes, and Licorice Decoction (*fú líng guì zhī bái zhú gān cǎo tāng*) 197
Pueraria Decoction (*gé gēn tāng*) 58, 151
Pueraria, Scutellaria, and Coptis Decoction (*gé gēn huáng qín huáng lián tāng*) 141, 197

Rambling Powder (*xiāo yáo sǎn*) 167
Red Bird Decoction (*zhū què tāng*) 39
Regulate the Middle Pill (*lǐ zhōng wán*) 236
Regulate the Stomach and Order the Qi Decoction (*tiáo wèi chéng qì tāng*) 162, 163
Rhei Radix et Rhizoma (*dà huáng*) 37, 162

Saposhnikoviae Radix (*fáng fēng*) 207
Scrophularia Decoction 39
Scutellaria Decoction (*huáng qín tāng*) 35, 36, 38
Scutellariae Radix (*huáng qín*) 36, 181, 182

Three-Unbinding Decoction (*sān ǎo tāng*) 207
True Warrior Decoction (*zhēn wǔ tāng*) 35, 37, 38, 141, 197
Two-Parts Cinnamon Twig Decoction with One-Part Ephedra Decoction (*guì zhī èr má huáng yī tāng*) 151

White Tiger Decoction (*bái hǔ tāng*) 35, 37, 38, 39
White Tiger plus Ginseng Decoction (*bái hǔ jiā rén shēn tāng*) 197

Zingiberis Rhizoma (*gān jiāng*) 36, 37, 67
Zingiberis Rhizoma Recens (*shēng jiāng*) 36, 37, 182, 192, 204, 206, 207

PINYIN INDEX

bàn biǎo bàn lǐ (半表半裡) 155
bàn zài lǐ bàn zài wài (半在裡半在外) 155
běn qì (本氣) 106, 107, 108, 110, 111, 113, 117, 120, 121, 122, 123, 125, 126, 132, 133, 137, 153, 228
  for jue yin 149
  for shao yang 144, 145
  for shao yin 146, 147
  for tai yang 140
  for tai yin 146
  for yang ming 142
  interaction with *zhōng qì* (中氣) 118–121
  qi transformation mechanisms 127–128
  zang-fu correspondences 124
biàn zhèng lùn zhì (辨證論治) 65
biāo qì (標氣) 106, 107, 108, 110, 111, 112, 113, 117, 118, 125, 126, 132, 133, 137, 153, 228
  for jue yin 148
  for shao yang 144, 145
  for tai yang 140
  for tai yin 146
  in shao yin 146, 147
  production according to weather change 121–126, 130–132
  qi transformation mechanisms 127–128
  zang-fu organ correspondences 124
bìng (病) 93
bō guà (剝卦) 220, 230

céng cì (層次) 90
chén (辰) 210, 211, 212, 222, 223, 224, 225, 226, 232
chǒu (丑) 210, 211, 212, 222, 223, 226, 227, 231, 233
chū (出) 186
còu (腠) 179
  as interstices 173
  relationship to three burners 175
còu lǐ (腠理)
  open with deficiency 175
  relationship to three burners 175

dà zhuàng guà (大壯卦) 219, 228, 232
dào (到) 215
dì zhī (地支) 210
dùn guà (遁卦) 220, 229

fǎ (法) 55
fǎn (反) 41
fāng zhèng (方證) 74
fù (復) 41
fu guà (复卦) 218, 231
fú yáng lùn tán (扶陽論壇) 77
fú yáng pài (扶陽派) 66

gòu guà (姤卦) 219, 229
guài guà (夬卦) 219
guān guà (觀卦) 220, 230

hài (亥) 210, 211, 222, 223, 226, 231
hán (寒) 18
hé (和) 156, 169, 200
  as appropriate, balance 159
  as balance 178
  as treatment method 163
  bamboo pipes pictogram 167, 168, 182
  Confucius' understanding of 159
  for nutritive and defensive qi 163
  in Difficult Questions 169
  in Yellow Emperor's Inner Classic 160, 161
  Zhang Ji's use of 160
hé fǎ (和法) 156, 169
  as harmonization 159, 184
huǒ shén pài (火神派) 65, 66, 77

jiě (解) 40
jiē duàn (階段) 91
jìn (盡) 215
jìn jì (盡劑) 215
jīng zhèng (經證) 52

kāi hé shū lǐ lùn (開合樞理論) 108
kūn guà (坤卦) 221, 231

lín guà (臨卦) 218, 231
liù jīng (六經) 51, 60, 65, 72, 79, 84
  41 opinions about 81
  absence in Zhang Ji's writings 80
  as complexity of channels 85
  as disease location method 89
  as five stages 90
  as group of syndromes 91, 92
  as layers 90
  as physiological functions 94
  as physiological structure 87
  as six anatomical systems 82
  as six channels 81, 82
  as six diseases 93
  as three yin and three yang 86, 93
  as twelve channels 87
  debates about 95
  in Yellow Emperor's Inner Classic 86
  modern importance to study 93
  qi transformation and 96
liù jīng biàn zhèng (六經辨證) 79, 95
  six conformations differentiation 96
liù jīng bìng (六經病) 79, 94
liù jīng xíng céng (六經形層) 60
liù qì (六氣) 109
lú huǒ shén (盧火神) 67

mǎo (卯) 210, 211, 212, 213, 222, 223, 224, 225, 226, 228, 232

pǐ guà (否卦) 220, 230

qì (氣) of herbs 180
qì huà (氣化) 106, 108
qián (前) 214
qián guà (乾) 217, 219, 229

rì bū (日晡) 235
róng rùo wèi qīang (營弱衛強) 200

shàng (上) 31, 186, 213, 214
shāng hán (傷寒) 17, 200
  broad sense 17, 18–19
  in women 21–22
  narrow sense 17, 20–23
  two types 17
  word order and meaning 21
shāng hán xué (傷寒學) 47, 48
shāng hán xué pài (傷寒學派) 46, 47
shāng hán zhòng fēng (傷寒中風) 21
shào pài shāng hán (紹派傷寒) 65
shēn (神) 198, 210, 211, 223, 224, 225, 226, 230, 234, 235
shí èr dì zhī (十二地支) 210
shí èr xiāo xī guà (十二消息卦) 216
shū (樞)
  absence from Discussion of Cold Damage 171
  as dynamic qi movement 170
  as pivot 169, 183
  for shao yang 169

sì (巳) 210, 211, 214, 217, 222, 223, 225, 230

tài guà (泰卦) 218, 228, 232
tài hé diàn (太和殿) 156
tài yáng (太陽) 21
tí gāng (提綱) 54
tiáo biàn (條辨) 54

wèi (未) 210, 211, 212, 214, 217, 222, 223, 225, 226
  as flavor 180
  in yang ming 99
wǔ (午) 210, 211, 217, 222, 223, 224, 225, 226, 230
Wǔ Fù Zǐ (吳附子) 67
wǔ yùn (五運) 109
wǔ yùn liù qì (五運六氣) 45, 107, 108

xià (下) 31, 186
xié (邪) 19
xíng shēng zì (形聲字) 157
xū (戌) 210, 211, 212, 222, 223, 224, 225, 226, 230, 234, 235

yáng fú yīn rùo (陽浮陰弱) 200
yáng yáo (陽爻) 217
yín (寅) 210, 211, 212, 213, 222, 223, 224, 225, 226, 228, 232, 233
yīn yáo (陰爻) 217
yǒu (酉) 210, 211, 224, 225, 226, 230, 234, 235
yù (愈) 40
yù jù shí (欲劇時) 234

zhèng (症) 58
zhèng huǒ shén (鄭火神) 67
zhòng fēng (中風) 200
  in women 22
zhōng qì (中氣) 106, 107, 108, 117, 119, 120, 121, 122, 123, 125, 126, 132, 137, 153, 228
  for jue yin 147–148
  for shao yang 144, 145
  for shao yin 146
  for tai yang 140
  for tai yin 146
  for yang ming 142, 143
  interaction with *běn qì* (本氣) 118
  qi transformation mechanisms 127–128
  six qi relationships 109, 111
  zang-fu correspondences 124
zhōng xī huì tōng (中西匯通) 63
zhōng xī huì tōng xué pài (中西匯通學派) 63
Zhù Fù Zǐ (祝附子) 67
zǐ (子) 210, 211, 222, 223, 224, 226, 231
zōng hé tí (綜合體) 86